What educators are saying about *Functional Anatoi*

At last, a textbook written by an OT, for OT education at every level. Throughout, this text guides the student's thought process towards occupation-based reasoning in every chapter. Anatomy has become functional and certainly more relevant to the entry-level OT and OTA student.

> ADA HOERL, MA, BS, AS IN OCCUPATIONAL THERAPY
> *Professor, Occupational Therapy Assistant Program,*
> *Sacramento City College, Sacramento, CA*

This is the first anatomy textbook that focuses on the specific requirements of the occupational therapy curriculum.

> JOYDEEP CHAUDHURI, MD
> *Professor, School of Occupational Therapy, Husson University, Bangor, ME*

Functional Anatomy for Occupational Therapy is an occupation-centered text where all the topics relate back to occupation and function. Embedding this meaning into the text will improve student learning and application of the knowledge.

> GABE BYARS, MS, OTR/L, LSVT-BIG, MSCS
> *Assistant Professor, Occupational Therapy Assistant Program,*
> *Salt Lake Community College, Salt Lake City, UT*

Excellent book to provide the foundations of functional anatomy for students and a great refresher for clinicians and academicians!

> CARRIE CIRO, PHD, OTR/L, FAOTA
> *Associate Professor of Occupational Therapy,*
> *University of Oklahoma Health Sciences Center*

This book is definitely needed and will hopefully become a staple in all OT programs.

> BETH ROROS, CHT
> *Assistant Professor, Delaware Technical Community College, Georgetown, DE*

This well-designed and beautifully illustrated textbook of functional anatomy will be an excellent resource for entry-level OT students.

> PATRICIA HENTON, OTD, OTR/L, ICA, CEIM
> *Assistant Professor, OTD Program, Huntington University, Huntington, IN*

Functional Anatomy for Occupational Therapy is the "just right challenge" to optimize learning for occupational therapy students. It includes the correct amount of depth with adequate detail, yet it does not oversimplify things. It is written specifically for occupational therapy students and puts occupation in the forefront. As always with Books of Discovery textbooks, the exceptional images add to the clarity of the concepts. I think occupational therapy students will engage with this text and enjoy learning the important foundational content.

> SUSANNE HIGGINS, OTD, OTR/L, CHT
> *Associate Professor, Occupational Therapy Program,*
> *Midwestern University, Downers Grove, IL*

FUNCTIONAL ANATOMY for Occupational Therapy

FUNCTIONAL ANATOMY for Occupational Therapy

Nathan Short

Joel Vilensky

Carlos A. Suárez-Quian

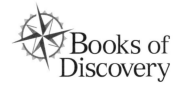

Books of Discovery

Published by Books of Discovery

Boulder, Colorado USA

booksofdiscovery.com

800.775.9227

ISBN: 978-0-9987850-1-1

Library of Congress Control Number: 2021934519

Printed in the United States

15   14   13   12   11   10   9   8   7   6   5   4   3   2   1

Managing editor: Alan Bernhard

Development editor: Brenda Hadenfeldt

Copy editor: Donna Polydoros

Designer: Jessica Xavier, Planet X Design

Disclaimer

Care has been taken to confirm the accuracy of the information presented in this publication and to describe generally accepted practices. However, the publisher, authors, and editors are not responsible for omissions or errors or for any consequences from application of the information in this textbook, and make no warranty, expressed or implied, regarding the completeness or accuracy of the contents of this publication. Application of the information in a particular situation remains the practitioner's professional responsibility.

For the Light of the world and
Creator of this amazing body,
and the lights of my life, Uma and Addy.

NATHAN SHORT

Contents

CHAPTER 10

Positioning, Postural Alignment, and Functional Mobility 337

Reviewers

Gabe Byars, OTR/L
Assistant Professor
Salt Lake Community College

Joydeep D. Chaudhuri, MD
Associate Professor
School of Occupational Therapy
College of Health and Pharmacy
Husson University

Carrie Ciro, PhD, OTR/L, FAOTA
Associate Professor
Elam-Plowman Chair of Rehabilitation Sciences
CAH Assistant Dean of Faculty Development
University of Oklahoma

Patricia Henton, OTD, OTR/L, ICA, CEIM
Assistant Professor
Doctor of Occupational Therapy Program
Huntington University

Susanne Higgins, OTD, OTR/L, CHT
Associate Professor
Occupational Therapy Program
Midwestern University

Ada Boone Hoerl, MA, COTA/L
Program Coordinator, Chair, Professor
Occupational Therapy Assistant Program
Sacramento City College

Jessica Sofranko Kisenwether, PhD, CCC-SLP, CIP
Former Associate Professor, Department of Speech-Language Pathology, Misericordia University
Manager, NASA IRB and Human Research Protection Program
NASA Office of Research Assurance

Beth A. Roros, OTR/L, CHT
Adjunct Professor, Masters Occupational Therapy Program, Wesley College, Dover, DE
Adjunct Professor, Occupational Therapy Assistant Program, Delaware Technical Community College, Georgetown, DE

Katherine Schofield, DHS, OTR/L, CHT
Assistant Program Director and Associate Professor
Occupational Therapy Program
Midwestern University

Lani R. Stockwell, OTD, MSOT, OTR/L, CSRS
Chair, Department of Occupational Therapy
Founding Director, Clinical Doctorate of Occupational Therapy Program
Clinical Associate Professor
College of Health Sciences
Marquette University

Kathy Swoboda, MLS, OTR/L
OCAT Program Director
Kent State University at East Liverpool

Orley A. Templeton, OTD, OTR/L
Assistant Professor
Occupational Therapy Department
Misericordia University

Acknowledgments

To Andrew Biel and Robin Dorn, the Trail Guide series is a work of art. Thank you for letting us ride on your coattails and build upon the foundation you laid. To Brenda Hadenfeldt, our development editor, your thoughtful feedback and attention to detail made this book what it is, and we cannot thank you enough for your consistent support and encouragement. To Rhoni Hirst, Tim Herbert, and the rest of the team at Books of Discovery, thank you for seeing the vision for this book and investing so much to see it come to fruition. Someone had to keep the many pieces of this complex puzzle together. Huge thanks go to Alan Bernhard of Boulder Bookworks for managing the process from beginning to end. Your hard work and attention to detail did not go unnoticed and were essential to the process. There was something transcendent that brought our personalities and skill sets together. It was a blessing to be part of that synergy with all of you.

NS and JV would like to specifically thank Sherilyn Emberton, Luke Fetters, and Ruth Ford of Huntington University for creating a culture where academic pursuits like this project can thrive. We would also like to acknowledge the faculty and students of the Huntington University OTD Program, who provided invaluable feedback along the way. Jill Trosper also graciously provided broad administrative support, allowing us to focus and commit time to this project.

NS is most grateful to Uma and Addy, who put up with a lot of late nights, early mornings, and general ranting. I love you both.

JV, as always, thanks his wife, Deborah, for putting up with him and his idiosyncrasies (such as still writing books at sixty-nine years of age) for more than forty years.

CASQ could not have done this without the incredible generosity of the body donors who make the teaching of gross anatomy possible, and Mark Zavoyna, manager of the Georgetown University Anatomical Donor Program, who embalmed all the cadaveric material exhibited in this book. He is a true master of the art. Finally, but always first in his life, he thanks his wife, Kathryn, for making life worth living every day.

Nathan Short, Joel Vilensky, and Carlos A. Suárez-Quian

Preface

Welcome to *Functional Anatomy for Occupational Therapy*. The impetus for developing this textbook was to create a comprehensive occupation-based functional anatomy resource for occupational therapy (OT) and occupational therapy assistant (OTA) students and future practitioners. Toward this ambitious goal, we include functional anatomy, cadaver figures paired with explanatory illustrations, clinical applications, and OT-based case studies, as well as goniometry and manual muscle testing (MMT) opportunities with the included *OT Guide to Goniometry & MMT* eTextbook. These complementary texts are intended for generalist-level education and as clinical resources for future practice.

Occupation, defined as purposeful activity meaningful to the individual, involves movement of the body generated by musculoskeletal structures applying coordinated force to joints. But this is only the motor component of occupational performance. While motor performance skills are collectively affirmed by the theories and framework of the profession, they represent an essential, but singular, component of a much more complex integrative process.[1]

Movement, in the context of occupation, is purposeful and guided by client factors such as values, motivation, and others. It is influenced by contexts, both environmental and personal.

In many ways, through the lens of occupation, motor skills are subordinate to the other factors that give them meaning. To appropriately frame the physical aspect of occupational performance, this textbook refers frequently to purposeful movement, indicating meaningful motion that is guided by the individual for an intended purpose.

Partly because OT is not merely a physical therapeutic practice, the level of anatomy taught varies significantly within occupational therapy programs, such as master of occupational therapy (MOT), doctor of occupational therapy (OTD), and OTA. Anatomy coursework in these programs ranges from complete cadaver dissection to almost no additional anatomy instruction beyond that provided in an undergraduate anatomy course.[2] This variance may be attributed to the broad scope of OT practice and differing perspectives on the importance of functional anatomy. A more consistent, thorough understanding of functional anatomy, appropriately framed in the context of occupation, can improve students' ability to analyze and promote occupational performance across practice settings.

It is challenging to design a textbook that covers the scope of functional anatomy for future practitioners across a variety of situations, such as bed mobility in an intensive care unit (ICU), performance of activities of daily living (ADLs) and instrumental activities of daily living (IADLs) in a rehabilitation setting, motor development milestones for children, and improving hand function in an outpatient setting.

In this text we aim not to cover comprehensive assessment and intervention for the broad scope of practice but to lay a foundation in functional anatomy from which to develop these skill sets to thrive in various practice settings. To that end, we give examples throughout of the clinical relevance and application to individuals across the life span, with specific pathologies, and in different practice settings.

Although OT and OTA programs are quite variable in the level of anatomical content taught, all include instruction on goniometry and MMT. These skills are ubiquitous to many practice settings, and demonstrated competency is mandated by educational standards.[3] The included *OT Guide to Goniometry & MMT* eTextbook thoroughly describes best-practice techniques for these assessments from a uniquely occupation-based perspective.

Teaching functional anatomy, goniometry, and MMT within the OT curriculum often requires multiple textbooks, which frequently overlap and are written by professionals in other disciplines. A practical goal of this text is to provide a comprehensive occupation-based approach in a single source.

We hope that this textbook is an accessible, useful, and clinically applicable resource for OT students and will ultimately improve their ability to promote occupational performance for individuals across the life span and throughout the spectrum of practice.

Notes

1. American Occupational Therapy Association, *Occupational Therapy Practice Framework: Domain and Process*, 4th ed. (Bethesda, MD: AOTA Press, 2020).

2. Katherine Anne Schofield, "Anatomy in Occupational Therapy Program Curriculum: Practitioners' Perspectives," *Anatomical Sciences Education* 7, no. 2 (March–April 2014): 97–106, https://doi.org/10.1002/ase.1378.

3. American Occupational Therapy Association, "2011 Accreditation Council for Occupational Therapy Education (ACOTE®) Standards," *American Journal of Occupational Therapy* 66, no. 6 (2011): S6–74, https://doi.org/10.5014/ajot.2012.66S6.

User's Guide

IN THIS TEXTBOOK you'll find a variety of approaches to explain complex content. Each approach offers a pathway to deeper understanding and frames the concepts within the context of occupational therapy (OT). To facilitate your learning of both the functional anatomy and its clinical relevance, several unique features and resources have been included. These features work together to support your retention of the material and the development of skills that will enable you to become an effective OT practitioner.

Sharpen Your Goniometry and Manual Muscle Testing Skills

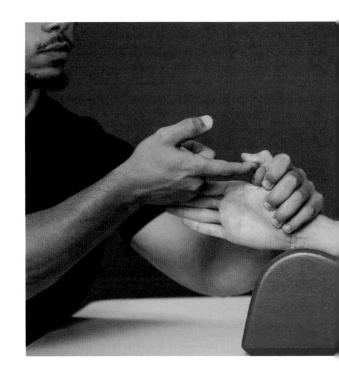

The included *OT Guide to Goniometry & MMT* eTextbook features photos and videos of best-practice techniques, as well as examples of documentation and occupation-based goals. The photos and narrated videos support visual and auditory learning.

Once you achieve cognitive understanding, you will use hands-on implementation of the techniques for a kinesthetic approach to linking content and making clinical connections. As you take time to practice these techniques, try describing the underlying anatomy that contributes to movement and strength, and consider the functional implications of deficits. Prompts to apply these clinical skills are provided in most chapters. Try out these techniques on classmates, friends, and family. Working with a variety of body types and conditions will better prepare you for future clinical practice.

The ability to accurately measure functional motion and strength will help you set goals, communicate with your future patients and other clinicians, track progress, and justify occupational therapy services. These clinical skills will become natural to you with experience. The more you refine your technique as a student, the better your future patients will be served.

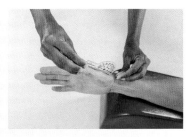
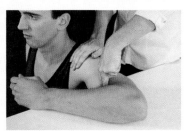
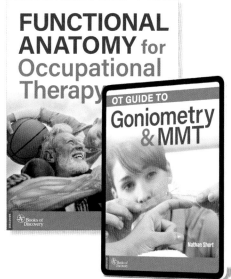

Learning Objectives and Key Concepts

Before beginning a chapter, consider the authors' and instructors' intentions for your learning journey. We've included two features that can help improve your retention and organize your learning:

- **Learning Objectives** help you prioritize and focus your reading on the key takeaway information within each chapter. They offer a road map that can help guide you to your destination.
- **Key Concepts** bring your attention to essential ideas and terminology that you'll encounter in each chapter. They are waypoints on your journey that help define the content that will be important to you.

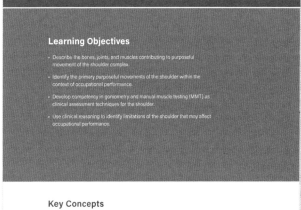

Learning Objectives

- Describe the bones, joints, and muscles contributing to purposeful movement of the shoulder complex.
- Identify the primary purposeful movements of the shoulder within the context of occupational performance.
- Develop competency in goniometry and manual muscle testing (MMT) as clinical assessment techniques for the shoulder.
- Use clinical reasoning to identify limitations of the shoulder that may affect occupational performance.

Key Concepts

adhesive capsulitis	scapular winging
bicipital tendinitis	scapulohumeral rhythm
dynamic stability	shoulder separation
fall on outstretched hands (FOOSH)	static stability
glenohumeral subluxation	subacromial impingement
hemiparesis	thoracic outlet syndrome (TOS)
rotator cuff	
scaption	
scapular dyskinesis	
scapular plane	

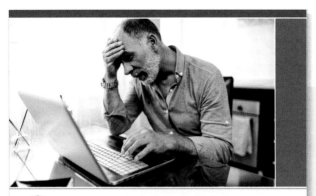

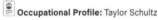

Occupational Profile: Taylor Schultz

TAYLOR SCHULTZ is a fifty-six-year-old account executive with a commercial insurance company. He spends the majority of his day, sometimes eight to ten hours, at his computer workstation. Recently, he began experiencing pain in his dominant (right) shoulder, particularly with overhead motion. He does not recall a specific injury, just gradually increasing pain.

The symptoms are now affecting his golf game—his primary leisure occupation—and, more importantly, the way he spends time with his teenage son. Additionally, he is having trouble with upper body dressing

and showering. He has also noticed an impact on his job performance. The pain is keeping him from sleeping at night, and he feels less productive and has lower energy levels. He has an annual report due next month, and his supervisor has been putting pressure on him to complete it.

Fortunately, Taylor's primary care physician (PCP) has referred him to occupational therapy in an outpatient setting—your office. Before he comes into the clinic, let's take a look at the underlying anatomy of the shoulder.

143

Occupational Profiles

Occupational Profile features appear in the body region chapters as a way to apply the content to a real-world clinical scenario. Specific information is included within each profile as components of a broader case study. These individuals are then revisited throughout the chapters to demonstrate the relationship of content to clinical practice. These features are intentionally general, highlighting individuals with specific diagnoses and related barriers to occupational performance in various settings across the life span. They are intended not as definitive guides to assessment and intervention, but as clinical perspectives to help you integrate your developing knowledge of functional anatomy.

TAYLOR SCHULTZ | Based on what you know so far, do you think targeted strengthening of the rhomboids and middle trapezius would have any value as an exercise to promote occupational performance for Taylor? Why or why not?

Clinical Applications

The **Clinical Applications** featured in many chapters describe clinical concepts or diagnoses to apply the specific functional anatomy within each chapter. These features provide a window into your future practice and emphasize the importance of developing your foundational knowledge base.

CLINICAL APPLICATION
Manual Scapular Mobilization

The borders and many of the bony landmarks of the scapula are easily palpated just beneath the skin and superficial trapezius muscles. Palpation and manual mobilization of the scapula are often used in assessment and intervention because scapular mobility is vital to overall upper extremity motion and occupational performance.

For instance, an individual who has had a CVA (stroke) may experience generalized weakness of the scapular muscles. . . .

Try Its

Try It features offer activities to help solidify an anatomical or clinical concept and are geared toward kinesthetic learning. When an abstract concept translates into an experience, you'll understand in a way that is both relevant and easily recalled.

▶TRY IT

To illustrate functional movement in the scapular plane, raise your arm overhead as if giving someone a high five. Now, note the position of the humerus. Is it in flexion (sagittal plane) or abduction (frontal plane)? Likely it is midway between in the scapular plane.

Put yourself in a future patient's shoes: You just had a painful shoulder surgery a few days ago and are coming to your first OT appointment. . . .

BICEPS BRACHII	
Purposeful Activity	
P	Combing your hair, eating an apple, washing your face (elbow flexion with the forearm supinated)
A	Flex the elbow (humeroulnar joint) Supinate the forearm (radioulnar joints) Flex the shoulder (glenohumeral joint)
O	Short head: Coracoid process of scapula Long head: Supraglenoid tubercle of scapula
I	Tuberosity of the radius and aponeurosis of the biceps brachii
N	Musculocutaneous C5 and C6

PAOIN Tables

We've included **PAOIN Tables** to help you understand a muscle's contribution to purposeful movement and occupational performance. Along with examples of activities that are enabled, these features identify the action, origin, insertion, and innervation for the muscles described. Each table begins with several purposeful activities (**P**) to analyze specific muscles using a top-down approach through the lens of occupation. Then we provide the actions (**A**), the attachment sites (**O, I**), and the nerve (**N**) innervation for that muscle.

Review Questions

Quizzes ask students to actively engage the material they've studied to reinforce their learning. Chapters end with a short set of review questions to help you measure your understanding. Answers to review questions are located in a separate section near the end of this book.

Review Questions

1. What portion of the extensor digitorum extends the proximal interphalangeal (PIP) joints of the fingers?
   a. sagittal bands
   b. terminal tendon
   c. central slip
   d. extensor carpi radialis

2. What muscle bifurcates and inserts on the middle phalanx of each finger to flex the proximal interphalangeal (PIP) joint?
   a. flexor digitorum profundus
   b. flexor digitorum superficialis
   c. palmaris longus
   d. flexor pollicis longus

3. Which aspect of your hand would be most effective to use when wringing out a washcloth for bathing?
   a. ulnar aspect (ring and small fingers)
   b. distal fingertips and thumb
   c. central aspect (middle and ring fingers)
   d. radial aspect (thumb and index and middle fingers)

4. Which of the following pinch patterns would be most affected by an injury to the ulnar nerve?
   a. tip pinch
   b. lateral (key) pinch
   c. three-jaw chuck pinch
   d. composite grasp

5. Simultaneous contraction of the extensor carpi ulnaris (ECU) and the flexor carpi ulnaris (FCU) would produce what movement at the wrist?
   a. extension
   b. flexion
   c. radial deviation
   d. ulnar deviation

6. What is the only muscle that can flex the distal interphalangeal (DIP) joint?
   a. palmaris longus
   b. flexor digitorum profundus
   c. flexor digitorum superficialis
   d. flexor carpi ulnaris

7. Place the tip of your right index finger on the letter J of a computer keyboard in QWERTY format. Without moving your wrist, move the tip of your finger to the letter H. Which of the following muscles enables this functional motion?
   a. flexor digitorum profundus
   b. extensor digitorum
   c. 1st palmar interosseous
   d. 1st dorsal interosseous

8. The majority of the motion at the wrist occurs between which of the following bones?
   a. ulna, lunate, and triquetrum
   b. radius, scaphoid, and lunate
   c. ulna, scaphoid, and lunate
   d. radius, trapezium, and lunate

9. Which of the following pairs of muscles is essential for the motions of the thumb and index finger for tip pinch, as when threading a needle?
   a. flexor digitorum superficialis and flexor pollicis brevis
   b. flexor digitorum profundus and abductor pollicis longus
   c. adductor pollicis and flexor digitorum superficialis
   d. flexor digitorum profundus and flexor pollicis longus

10. Collectively, the interossei muscles of the hand contribute to all of the following movements except
    a. abduction of the fingers.
    b. adduction of the fingers.
    c. flexion of the distal interphalangeal (DIP) joints.
    d. flexion of the metacarpophalangeal (MCP) joints.

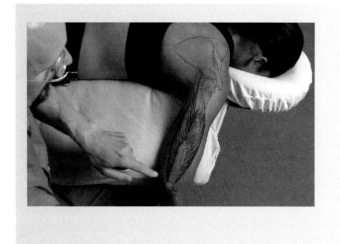

▶ Online Palpation Videos

Digital anatomy and palpation resources are provided as online supplements to this textbook and available at **booksofdiscovery.com/for students/**. Palpation is an essential clinical skill because it helps you identify specific anatomical structures beneath the surface of the skin. Clinically, accurate palpation is necessary to identify anatomical landmarks for assessments like goniometry and MMT, to inform differential diagnosis, and to guide manual therapy interventions.

Expand Your Learning with the Big Picture in Mind

It takes time to master functional anatomy and its clinical application. Here are a few study tips that we recommend:

- Although memorization is involved with anatomy, the goal is understanding and application. As you examine muscle origins and insertions, think about the purposeful movement produced when a muscle applies force to these attachment sites. Then think through this motion from a functional perspective.
- Examine and analyze anatomy using a variety of resources, such as illustrations, cadaver images, and digital resources. Being able to identify and apply anatomy in different contexts will help solidify your understanding.
- After you have read and digested the content on your own, teach the content to a classmate or family member. Consider occupations that you or they enjoy, and analyze and describe the functional anatomy, biomechanical principles, and specific movements involved. By explaining a concept to someone else, you demonstrate a higher level of understanding.
- The purpose of an anatomy course for an OT or OTA student is its functional application. This book is filled with functional examples involving specific structures, but you should also think of your own. What muscles and movements are required for

self-feeding, toileting, or functional mobility? How would a deficit in motion or strength affect the performance of the specific occupation?

- Practice, practice, practice your clinical skills, such as goniometry and manual muscle testing, on as many different people as you can. Mastering these basic assessment skills now will pay dividends in the future when you are a practitioner to help you better serve your patients. As you practice, describe

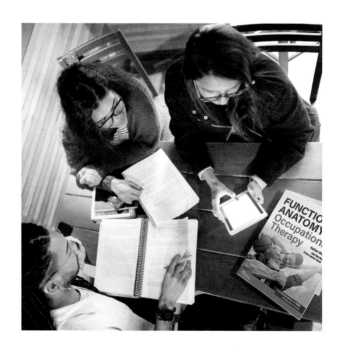

the underlying anatomy, its relevance to purposeful movement, and its contribution to occupational performance.

Think Like an OT Practitioner

There are many questions posed throughout this book that are intended to help you begin to think like an occupational therapy practitioner. The questions relate to functional anatomy, application of the *Occupational Therapy Practice Framework*, fourth edition (OTPF-4), and general problem solving and clinical reasoning. You will notice that answers to many of these questions are not included; this is intentional. Often in occupational therapy practice, there are multiple evidence-based creative methods of assessment and intervention. Also, research is continually supporting new and unique clinical techniques. Most of these questions are meant not to lead you to concrete, static answers, but to provide a starting point for further critical discussion and examination of the latest evidence, which will evolve over time.

In addition, your instructors will provide unique perspectives based on their clinical experiences, and you will develop your own evidence-based preferences. As prac-

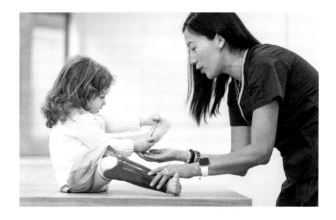

titioners, we are lifelong learners, often finding different or better answers to the same questions as we develop clinical expertise and integrate research into practice.

This book was written with you, a future occupational therapy practitioner, in mind. We have combined and presented our collective anatomical and clinical knowledge in the hope that it will lay a strong foundation. As you begin this journey, keep your future patients in mind; they will be the beneficiaries of your hard work and commitment.

PART I

Foundational Concepts of Occupational Anatomy

CHAPTER 1

Introduction to Occupation-Based Anatomy

Learning Objectives

- Describe functional anatomy within the broader context of occupational therapy theory and practice.

- Explain foundational concepts of kinesiology, physics, and biomechanics as they apply to purposeful movement and occupational performance.

- Recognize the relationships between the design and function of anatomical structures of the human body.

Key Concepts

arthrokinematics	kinetic chain	performance skills
axis of motion	length-tension relationship	planes of motion
biomechanics	mechanical advantage	purposeful movement
closed-chain movement	moment	second-class lever
elasticity	moment arm	strain
end-feel	motor skills	stress
first-class lever	occupational performance	surface anatomy
force	occupations	third-class lever
functional anatomy	open-chain movement	torque
functional mobility	osteoarthritis	Young's modulus
joint reaction force	osteokinematics	
kinesiology	performance patterns	

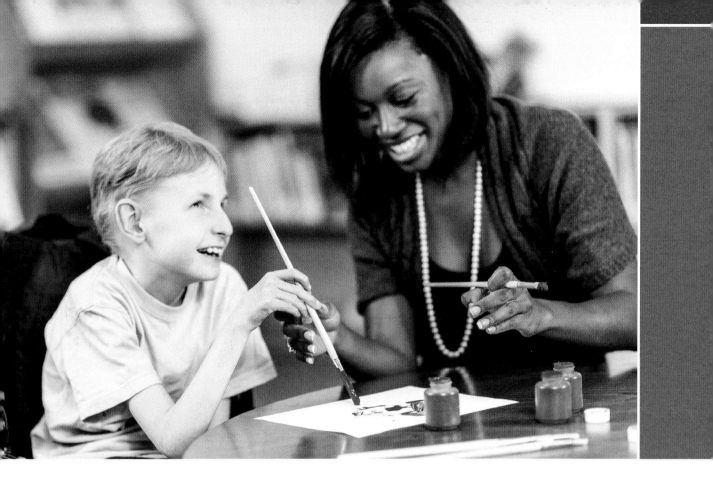

Getting Oriented

If you are reading this book, you are likely beginning your journey as an occupational therapist (OT) or occupational therapy assistant (OTA). Like many OTs or OTAs, you may feel a sense of calling or higher purpose to serve others and see them achieve their full potential. Perhaps you want to work with children, using play-based interventions to help them reach developmental milestones. Or your journey could lead to a rehabilitation setting, helping individuals recover the ability to complete their **activities of daily living (ADLs)** and **instrumental activities of daily living (IADLs)**.

Regardless of the setting or population, you will be part of a distinct profession with the common goal of helping people do the things they love and live their lives to the fullest.

What purposeful activities are most meaningful to you? As a full-time professor and parent, I enjoy recreational cycling as an opportunity to be outdoors and exercise. Biking to work on a nice day combines several occupations—leisure, community mobility, and health management—and it saves gas money! While the physical act of cycling involves muscle coordination, strength, and balance, the personal meaning and intrinsic motivation are what get me out of bed early to ride, distinguishing *occupation* from merely physical function.

The Language of Occupation

As an occupation-based student and future clinician, you will need to be familiar with some language specific to the profession. While you might not use these exact terms when talking to a patient, having a shared understanding of these words and concepts is key to facilitating professional discussion. The definitions that follow are adapted from the *Occupational Therapy Practice Framework*, fourth edition (OTPF-4).[1]

Occupations, or everyday activities that people do to bring meaning and purpose to life, include ADLs, IADLs, rest and sleep, education, work, play, leisure, health management, and social participation (**1.1**).[2] **Occupational performance** is the act of completing these meaningful activities by a person (such as an individual patient or caregiver), group(s) (several individuals with shared characteristics, such as a support group), or population(s) (an entire community of persons, such as all employees of a business). **Performance skills** are goal-directed actions that contribute to occupational

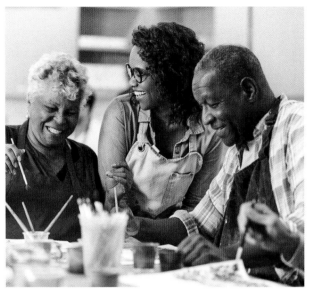

1.1 Occupations are the everyday activities that people do to give meaning and purpose to their lives.

performance. They comprise motor, process, and social interaction skills.

Motor skills include reaching, stabilizing, manipulating, and walking, to name a few.[3] Motor skills rely on underlying musculoskeletal structures that apply coordinated force to joints throughout the body. Learning how the muscles, joints, ligaments, and tendons work together to animate (move) the body is essential to a holistic understanding of occupation. However, this is only the *physical* contribution to occupation. Cognitive, emotional, and psychosocial function are essential to **process skills** like navigating and organizing and **social interaction skills** like speaking.[4] Collectively, the underlying performance skills—motor, process, and social interaction skills—support occupational performance in specific environmental contexts (**1.2**).

This text focuses on **functional anatomy**, or the underlying body structures that contribute to movements involved in daily function. Functional anatomy in the context of occupational therapy relates primarily to motor performance skills.

Occupational therapy addresses all of the motor performance skills involved with occupational performance, including **functional mobility**, or moving from one position or place to another. Examples include changing positions in bed (in-bed mobility), transferring to various functional surfaces (such as a bed, car, or shower chair), using a wheelchair to move, or walking through a home or community setting.

To emphasize the nature of movement involved in occupational performance, we will use the term **purposeful movement** when presenting the functional motion available at various joints of the body. For example, the shoulder can flex without any guiding purpose. In contrast, purposeful movement might involve shoulder flexion for bathing or dressing. Purposeful movement emphasizes the meaning behind the motion, recognizing movement as an outflow of individual **volition**, or will.

Additionally, occupational therapy addresses an individual's **performance patterns**, or the habits, routines, roles, and rituals that create the rhythms and expectations of daily life.[5] Through **activity analysis**, OTs and OTAs identify and address the various performance skills and patterns that facilitate or inhibit occupational performance.

As a future occupation-based therapist, you will want to avoid focusing on only one aspect of occupational performance (also known as reductionism). Consider a father who recently sustained a stroke learning to walk again in order to walk his daughter down the aisle at her wedding. As a practitioner, you could analyze his gait pattern, address loss of motion or weakness, or perhaps recommend a mobility device such as a walker or cane. However, in this instance, functional mobility is much more than just a gait pattern; it is facilitating a sacred moment between this father and daughter. Thorough evaluation and collaborative goal-setting can help you channel personal motivation toward the desired occupational outcome (**1.3**).

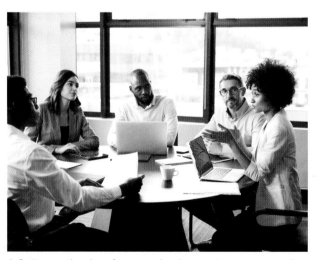

1.2 Occupational performance involves motor, process, and social interaction performance skills.

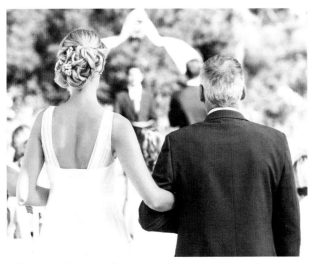

1.3 Occupational performance involves much more than movement.

Theoretical Foundations of Occupation

As an OT or OTA student, you will learn about the theories, models of practice, and frames of reference that provide the theoretical foundation for occupational therapy and guide practice. While each approach conceptualizes occupational performance with a unique perspective and emphasis, all affirm the physical aspect of occupation.

For example, the Model of Human Occupation (MOHO) identifies motor skills as a component of volitional (chosen) performance of roles, habits, and routines.[6] Similarly, the Canadian Model of Occupational Performance and Engagement (CMOP-E) and Person-Environment-Occupation (PEO) Model describe physical performance as components of the person. Additionally, the sensory integration frame of reference describes postural control and bilateral coordination as outcomes of the integrative process, combining and responding appropriately to sensory input for optimal motor functioning.[7]

The commonality among these approaches is that motor skills are *essential* but *subordinate* to the volitional, environmental, and cognitive aspects of occupation. By definition, occupation emphasizes the purpose behind the motion. Bones, joints, and muscles serve the will of the individual within a specific environmental context. This text does not advocate a particular model or frame of reference. Rather, the goal is to provide a comprehensive resource for understanding functional anatomy as a contributor to motor performance skills and occupational performance.

Anatomical Terminology

Knowing the language of anatomy helps in navigating the human body and communicating clearly and effectively in clinical practice. As an OT or OTA, you will communicate regularly with therapists, physicians, and other health care providers. You will also read research manuscripts, clinical documentation, operative notes, and imaging reports (such as an X-ray or MRI scan). Understanding and using standard anatomical terminology is essential for clear communication to optimize patient care.

The following sections give basic definitions of terms used throughout this text in relation to functional anatomy and movement.

It's All about Perspective

To understand anatomy, be it in an illustration, X-ray, or actual human body, we need to know the specific perspective, or viewpoint, that is being presented. In anatomical language, the starting perspective is the **anatomical position**: the human body standing upright with feet slightly apart, head facing forward, arms down to the sides, and palms facing forward (**1.4**, left).

Anatomical position serves as a reference point for further description:

- The **posterior** aspect, or back, of an anatomical region is also referred to as **dorsal**. The dorsal aspect of the hand refers to the perspective opposite the palm.

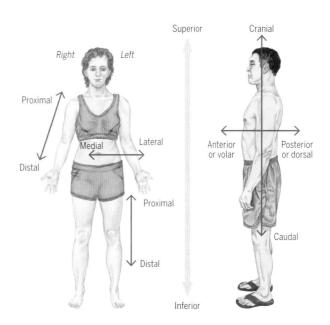

1.4 Anatomical terms of location

- The **anterior** aspect, or front, of an anatomical region is commonly referred to as **volar** (or **ventral**). The volar aspect of the hand refers to the palm.
- **Medial** and **lateral** are relative terms for an anatomical position closer to or farther from (right or left) the body's **midline**—the midsagittal plane, or the sagittal plane exactly in the center of the body. For example, in the anatomical position, the thumb is lateral to the small finger.
- **Proximal** and **distal** indicate position relative to the trunk. For example, the foot is distal to the knee, while the knee is proximal to the foot.
- **Radial** and **ulnar** indicate relative position on the forearm, wrist, and hand, with the radius and ulna bones serving as the reference point. For instance, the thumb is on the radial aspect of the hand, while the small finger is on the opposite ulnar aspect (look for these terms in Chapters 6 and 7).
- **Superior** indicates above, and **inferior** indicates below.
- **Cranial** refers to the direction of the skull, while **caudal** indicates beneath, or toward the "tail."
- **Ipsilateral** refers to the same side of the body, and **contralateral** refers to the opposite side. These terms are used in reference to muscle function. For example, the upper trapezius contributes to ipsilateral (same-side) flexion and contralateral (opposite-side) rotation of the head and neck.

Musculoskeletal Terms

This text uses many terms related to the musculoskeletal system that you will commonly use in clinical practice.

Skeletal muscles generally have two or more attachments to bones of the body. Typically, the attachment that moves the least upon muscle contraction is referred to as the **origin** of the muscle, and the more movable attachment is referred to as the **insertion**. Often, but not always, the origin is proximal (closer to the trunk) and the insertion is distal (farther from the trunk, relative to the origin). When a muscle contracts, the origin and insertion are brought closer together. For example, the biceps brachii flexes the elbow, bringing its insertion (radial tuberosity) on the forearm toward its origins (coracoid process and supraglenoid tubercle) at the shoulder. **Attachment** is also used as a more general term, not specifying origin or insertion, for a muscular connection to bone.

In clinical practice, the use of physical touch, or **palpation**, often helps to identify musculoskeletal

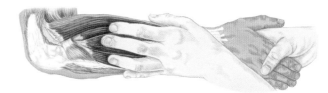

1.5 Palpation is a valuable clinical skill used to identify anatomical structures beneath the skin.

structures beneath the surface of the skin and provide valuable information about the state of underlying tissues (**1.5**). For example, a hand with impaired circulation or innervation may feel cold and lifeless, while an acute soft tissue injury may cause skin temperature to increase due to inflammatory activity. Palpating specific muscles or their tendinous attachments also helps to identify weakness or a site of painful tendinitis. Digital palpation resources have been included with this text to help you develop this valuable clinical skill.

Surface anatomy describes the features of anatomy that are palpable or visible on the surface of the skin. A specific component of a bone that protrudes beneath the skin is termed a **bony landmark**. An example is the ulnar head on the dorsal/ulnar aspect of your wrist. Identifying bony landmarks also guides the goniometry and manual muscle testing (MMT) techniques described in the *OT Guide to Goniometry & MMT* eTextbook. These clinical assessments are used across the spectrum of practice.

The skilled occupational therapist uses visual examination and palpation to guide clinical assessment and reasoning. What would the loss of wrinkles on the back of the joints of the fingers (knuckles) indicate? What would pain with palpation of the extensor tendon at the lateral elbow suggest? These clinical observations are often an important part of the assessment process, so each chapter highlights key surface anatomical landmarks.

Other terms describe detailed features of the musculoskeletal system, such as *condyle*, *tuberosity*, and *fossa*. These terms are defined within each chapter as they relate to structures within each body region.

Kinesiology

Kinesiology is the study of anatomy and mechanics in relation to human movement. Many of the terms for describing motion in kinesiology are used across disciplines. Occupation-based clinicians need to have a conceptual understanding of kinesiology and human movement as a component of activity analysis and occupational performance.

Keep in mind that kinesiology is a broad and complex area. For instance, some researchers focus solely on the mechanics of joint movement. This text is not a comprehensive kinesiology source, but it does include some foundational terms and concepts you will want to know. Learning to formally describe movement in this common language will improve your communication with other professionals, your documentation skills, and your understanding of medical records and research.

Planes and Axes of Motion

Any motion at a particular joint in the human body can be described by the plane(s) in which it occurs and the axes around which it rotates when the body is in the anatomical position. The **planes of motion** are described as sagittal, frontal (coronal), and transverse (**1.6**).

- The **sagittal plane** divides the body into right and left sides. Most flexion and extension movements occur in this plane. The midsagittal plane is exactly in the center of the body, passing through the nose and navel and between the legs. Clinically, the midsagittal plane is referred to as the midline of the body.

- The **frontal plane**, sometimes referred to as the coronal plane, divides the body into anterior and posterior portions and usually involves abduction and adduction.

- The **transverse plane** divides the body into inferior and superior portions, with most rotatory motion occurring in this plane.

Pure planar motion is rare with functional movement, as the body does not usually remain in a single plane. Consider putting on a seat belt: your shoulder flexes in the sagittal plane while simultaneously horizontally adducting across your chest in the transverse plane.

Therapy interventions sometimes begin in a single plane of motion—for example, after a joint replacement, to limit musculoskeletal strain. But interventions should progress to the multiplanar movements that are more common to occupational performance.

While human motion takes place *in* these various planes, rotary movement of joints also occurs *around* various **axes of motion** that are aligned perpendicularly to the planes of movement (**1.7**).

Think of an axis of motion as a straight line, or dowel rod, around which the joint rotates. This axis is the joint's **center of rotation**. The **frontal axis** is positioned medial to lateral, the **sagittal axis** is anterior to posterior, and the **vertical axis** is inferior to superior.

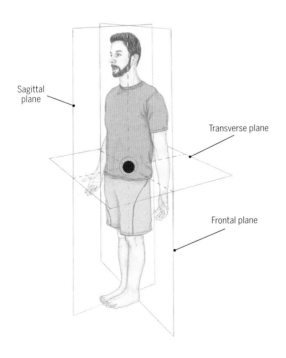

1.6 Planes of motion

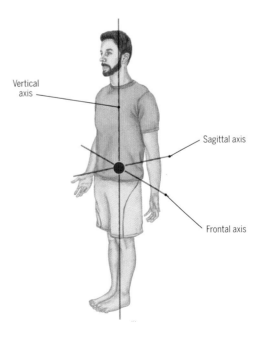

1.7 Axes of motion

Practice applying these terms to joint motions. For example, can you describe the plane and axis of motion for knee flexion? Think generally at this point. We will be more specific later on.

Kinetic Chains

The cooperative, interdependent movement of the segments and joints of the body is referred to as a **kinetic chain**. Kinetic chains occur in both closed-chain and open-chain movement patterns, depending on the activity.

Closed-chain functional movement involves the proximal joint(s) moving in relation to a fixed (nonmoving) distal segment. For example, imagine squatting down to pick up a box from the floor. Your feet are firmly planted on the ground, creating closed kinetic chains in the lower extremities as your hips and knees flex to lower the body toward the fixed position of the feet. Pushing a grocery cart is an example of closed-chain function of the upper extremities (**1.8**). Closed-chain patterns promote stabilization of joints and generally recruit more muscles to support the various joints in the chain.

In contrast, **open-chain** motions involve free movement of the distal body segment in space, allowing joints to move together or independently of the others. Imagine a maestro energetically waving a baton to conduct a symphony orchestra. As the hand moves freely in space, the proximal joints of the arm can move together or independently (**1.9**). Open-chain kinetic patterns require less muscle recruitment, as mobility is prioritized over stability for these types of functional movements.

Many ADL tasks include a combination of both open and closed kinetic chains. Suppose you are standing at

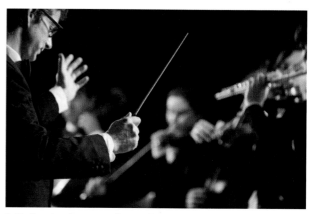

1.9 Conducting an orchestra is an example of open-chain function of the upper extremities.

the sink to complete hygiene tasks. The lower limbs are in static weight-bearing position (closed-chain), in which movement of any segment of the leg requires movement of the adjacent joints. Meanwhile, the upper limb demonstrates open-chain movement, allowing the hand to freely move in space to comb hair and brush teeth to prepare for the day.

As a clinician, you will address both open-chain and closed-chain functional activities, as both are essential to occupational performance.

Let's try to link some of the language and concepts of functional anatomy and kinesiology using the lens of occupational performance. Answer the following questions:

- Describe the axis and plane of motion for elbow flexion and extension. What ADLs or IADLs would feature this specific motion? Answer the same questions regarding knee flexion and extension.
- What closed-chain and open-chain kinetic patterns of movement can you identify and describe from your morning ADL routine?
- Choose a favorite leisure occupation. What joint movements, planes of motion, and kinetic chains are involved?

Principles of Physics: Forces and Levers

Force, moment arms, levers—all are concepts from physics that lay theoretical foundations for understanding human movement and function. Understanding these concepts is essential when considering the musculoskeletal forces acting internally on the body or when designing custom orthotics or adaptive equipment that exerts external force.

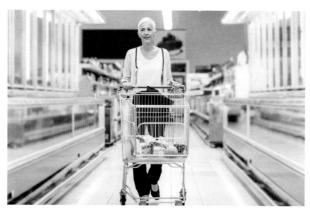

1.8 Pushing a grocery cart is an example of closed-chain function of the upper extremities.

Force

Force is any push or pull of matter. In humans, force occurs in the form of **tensile force** (pulling) or **compressive force** (pushing) between anatomical structures in the body (**1.10**). Tensile force is applied with joint motion as the tendon attachment transfers force from contractile muscle tissue to bone. Compressive force is present in the spine and lower extremities while sitting or standing.

Motor performance skills like reaching, lifting, and transporting involve external **resistance** in the form of the weight of the body or object being carried. This resistance must be overcome by **effort**, or the internal force generated by muscles. Resistance is also described as **resistive force**, and effort may be referred to as **exerted force**.

For example, moving a box from the floor to a countertop requires the muscles of the body to exert enough force to overcome the weight of the box. When the resistive and exerted forces are equal, the body or body segment is held in a static (nonmoving) position, such as when cradling a newborn in your forearms with your elbows flexed.

Occupational performance involves summative forces—the total force generated by multiple muscles—contributing to multiple simultaneous movements for specific tasks. Say you are drinking a cup of hot coffee. The muscles of the core, from which all human motion emanates, stabilize the body, while the muscles surrounding the scapula contract to provide a stable base for shoulder movement. Grossly positioned and stabilized proximally, the elbow, wrist, and hand can now supply the steady, precise motion needed to safely bring the cup to your mouth without spilling a drop. This illustrates the concept of a kinetic chain in the context of occupational performance.

In physics, a **moment** refers to the turning effect of force (the ability to rotate an object around an axis) and is synonymous with **torque**. Biomechanically, a muscle's moment, or torque, is its ability to rotate a joint

For example, the biceps brachii may exert a moment to rotate the forearm around the elbow, producing flexion—an important purposeful movement for hygiene and self-feeding. The quadriceps may exert a moment at the knee for extension to stand or walk.

The specific motion that a muscle is able to generate at a particular joint is referred to as its **action**. This term is sometimes used synonymously with *moment*.

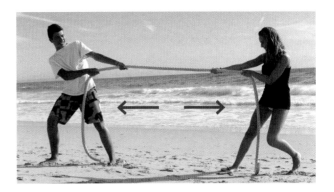

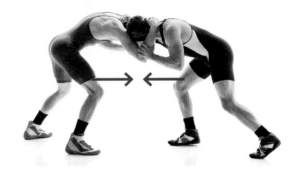

1.10 Tensile (*top*) and compressive (*bottom*) forces

The moment (action) of a muscle is affected by the distance between the muscle force and the joint it is acting upon. A **moment arm**, or lever arm, is a mathematical concept indicating the distance from an axis (joint) to the force acting upon it (muscle) (**1.11**).

In the human body, the farther the position of the muscle and its generated force are from the axis of rotation (joint), the greater the **mechanical advantage**, or leverage, the muscle will have on the joint.

Look again at Figure **1.11**. If the muscle from bone 1 were to attach at the distal end of bone 2, as opposed to

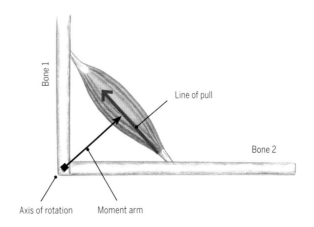

1.11 Muscles generate rotational force (moments) at the joints of the body.

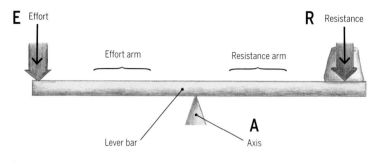

1.12 Components of a lever

at its current attachment site, how would this change the muscle's ability to generate force at the joint (axis)? Would the force applied at the joint increase or decrease?

Imagine a child sitting on a seesaw with someone much larger on the opposite side. In order to lift the larger individual, would it be better for the child to be closer to or farther away from the axis of the seesaw?

While increasing the distance from the axis enhances the mechanical advantage of the applied force, it also decreases its velocity (speed) of motion. Some muscles are arranged to optimize force, attaching farther from the joint, while others attach closer, enhancing velocity of movement.

Levers in the Body

Levers, or pulley systems, in the body provide mechanical advantage and generate functional motion. Levers are classified by the arrangement of the effort (muscle-exerted force), axis (joint), and resistance (the resistive force of the weight of a limb or object against gravity) (**1.12**).

In a **first-class lever**, exerted force and resistive force are on opposite sides of an axis, such as in a seesaw. The human neck is an example of a first-class lever: the anterior and posterior musculature contributes to opposing flexion and extension forces across the cervical vertebrae, which act as the axis in this lever system (**1.13**).

Second-class levers and **third-class levers** are configured with exerted and resistive forces on the same side of the axis, but each class has a different order (**1.14**).

A second-class lever is characterized by the resistive force being closer to the axis than the exerted force, such

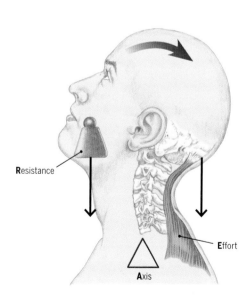

1.13 The cervical spine is an example of a first-class lever.

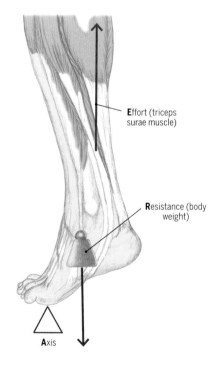

1.14 The ankle is an example of a second-class lever.

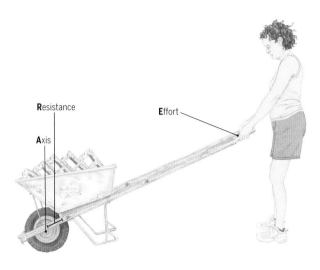

1.15 Using a wheelbarrow demonstrates a second-class lever.

as in a wheelbarrow (**1.15**). A third-class lever reverses the order, such as with a shovel (**1.16**).

Third-class levers are the most common in the human body. The biceps, for instance, exerts tensile force just distal to the axis of the elbow, while the resistive force is the weight of the extremity or object being carried by the forearm or hand (**1.17**). Whereas the second-class lever configuration often optimizes mechanical advantage, the third-class lever allows for higher-velocity movements of the limbs.

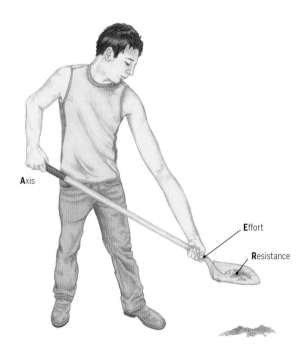

1.16 Shoveling is an example of a third-class lever, the most common type found in the human body. Quite a moment arm!

CLINICAL APPLICATION
Joint Reaction Force[8]

Newton's third law states that for every action, there is an equal and opposite reaction. Take a look at Figure **1.17**. The biceps is generating an internal (exerted) force at the elbow to lift the object, and the weight of the object against gravity is generating an opposing external (resistive) force at the elbow.

The force generated within the joint in response to external forces acting upon it is called the **joint reaction force**. As the muscles of the body generate an internal force at a specific distance from the joint (internal moment arm), the external weight of the object applies a resistive force at a particular distance from the joint (external moment arm).

Take note of the relative length of the internal moment arm (distance from biceps insertion to the elbow joint) and the external moment arm (distance from the weight of the object to the elbow joint) in the figure. We already know that the length of the moment arm determines the mechanical advantage, or leverage, of force. The mechanical advantage can be calculated as a ratio by dividing the external moment arm (28 cm) by the internal moment arm (4 cm), resulting in a ratio of 7:1. Because the external moment arm is seven times longer than the internal moment arm, the biceps has to generate 70 lb. of force to hold the 10 lb. weight.

Suppose the weight is a heavy functional object—perhaps a large purse or heavy box. How could you decrease the joint reaction force on the elbow when carrying these objects? Reducing joint reaction forces decreases wear and tear and is a key principle when implementing joint protection techniques to prevent symptoms associated with osteoarthritis.

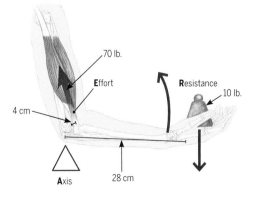

1.17 The ratio of the internal and external moment arms is used to analyze joint reaction force.

▶TRY IT

Mechanical advantage should be considered when designing custom orthotics or adaptive equipment to facilitate occupational performance. An orthosis exerts force on a joint to stabilize or mobilize it. The length of the orthosis relative to the joint it crosses is a key determinant of the amount of force it applies. An orthosis to stabilize the wrist or hand will benefit from a longer forearm component, increasing the joint's external moment arm and mechanical advantage.

Additionally, adaptive equipment can be designed to increase leverage and decrease joint reaction force. Take a look at the adaptive jar opener in Figure 1.18. What impact would the length of the opener have on the force exerted on the lid and joint reaction forces in the hand?

Try some different jar or bottle openers as examples of adaptive equipment and pay attention to the amount of stress you feel in the joints of your wrist and hand. Consider the relative length of these adaptive aids as a factor

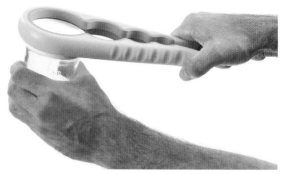

1.18 Using an adaptive jar opener. How does the length of the opener affect its mechanical advantage?

in increasing mechanical advantage. Think about how you might decrease these forces and their impact on the joints of your future patients.

Stress and Strain

Applied forces cause changes in the materials to which they are applied. For example, a muscle typically elongates under a tensile load. The collagen base of soft tissues allows for varying degrees of **elasticity**, or the ability to stretch and return to the original shape after tensile force is removed.

Stress is the amount of applied force per area, such as pounds per square inch, whereas **strain** describes the amount of material displacement under a specific amount of stress. For example, pizza dough undergoes stress in the form of pressing, rolling, and stretching (tensile and compressive forces), and it responds to this stress by changing its shape (strain).

A stress-strain diagram illustrates **Young's modulus**, or the stiffness of a particular material—how much it strains, or displaces, under increasing stress (force) (1.19). The slope of the line (rise over run) indicates the flexibility of the material. A higher slope indicates more brittle behavior, while a lower slope suggests more elasticity.

Compare rubber bands of different sizes. A large, thick rubber band will displace less than a small, thin rubber band under the same amount of stress. Similarly, body tissues demonstrate relative strain under stress that varies based on biological composition, structure, and functional purpose.

Bone, the scaffolding of the body, is more brittle in nature to provide structural support for functional move-

ment and mobility. Ligament and tendon, by contrast, are much more extensible—or able to stretch under force—to provide a balance between stability and mobility.

Most forces related to functional activity are well below the limits soft tissues can withstand, as demonstrated by the return to normal shape after strain, called **elastic deformation**. However, forces can exceed the capability of tissue for elastic deformation, causing **load to failure** in the form of permanent rupture or deformation. As stress increases, tissues strain, or displace, to their **yield point**, the maximum stress that can be sustained before tissue failure.

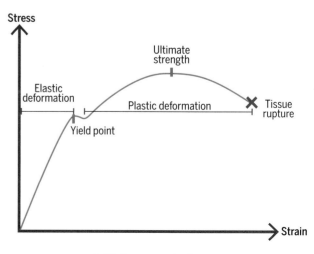

1.19 Stress-strain diagram

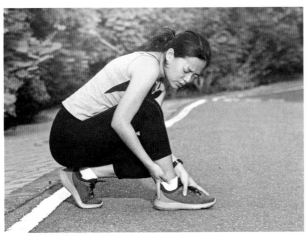

1.20 Forces imposed on body tissues can exceed their ability to elongate and return to normal length (plastic deformation).

Response of tissue beyond the yield point depends on its relative **stiffness**. Brittle tissue (such as bone) will fracture or rupture. More malleable tissue (such as ligaments) will undergo **plastic deformation** (sprain) or permanent deformation but retain continuity (**1.20**). This restructuring and permanent loss of baseline tissue length may contribute to **joint instability**, as in the case of recurrent shoulder dislocation that affects the integrity of the joint capsule.

We have all experienced musculoskeletal pain or a specific injury. Perhaps you can recall a time when you or someone you know injured a joint. Think about the external force that was applied—its direction, magnitude, and speed.

- Was the person in an open-chain or closed-chain position?
- How did the body tissues respond to the force? Did they elongate (plastic deformation) or rupture completely?
- How was the injury treated?

Understanding the mechanics of traumatic injuries will inform your clinical perspective during the rehabilitation process.

Biomechanical Properties of Body Tissue

You've probably heard the saying "form follows function," meaning that the design of an object or building is often essential to its intended purpose. Likewise, the tissues of the human body are uniquely designed to contribute to particular types of movement and function.

Biomechanics examines the structure, function, and motion of the biological systems that make up a living organism. Consider how the body would move if bones were made up of the same flexible collagen as tendons. Standing would be impossible. Instead, bones and soft tissues (muscles, tendons, and ligaments) are composed of different materials with just the right amount of rigidity, flexibility, and contractibility to facilitate movement.

To develop an in-depth understanding of the motor skills involved in occupational performance, let's take a look at the biomechanical properties of these functional tissues.

Biomechanics of Bone

Bone is primarily made up of collagen and a calcium mineral base called hydroxyapatite. This **bony matrix** has variable proportions of these key ingredients depending on its location and function within the body. Dense **cortical bone** has greater mineral content than collagen, while **cancellous (spongy) bone** is higher in collagen content (**1.21**).

Cortical bone is found in the shaft of long bones like the humerus and femur. It supplies rigid support to sustain various force demands of the extremities with activity. Cancellous (spongy) bone, by contrast, is found within the marrow cavity and at the ends of the long

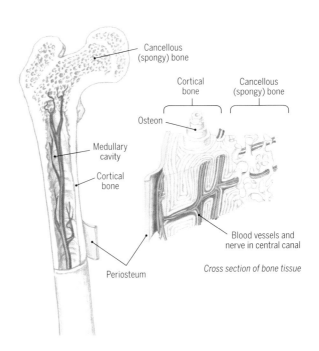

1.21 Interior detail (*left*) and cross section (*right*) of adult femur bone tissue

bones—for example, the femoral head. Cancellous bone is composed of ribbons of bone, referred to as the bony trabeculae, which increase its ability to absorb compressive loads.

Weight-bearing bones like the femur—more specifically, the femoral head—are designed to absorb ascending and descending forces associated with activities like ambulation (walking or running) or lifting. Ascending force is generated by the foot coming into contact with the ground and moves upward through the legs into the trunk. Descending force is generated by the weight of the body or an object being lifted and moves downward through the trunk into the lower body.

The articulating (connecting) ends of long bones are covered with **articular (hyaline) cartilage**, dense connective tissue that supplies a cushion to absorb repetitive compressive forces between bones (**1.22**). Articular cartilage is composed of a dense extracellular matrix (ECM)—made up of water, collagen, and proteoglycans—as well as specialized cells called chondrocytes, which play a role in the development and maintenance of the ECM.

Around two to four millimeters thick, this protective tissue is divided into distinct layers, or zones (superficial, deep, and calcified), which feature a progressive increase in density of collagen and resistance to compression.

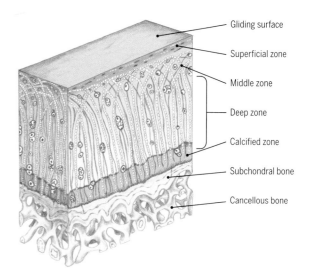

1.22 Distinct layers of cartilage provide a protective cushion for articular ends of bones.

With prolonged joint compression (as when standing), the layers of tissue compress, increasing their firmness and resistance. During an activity that requires extended standing, such as waiting in line for a concert or singing in church, the weight-bearing joints of the body accommodate to extended compression by becoming firmer, thereby protecting joints from prolonged force.

Mature cartilage is avascular (lacking blood vessels) and aneural (lacking innervation), which limits its ability to heal after injury. Also, because cartilage lacks nociceptors (pain receptors), it is often already severely compromised once joint pain is present.

Osteoarthritis (OA), for example, is a common musculoskeletal pathology that involves the degeneration of cartilage within a joint. Conservative interventions may involve adaptive equipment or activity modifications like the joint protection techniques discussed earlier. However, severe degeneration of the joint might require a joint arthroplasty (replacement) for long-term relief and restoration of function.

Biomechanics of Ligaments and Tendons

Ligaments and tendons are composed of dense connective tissue (mainly collagen fibers) that result in high resistance to tensile forces. **Ligaments** connect bone to bone, and **tendons** connect muscle to bone. Ligaments contribute stability to the joints of the body, whereas tendons transfer the force of muscle contraction to bone for joint movement.

CLINICAL APPLICATION
Low-Load Prolonged Stress

The soft tissues of the body (ligaments, tendons, and muscles) adapt to the forces placed on them, undergoing physical changes (plasticity) based on external force and positioning. These types of changes, such as when soft tissues lose their ability to lengthen normally (adaptive shortening), can result in limited functional motion. How do clinicians address such tissue barriers to occupational performance?

Shortened soft tissues respond best to low-load prolonged stress as opposed to aggressive, quick stretching, which could lead to further inflammation or tissue damage. Clinically, mobilization orthoses or manual therapies can provide this low-load prolonged stress to restore tissue length and related joint mobility in preparation for occupational performance. Can you think of other ways to encourage low-load prolonged stress to safely elongate contracted soft tissues?

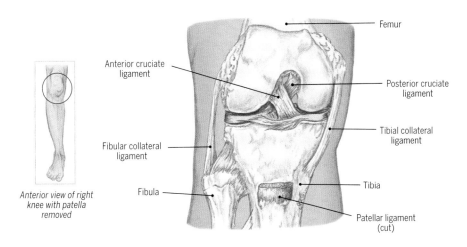

Anterior view of right knee with patella removed

1.23 Major ligaments of the knee

Ligaments are found surrounding, or sometimes within, joints, such as the collateral (surrounding) and cruciate (within) ligaments of the knee (**1.23**). They support the joints and often limit movements in specific planes.

A **joint capsule** forms a dense fibrous sleeve around a synovial (moving) joint, giving it a degree of passive stability and a sealed compartment that contains lubricating synovial fluid. Often, joint ligaments are thickened portions of the joint capsule itself—for example, the medial collateral ligament of the knee.

An **aponeurosis** is a broad fibrous insertion that often connects adjacent muscles. An example is the aponeurosis of the abdominal muscles that forms the rectus sheath (**1.24**).

The bones, ligaments, and tendons described in the previous sections are passive structures. They do not actively generate force. Rather, they convey and stabilize forces applied by muscle contraction. The following section describes the composition and function of muscles.

Biomechanics of Muscle

Muscles provide force for functional movement of the skeleton. They also alter the shape of internal organs and vessels (ducts, arteries, and veins), facilitating the function of various body systems.

There are three types of muscles: skeletal (striated) muscle; cardiac (heart) muscle, which is also striated; and smooth (visceral) muscle (**1.25**). In this text we are

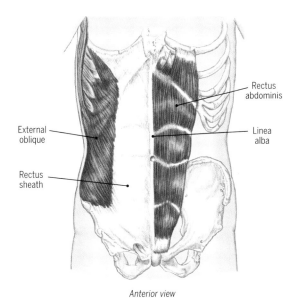

Anterior view

1.24 Rectus sheath

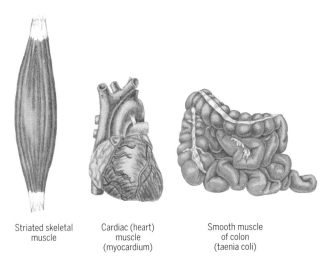

Striated skeletal muscle

Cardiac (heart) muscle (myocardium)

Smooth muscle of colon (taenia coli)

1.25 Types of muscle

concerned primarily with skeletal muscle, as it generates force for purposeful movement and occupational performance.

Skeletal Muscle

Skeletal muscles move the bones of the skeleton, supplying force for purposeful movement of the body. They have a fleshy belly made up of contractile tissue and are connected to a bone by the dense noncontractile tendons. However, not all muscles attach to bone. Skeletal muscles also move the skin of the face for expression and control eye motion to scan the environment for safe functional mobility.

Histologically (microscopically), skeletal muscles appear striated, with alternating bands of fibers, so skeletal muscle is also referred to as striated muscle (**1.26**).

Some muscles have fibers arranged in a parallel, linear pattern to produce specific motion, such as the flexor and extensor muscles of the wrist. Other muscles contain fibers with multiple orientations within the same interconnected group of tissue. For example, the trapezius has three distinct groups of fibers—upper, middle, and lower—each with unique actions on the scapula. Closely examining the orientation of a muscle's fibers, along with its attachments, should give you enough information to determine its action(s), or what movement(s) the muscle is capable of producing.

As noted, tendinous attachments to bones are commonly referred to as the origin and the insertion. In many cases, the origin is more proximal and stable, and the distal insertion is more mobile.

Consider the biceps brachii. As it contracts, the elbow flexes, bringing the insertion on the forearm (radial

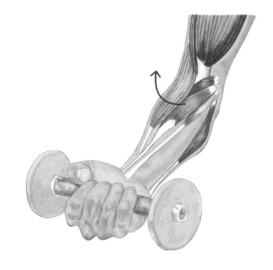

Anterior/medial view

1.27 The biceps contracts to bring the forearm toward the shoulder.

tuberosity) toward its origins at the shoulder (the coracoid process and supraglenoid tubercle) (**1.27**). The mobile forearm segment is pulled toward the static upper body and shoulder.

In some instances, a muscle can act in each direction, pulling a bone toward either attachment. An example is the upper trapezius. When the scapula is stable, the upper trapezius can flex the cervical spine laterally. But when the cervical spine is stable, it can also elevate the scapula (**1.28**).

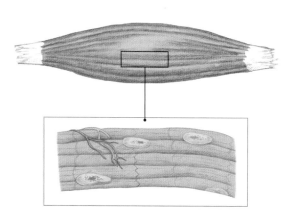

1.26 Striated appearance of skeletal muscle

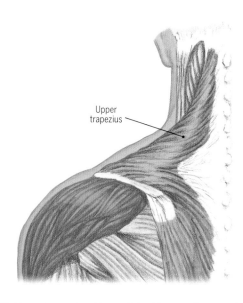

Upper trapezius

1.28 Upper trapezius. How might this muscle move both the neck and scapula?

As you study functional musculoskeletal anatomy, keep in mind that some distinctions are based on function and others are arbitrary. In other words, although we delineate and define structures in the body to study them, the ultimate learning objective is to have a holistic (not segmented or compartmentalized) understanding of how the body functions. While it's important to study the individual bones, muscles, and joints of various body regions, occupational performance involves their integrated and coordinated function.

Cardiac Muscle

Cardiac muscle tissue forms the muscular components (myocardium) of the heart (**1.29**).

Similar to skeletal muscle, cardiac muscle is striated and organized into segments (sarcomeres). But cardiac muscle fibers are shorter than skeletal muscle fibers and usually contain only one nucleus, whereas skeletal muscle cells are multinucleated.

Cardiac muscle fibers cells also are interconnected, allowing the cells to contract in a wavelike pattern and facilitating the function of the heart as a pump.

Smooth Muscle

Smooth muscle tissue, also called involuntary muscle, is the musculature within internal organs, such as the intestines and vessels (**1.30**). It can remain contracted for long periods, regulating body processes like digestion.

Smooth muscle is nonstriated, lacking cross stripes under microscopic magnification, and consists of uninucleated spindle-shaped cells. In contrast to striated muscle, smooth muscle contracts slowly and automatically (generally without voluntary control).

Skeletal Muscle Histology

Histology is the microscopic study of body tissue, including its chemical composition and design. The muscles of the human body have some common components but, as noted earlier, are also designed to serve different functional purposes. For our focus on how functional anatomy contributes to purposeful movement, exploring the composition of skeletal muscle in particular is helpful.

Muscles are composed of individual muscle fibers (cells). Each individual fiber is surrounded by a connective tissue layer called the **endomysium** (**1.31**). The endomysium contains capillaries and nerve fibers that innervate and supply individual muscle fibers.

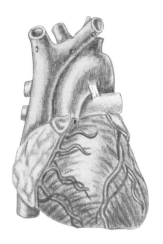

1.29 Cardiac muscle

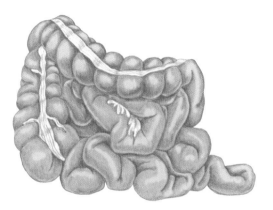

1.30 Smooth muscle of the colon

Groups of muscle fibers (fascicles) are similarly wrapped in a connective tissue sleeve, the **perimysium**. A final layer of connective tissue, called the **epimysium**, surrounds groups of fascicles, forming the entire muscle.

The perimysium and epimysium provide muscle extensibility, or the ability to be stretched. The fibers of the epimysium converge at the end of the muscle to form tendons, transferring the force of muscle contraction to bone and generating motion.

A cross-sectional magnified view of a single skeletal muscle fiber shows that each fiber is composed of hundreds of long cylindrical strands of contractile proteins, called **myofibrils**. Myofibrils are divided into segments called **sarcomeres**, the contractile units of a muscle (**1.32**). The thicker filaments are composed of the protein **myosin**, and the thin filaments are composed of the protein **actin** (**1.33**).

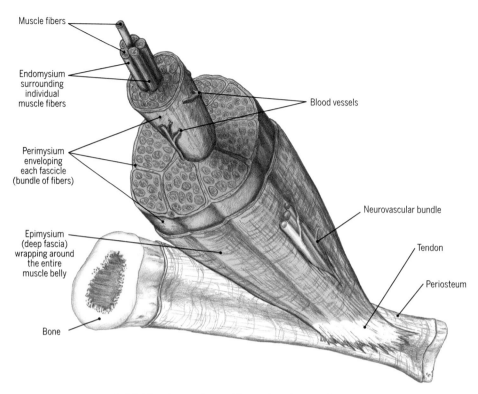

Muscle fibers

Endomysium surrounding individual muscle fibers

Blood vessels

Perimysium enveloping each fascicle (bundle of fibers)

Neurovascular bundle

Epimysium (deep fascia) wrapping around the entire muscle belly

Tendon

Periosteum

Bone

1.31 Muscles are formed by various layers of tissue.

The thick myosin filaments form the central horizontal shaft of each sarcomere, with the **M line** noting their midpoint. Coiled **titin filaments** form a stabilizing border around the myosin, limiting their excursion and contributing to passive tightness of the entire muscle. Thin actin filaments lie on either side of each myosin filament, overlapping to provide surface contact to generate the force of muscle contraction. **Z discs** at opposing ends of the sarcomere connect the actin filaments and delineate one sarcomere from the next.

Myosin generates the force in a muscle contraction in a manner similar to the stroke of an oar. The myosin protein has a head and a tail region. The tails of approximately three hundred myosin molecules constitute the shaft of the thick filament. The myosin heads are directed outward toward the thin actin filaments, similar to the oars of a rowboat, creating a crossbridge, or link, between the two filaments. When a muscle contracts, calcium is released, sliding the actin filament along the myosin filament toward the center of the sarcomere.

Skeletal muscle fibers are divided into many individual **motor units**, each composed of a single motor neuron and the muscle fibers it innervates. Motor commands from the motor unit to the muscle fibers are all-or-none signals, meaning that the sarcomeres either contract completely or not at all. The strength of muscle contraction depends on the amount of motor units that contract, not on the strength of an individual signal.

1.32 Myofibrils are formed by parallel sarcomeres.

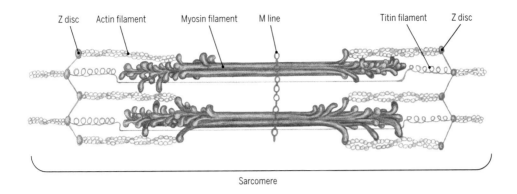

Z disc   Actin filament   Myosin filament   M line   Titin filament   Z disc

Sarcomere

1.33 Gliding filaments form individual sarcomeres.

Muscle Design and Strength

Many factors contribute to the amount of force a muscle can generate, including its size, fiber length and orientation, and the position of the joint and length of the muscle when activated.

Physiological cross-sectional area (PCSA) refers to the area of a cross section of muscle at its widest point (**1.35**). The PCSA of a muscle, along with its length, is a proportional indicator of its strength. The wider a muscle is, the more muscle fibers are available to contract. The longer the fibers are, the more potential they have to shorten.

Each muscle in the body has a unique design and orientation of fibers that directs the magnitude and direction of applied force for movement (**1.36**). Muscles in which the fibers are oriented obliquely (slanted) to the tendon are referred to as **pennate** muscles. These muscles are further categorized as **multipennate** muscles (such as

▶TRY IT

Lace your fingers together to represent myosin and actin filaments (**1.34**). Pull your fingers apart so that only the fingertips are touching. This represents a stretched muscle with minimal surface contact between the filaments, limiting contractibility and force production. Now push your fingers together as far as possible. In this position, the monofilaments have contracted to their potential, with no further room to glide (contract). At what point is the muscle the strongest?

Typically, a muscle is strongest in a midrange position, where the filaments have the greatest cross-linking (connection). This explains why most manual muscle testing is done in a midrange joint position, which for the biceps occurs in 90° elbow flexion.

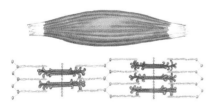

Relaxed muscle

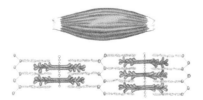

Partially contracted muscle

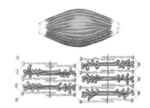

Fully contracted muscle

1.34 Muscle length and force production. How does the length of a muscle at the time of contraction affect its strength?

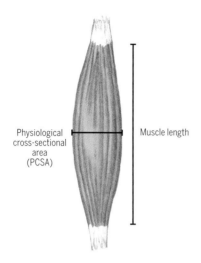

1.35 Physiological cross-sectional area and fiber length contribute to muscle strength.

CLINICAL APPLICATION
Length-Tension Relationship

Clinically, you will find it important to understand a muscle's strength relative to its length and position when activated or with formal strength testing. The idea that a muscle's strength is relative to its length at the time of contraction is referred to as the **length-tension relationship**.

Let's use the biceps as an example. Is it strongest when it is elongated (with the elbow fully extended) or shortened (flexed)? The answer lies in the design of the gliding sarcomeres. Recall that the sarcomeres tend to have the most overlap and interconnection with the joint in a midrange position. For the elbow, this is around 90° of flexion. The force produced by sarcomeres gliding translates to individual muscle fibers, and eventually the entire muscle, contracting in order to flex the elbow—perhaps to take a first drink of morning caffeine.

Take a look at the joint positions recommended for MMT in the *OT Guide to Goniometry & MMT* eTextbook. Most often, the joint is in a midrange position to optimize strength based on the length-tension relationship of the muscle fibers and underlying sarcomeres.

the deltoid), **bipennate** muscles (such as the lumbricals), and **unipennate** muscles (such as the semimembranosus). **Fusiform** muscles have fibers arranged parallel to the line of force, such as the sternocleidomastoid.

Pennate muscles have shorter fibers that do not run the entire length of the muscle but feature angular alignment toward a central tendon. As a result, they can exert more force than an equivalently sized parallel muscle.

Fusiform muscles, with longer fibers, can apply force over a much greater range of movement than pennate muscles. Think of a tug-of-war: a fusiform muscle is like twenty people pulling on a single rope, while a pennate

muscle resembles the same twenty people pulling on four different ropes.

Muscle fibers may also be configured in a circle around a structure. For example, the orbicularis oculi is a sphincter muscle for forceful closure of the eye.

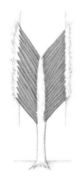
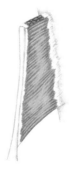
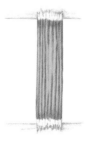
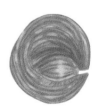

Multipennate (deltoid, infraspinatus) | Bipennate (lumbricals, rectus femoris) | Unipennate (semimembranosus, tibialis posterior) | Fusiform (supinator, sartorius) | Sphincter (orbicularis oculi)

1.36 Muscle designs and fiber orientations

Neuromuscular Control

Remember that a single muscle is made up of many individual motor units that send separate all-or-none signals to groups of sarcomeres (**1.37**). In other words, muscles are not activated by a single impulse from a single nerve ending but by the summation of many nerve endings signaling different groups of fibers to contract. A strong muscle contraction is the sum of many motor units firing, whereas a weak muscle contraction recruits fewer motor units.

In large postural muscles, such as the gluteus maximus, each motor neuron within the nerve that innervates that muscle (inferior gluteal nerve) innervates as many as two hundred muscle fibers. This provides significant functional movement from a small nerve.

In contrast, in small, delicate muscles such as the intrinsic muscles of the hand, the motor neuron will innervate only a few muscle fibers. For these muscles, the nervous system exerts exquisitely fine control of movement. Chapter 2 explains motor units in greater detail.

Even at rest, within any skeletal muscle, some motor units are always active. These low-grade motor signals coupled with tension from **fascia**—the noncontractile (passive) tissues within the muscle—contribute to **resting muscle tone**.

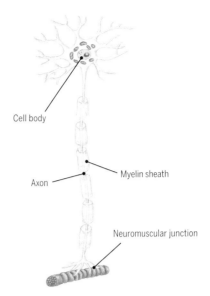

1.37 Motor unit

Loss of innervation to a muscle, commonly a result of a peripheral nerve injury, results in a **flaccid** (limp) muscle, which feels like a mass of dough with no elasticity when palpated. Conversely, a muscle may have increased tone, or **hypertonia**, with unregulated contractile signals coming from the central nervous system (CNS), such as in a child with spastic cerebral palsy. A limb with

---

 CLINICAL APPLICATION
Adaptive Shortening

Earlier we mentioned that soft tissues (ligaments, tendons, and muscles) adapt to forces placed on them and can physically change as a result. Let's look at an example.

If the elbow is casted (immobilized) in a 90° position after an injury (**1.38**), the surrounding soft tissues undergo **adaptive shortening**, decreasing in length because there is no force requiring elongation.

Once the cast is removed, the shortened tissues can significantly limit motion. This condition may also occur with hypertonia if increased tone positions a joint in flexion. Not only is the muscle now hyperactive (hypertonic), but the local soft tissues also have physically shortened. If unaddressed, this can lead to loss of passive motion at the joint, clinically known as a **joint contracture**.

Prevention is key. Maintaining soft tissue extensibility (length) will limit secondary contracture after injury. Once a joint contracture has set in, static progressive orthotics or serial casting may be used to restore motion. Some

contractures do not respond to conservative measures and may require surgery.

Think about the elbow flexion contracture again. If the loss of motion is permanent, what adaptive or compensatory strategies could be beneficial for performing ADLs and IADLs?

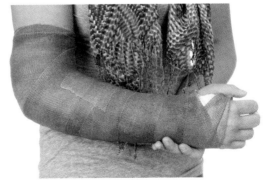

1.38 Elbow casted in a 90° position. What effect will this have on the joint and surrounding soft tissues?

hypertonia will demonstrate increased resistance to passive stretch.

Abnormal tone interferes with the voluntary use of the arms and legs and often presents a significant barrier to occupational performance. Dressing yourself, for instance, would be very difficult if the joints of your arms and hands were flexing uncontrollably.

Regulation of Muscle Tone

Muscle spindles are elongated encapsulated structures (3–4 mm in length) located within muscle fibers (**1.39**). They signal changes in muscle length, informing the brain as to the rate and amount of strain, and contribute to proprioception (the sense of position in space).

Functionally, the spindles also serve to protect muscles, triggering a **phasic stretch reflex** that activates the **agonist**, or muscle producing the desired motion, to contract if the muscle is overstretched. This is the reflex that is elicited by tapping a tendon with a reflex hammer (**1.40**).

Golgi tendon organs are slender encapsulated structures located at the junction of muscle and tendon (**1.41**). Because of their location in tendon (versus muscle), Golgi tendon organs are more sensitive than muscle spindles to tensile force within the tendon when a muscle contracts. They inform the brain of muscle force contraction and may trigger a protective reflex with overstretch, relaxing the agonist muscle to prevent damage to the tendon.

Fast- and Slow-Twitch Fibers

Muscles are composed of hundreds of thousands of fibers that produce purposeful movement for occupational performance. **Slow-twitch fibers**, also known as Type I fibers, are capable of low force sustained over a long period of time and are more resistant to fatigue. In contrast, **fast-twitch fibers**, or Type II fibers, are

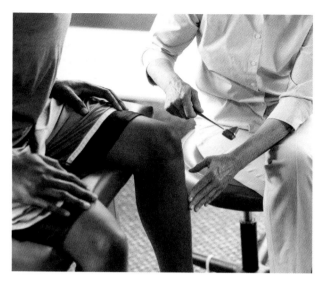

1.40 A reflex hammer stimulates the muscle spindle, which generates a phasic stretch reflex.

capable of generating powerful contraction for intense, focused movements but fatigue more quickly.

The muscles of the body are made up of approximately half of each type of muscle fiber. Both are equally important to purposeful movement. Imagine writing your next paper at a computer workstation. The slow-twitch muscle of the trunk sustains low-intensity contraction to maintain your body in an upright posture. With the core stabilized, the fast-twitch muscles of the fingers rapidly fire, typing your thoughts into words on the page.

Many of the concepts related to neuromuscular control are discussed further in Chapter 2. Continue to apply these concepts as you analyze the motor skills contributing to occupational performance.

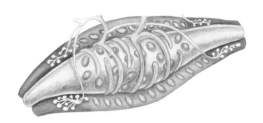

1.39 Muscle spindle

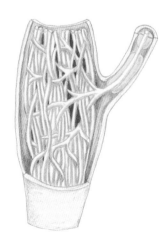

1.41 Golgi tendon organ

Muscle Function

A muscle's composition, design, and interaction with the nervous system affect the way it exerts force to produce motion. Now that we understand these underlying contributors, let's zoom out and examine the way muscles supply the forces of purposeful movement.

Muscles and Movement

Virtually all human movement results from the interaction of multiple muscles. As power requirements increase, more muscles and their motor units are recruited, or activated, to generate force for movement.

The brain generates learned patterns of motion, or **motor memory**, sending motor signals simultaneously to different parts of the body for integrated, coordinated functional movement. To better understand the function of any one muscle for a certain movement, think of individual muscles acting in one of four ways:

1. **Prime mover (agonist)**. Within a group of muscles producing a specific movement, the prime mover generates the most force to produce the motion. For example, the brachialis is the prime mover for elbow flexion (**1.42**).

2. **Antagonists**. Whenever there is movement, the muscles that would normally act to produce the contrary movement need to relax. These muscles are the antagonists. So when the triceps brachii contracts to produce elbow extension, we do not want strong contraction in the antagonists, the biceps brachii and brachialis. A stroke (cerebrovascular accident, or CVA) may result in increased muscle tone or spasticity of agonist muscles, limiting the counterbalancing action of the antagonists.

3. **Fixators**. Whenever a muscle contracts from its origin, that origin needs to be relatively stable. For example, in order for the levator scapulae to elevate the scapula, the cervical spine needs to be relatively stable, or fixed. Muscles that perform this function are fixators (stabilizers). Stability of motion begins in the pelvis and trunk (proximal), and motion becomes more precise through the extremities into the hands and feet. Think about an artist painting fine detail while sitting on a stool at an easel. The muscles of the core and proximal arm would all be considered fixators, stabilizing the wrist and hand for precise, controlled movement.

4. **Synergists**. As noted earlier, movements almost always require more than a single muscle. Muscles

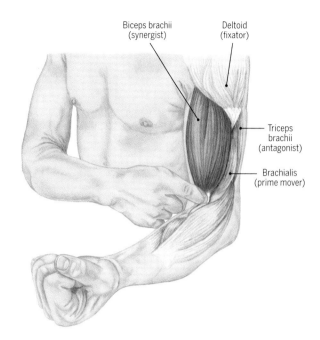

1.42 Muscle actions during elbow flexion

that assist the prime mover are known as synergists. For example, the brachialis is the prime flexor of the elbow joint, but with continued resistance, the biceps brachii is also recruited.

The term **force couple** also describes muscles working together, though acting in different directions, to produce the same motion or stabilize a joint. For example, scapular upward rotation, an important component of upper extremity motion, involves forces generated in different directions—as a force couple in synergy—by the upper trapezius, serratus anterior, and lower trapezius (see Chapter 5).

Some muscles cross only a single joint, while others cross multiple joints but, regardless, are able to move any joint they cross. The brachialis crosses only the elbow and therefore can solely flex the elbow. However, the flexor digitorum profundus (FDP) crosses the wrist and the three joints of the fingers—metacarpophalangeal (MCP), proximal interphalangeal (PIP), and distal interphalangeal (DIP)—contributing to flexion for all (**1.43**).

In order to isolate digital flexion (flex the fingers without flexing the wrist), the wrist extensors must activate to stabilize the wrist, directing the force of the FDP to the fingers. As they contribute to the desired motion, these stabilizing muscles (in this case, the wrist extensors) are considered synergists to digital flexion. This

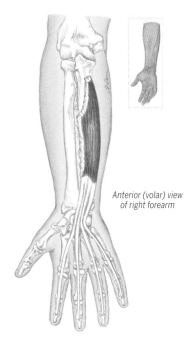

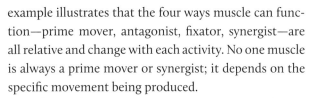

*Anterior (volar) view
of right forearm*

1.43 Flexor digitorum profundus crosses and acts on the wrist and all joints of the fingers.

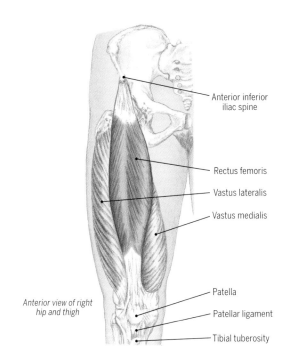

Anterior inferior
iliac spine

Rectus femoris

Vastus lateralis

Vastus medialis

Patella

Patellar ligament

Tibial tuberosity

*Anterior view of right
hip and thigh*

1.44 Rectus femoris is a two-joint muscle. What motions can it produce at the hip and knee?

example illustrates that the four ways muscle can function—prime mover, antagonist, fixator, synergist—are all relative and change with each activity. No one muscle is always a prime mover or synergist; it depends on the specific movement being produced.

Students often memorize origin, insertion, and muscle function from various charts. But memorization alone does not demonstrate an understanding of muscle function. In isolation, muscles can do only one thing: shorten. In order to determine the action of any single muscle in isolation (theoretically), you should look at the muscle's attachment sites and visualize in 3D what would happen if that muscle shortened.

For example, let's look at the rectus femoris muscle. Its origin and insertion (anterior inferior iliac spine and tibial tuberosity) are almost in the same sagittal plane (**1.44**). If this muscle contracts in isolation, it will shorten, resulting in only flexion of the hip and extension of the knee. This is fairly easy to visualize.

Muscle actions become harder to visualize when they cross multiple joints and multiple planes. Probably the most difficult muscle action to visualize is that of the sartorius because it crosses two joints and multiple planes (**1.45**). This muscle originates on the anterior superior iliac spine and inserts on the upper medial tibia. When the sartorius contracts in isolation, it causes

hip flexion and external rotation as well as knee flexion and internal rotation.

Try to visualize this muscle within your own body and imagine how its contraction could create all of these movements. If you can understand the action of the

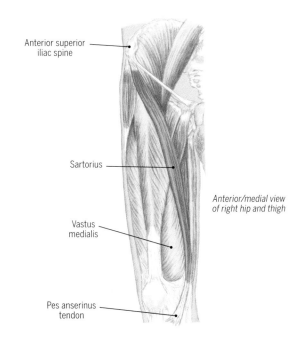

Anterior superior
iliac spine

Sartorius

*Anterior/medial view
of right hip and thigh*

Vastus
medialis

Pes anserinus
tendon

1.45 Analyze the actions of the sartorius muscle based on its attachments and pathway across the hip and knee.

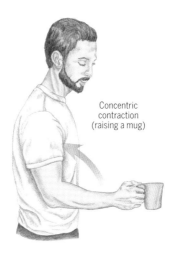
Concentric
contraction
(raising a mug)

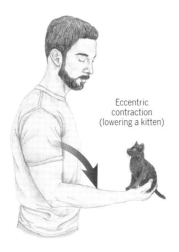
Eccentric
contraction
(lowering a kitten)

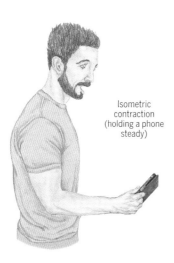
Isometric
contraction
(holding a phone
steady)

1.46 Types of muscle contraction

sartorius, you can understand the actions of any muscle in the body simply by looking at its attachments and remembering that in isolation, muscles can only shorten.

Types of Muscle Contraction

Muscles are able to generate force when contracting (shortening), while maintaining their normal length (statically), or when elongating (**1.46**). Muscle contractions without a change in length (and without joint motion) are referred to as **isometric** contractions. Contractions with a change in muscle length and joint motion are referred to as **isotonic**, including **eccentric** (lengthening) and **concentric** (shortening) contractions.

For example, holding a mug of coffee in your hand with a flexed elbow (90°) involves an isometric contraction of the brachialis to stabilize the mug in a static position. Bringing the mug to your lips requires further elbow flexion, with a concentric contraction of the brachialis (**1.46**, left). Lowering the mug back to a tabletop requires elbow extension, with the elbow flexors elongating with some degree of contraction to stabilize the hand and keep the cup level. This illustrates an eccentric contraction, with the muscle generating force while lengthening.

Load Rate

ADLs, IADLs, work, and leisure place various force demands on the musculoskeletal system. **Load rate** describes how quickly force is applied to tissue. The load rate of force applied to body tissue impacts how the tissue responds or, in cases of excessive force, the type of injury that occurs.

Although tendons and ligaments are extensible, they need time to adapt to force demands. Rapid application of force limits the ability of the tissue to accommodate through elongation and may result in failure of the central portion of the tissue. For example, high-speed lateral force applied to the knee with the foot planted during a soccer match could result in a medial collateral ligament (MCL) rupture.

Soft tissues are better able to adapt to forces that are applied gradually. However, excessive force applied at a low rate may result in a bony avulsion, or a small piece of bone pulled away at the attachment site of a tendon or ligament. Weightlifters experience these types of injuries with maximal tissue loading during a heavy lift with gradual, sustained force application.

Muscle sufficiency involves its ability to elongate and shorten to produce motion at joints. **Passive insufficiency** describes the inability of a muscle to elongate enough to allow a joint to move through its full range of motion (**1.47**). For example, try standing while trying to touch your toes and keeping your knees extended. While some people are flexible enough to do this without any problem, many find it impossible due to the passive insufficiency (tightness) of the hamstrings limiting hip flexion.

Joint motion is also limited by the finite capacity of muscle fibers to glide relative to one another. Once adjacent fibers have maximally shortened, the muscle cannot contract any further, even though the joint may not have reached its full range of motion. This phenomenon is known as **active insufficiency**.

Muscle in three phases of excursion

Stretched, 9" in length

Relaxed, 6" in length

Contracted, 3" in length

Passive insufficiency

Try to make a fist with your wrist flexed.

How might the extensor tendons (red line) limit flexion?

How might the flexor tendons (green line) limit flexion?

1.47 Muscle insufficiency. How might passive and active insufficiency affect motion of the wrist and fingers?

The muscles, tendons, and ligaments of the body are uniquely designed to stabilize and mobilize the bones around joints. The next section outlines several concepts related to joint function and describes common types of joints you will encounter throughout the rest of the text.

▶**TRY IT**

Examining the combined movements of the wrist and hand is an opportunity to appreciate active and passive insufficiency (**1.47**). To demonstrate active insufficiency, extend your elbow and flex your wrist as far as you can. Now try to make a tight fist with your fingers. What do you notice? What do you feel in your wrist flexor and extensor muscles?

In this position, the muscle fibers of the wrist and finger flexors have shortened as far as they can, and the muscles cannot contract any further, limiting your ability to make a full fist.

You might also feel some stretching of the extensor muscles on the opposite side of the forearm and hand as these muscles passively elongate. This restriction due to muscle tightness, or limited ability to elongate, illustrates passive insufficiency.

Whereas passive insufficiency may be improved by stretching the muscle, active insufficiency demonstrates anatomical limits of the muscle. What are some interventions that might decrease passive insufficiency to improve motion?

Joints: Design and Function

A **joint (articulation)** is simply the connection—synovial, fibrous, or cartilaginous—between two bones.

Synovial joints are the mobile joints of the body that allow for purposeful movement. **Fibrous joints** (such as the sutures of the skull) and **cartilaginous joints** (such as the pubic symphysis of the pelvis) feature little or no mobility and are designed for stability.

The synovial joints of the body demonstrate a variable balance of stability and mobility. Some joints feature significant surface contact and congruence between their articular surfaces, which enhances stability but limits mobility. The talocrural portion of the ankle is an example of a joint with significant bony stability, which increases its ability to support the weight of the body. Conversely, the glenohumeral (shoulder) joint supplies the vast mobility needed to position the arm in space, but it is inherently unstable, with minimal contact between its joint surfaces.

Stability also depends on the position of the joint and tension on the surrounding capsule and ligaments. A **close-pack position** is the specific position of a joint in which there is maximal contact between articular surfaces and maximal tension on the surrounding ligaments. This position creates a temporary functional fusion of the joint, forcing the two bones to act as a single functional unit. For example, the close-pack position of the knee is full extension, which provides the stability necessary for standing while showering or during the stance phase of ambulation.

An **open-pack position** describes the position of least surface contact and laxity of the surrounding ligaments, enhancing the mobility of the joint. The open-pack position of the humeroulnar portion of the elbow, for example, is near the middle of its range, or midrange. This is the specific joint position a clinician may want when using manual therapy to increase joint mobility, as there will be less resistance of the stabilizing ligaments.

There are different ways to classify the joints of the body. Commonly, they are classified by their structural (anatomical) design and the functional (mechanical) motion they permit. For example, a hinge joint (structural classification), such as the humeroulnar joint of the elbow (see **1.50**), allows for two motions: flexion and extension around a single axis. As such, hinge joints are also described as **uniaxial** (functional classification). **Degrees of freedom** refers to the number of axes around which a joint moves.

Synovial joints have six common structural classifications: ball-and-socket, ellipsoid, hinge, saddle, gliding, and pivot.[9]

In a **ball-and-socket joint**, a spherical surface of one bone fits into the concave depression of another bone. This type of joint is the most mobile, able to rotate around at least three distinct axes. The glenohumeral (shoulder) joint is a common example (**1.48**).

An **ellipsoid joint** consists of the oval-shaped convex end of one bone articulating with the elliptical concave basin of another bone. This type of joint permits flexion/extension and abduction/adduction (or radial/ulnar deviation) around two axes of motion. An example is the wrist (radiocarpal) joint (**1.49**).

A **hinge joint** permits only flexion and extension around a single axis, similar to the movements of a door hinge. Hinge joints tend to have collateral ligaments that limit medial and lateral movement. An example of a hinge joint is the elbow (humeroulnar) joint (**1.50**).

A **saddle joint** is a modified ellipsoid joint composed of convex and concave articulating surfaces—like two saddles—moving around two axes. The carpometacarpal (CMC) joint of the thumb is a classic example of a saddle joint (**1.51**).

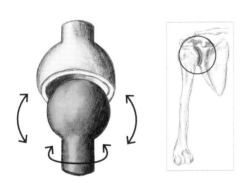
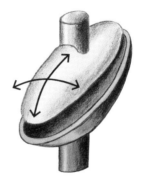
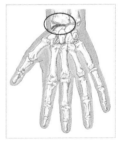

1.48 Ball-and-socket joint

1.49 Ellipsoid joint

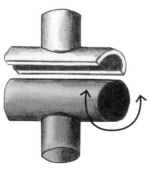
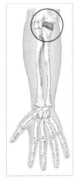

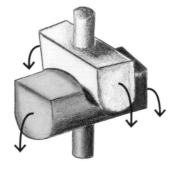
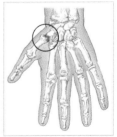

1.50 Hinge joint

1.51 Saddle joint

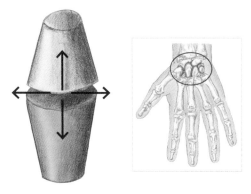
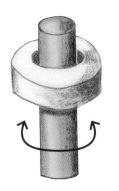
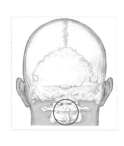

1.52 Gliding joint

1.53 Pivot joint

A **gliding joint** is typically found between two flat surfaces of adjacent bones and allows the least movement of all synovial joints. This type of articulation does not rotate around an axis but instead demonstrates translation (gliding) movements between bone surfaces, such as between the carpal bones with motion of the wrist (**1.52**).

A **pivot joint** features a single axis with one bone rotating around another. The atlantoaxial joint is formed by a pivot joint between the first and second cervical vertebrae, providing rotation of the head and neck (**1.53**).

Think about specific joints of your body. Some are simple enough to classify by observing the external appearance and motion. For example, look at your MCP joints (the knuckles at the base of each finger) while making a fist.

- What movements are these joints capable of and around how many axes?
- Which of the structural classifications would best describe these joints from their outward appearance and movement?

We'll discuss each joint in detail in future chapters, but you can begin to think about the various joints of the human body in terms of their structural design and functional classification.

Osteokinematics and Arthrokinematics

Osteokinematics refers to the gross movement of bones in relation to one another and is usually visible externally. For example, you can easily see the forearm move in relation to the humerus as the elbow flexes and extends.

Synovial joints of the body often primarily feature rotational motion, meaning that every point on the bone moves around a center of rotation (joint). For example, as the wrist is flexed and extended, the palm and fingers rotate around the same axis of motion at the midpoint of the wrist joint (**1.54**). Clinically, when discussing the specific movement patterns of a joint, the term **roll** may also be used as a less formal term to describe rotation.

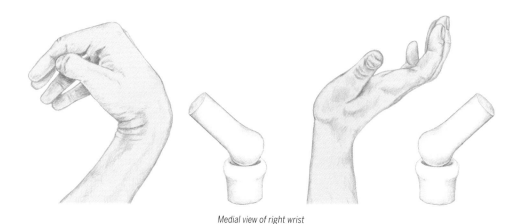

Medial view of right wrist

1.54 As the wrist flexes and extends, the carpal bones glide in the opposite direction of joint rotation.

Gross rotational motion between bones also involves smaller movements between the surfaces of the bones that form the joint. These internal joint patterns are described as **arthrokinematics** and involve **accessory motions** that cannot be achieved by voluntary muscle force alone.

Along with gross rotation, arthrokinematic patterns often include translation, or movement of all points on the joint surface in the same direction. For example, joint surfaces come closer together (**compress**), pull away (**distract**), or move parallel to one another (**glide**). A joint might also exhibit axial rotation, referred to as **spin**. While these patterns of movement tend to be small and not externally visible, they are essential to the broader osteokinematic pattern of joint motion.

An example of the clinical application of arthrokinematics is the convex-concave rule. This rule suggests that if a convex surface articulates with a proximal concave surface (convex-on-concave)—the wrist, for example (as in **1.54**)—then the distal bone glides in the opposite direction of rotational motion. Conversely, if a concave surface articulates with a proximal convex surface (concave-on-convex), like the MCPs discussed previously, then the distal bone glides in the same direction as rotational motion (**1.55**).

Let's examine the wrist in greater detail to better understand the convex-concave rule. As the wrist (radio-carpal joint) flexes and extends (rolls), the carpal bones (scaphoid and lunate) translate (glide), allowing the joint to achieve full end-range motion. Look at the surfaces of the joint (**1.56**). Take note that the distal end of the

radius is concave, while the proximal carpal bones—the scaphoid, lunate, and triquetrum—are convex. The convex carpals are positioned on the concave distal radius, a convex-on-concave design in which rotation (rolling) and translation (gliding) occur in opposite directions.

This means wrist flexion includes dorsal (opposite-direction) translation of the carpals, while extension involves volar translation. Without this translational motion, full rotation could not be achieved, as bone endings would compress, or impinge, against one another.

Clinically, understanding the arthrokinematic pattern of each joint is important. For example, say you are working with a patient who sustained a distal radius fracture and was immobilized in a cast for six weeks. Without the force demands of routine motion, the soft tissues of the wrist will have atrophied (decreased in size and weakened), including the wrist ligaments and joint capsule, affecting the arthrokinematics of the joint. To restore normal arthrokinematics of the wrist, you might use joint mobilization techniques, producing accessory motions to restore joint mobility to support occupational performance. For instance, applying external force with your hands to gently distract the carpal bones from the radius may help elongate the shortened capsule and restore joint mobility.

Some arthrokinematic patterns for specific joints are well studied and widely accepted, while others are less clear or even disputed. This text describes the generally accepted osteokinematic and arthrokinematic patterns as applicable to the specific joints of the body.[10]

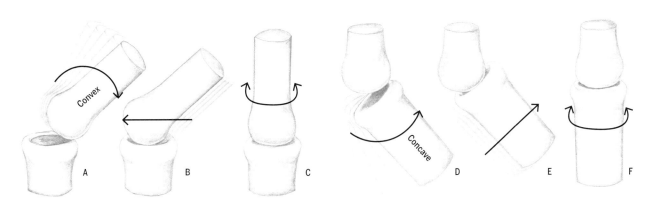

Convex-on-concave movements:
A–rolling, B–gliding, C–spinning

Concave-on-convex movements:
D–rolling, E–gliding, F–spinning

1.55 Arthrokinematic patterns

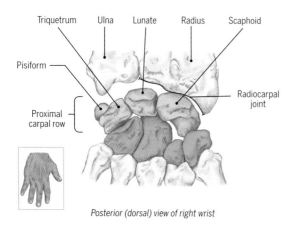

Triquetrum   Ulna   Lunate   Radius   Scaphoid

Pisiform

Proximal
carpal row

Radiocarpal
joint

Posterior (dorsal) view of right wrist

1.56 Articular surfaces of the wrist

The osteokinematic and arthrokinematic patterns of joint movement are often complex. It will take time and experience to learn to apply these concepts clinically. Take the opportunity to read and think through this section again. Once you feel you have a basic under-

standing of these concepts, consider the PIP joint of the finger and answer the following questions:

- Are the surfaces of this joint arranged as convex-on-concave or concave-on-convex? If you are not sure, make a fist and observe the distal end of your proximal phalanx (second knuckle). Is it convex or concave?
- Which direction does the distal bone (middle phalanx) glide as it flexes or extends on the proximal phalanx?
- How does the joint feel when passively moved to its end range of flexion or extension? Why? What prevents further passive motion at its end range?

Developing an Occupational Lens

As you can see, occupational therapy integrates principles from many other disciplines for a unique, holistic perspective—the lens of occupation. The foundational concepts in this chapter will be applied repeatedly throughout this book and in your future clinical practice. The information may seem somewhat abstract and overwhelming now, but basic knowledge of these principles will help you solidify your understanding of the physical aspect of occupation.

Whether you are planning to work with children in the school system, provide ergonomic assessments for the adult population, or address fall prevention with older adults, the ability to conceptualize and analyze the underlying anatomy is essential to promoting occupational performance.

Practice using the new language and concepts from this introductory chapter—performance skills, planes of motion, moment arm, joint reaction forces, arthrokinematics—as you continue your study of the various joints and regions of the human body. Work toward a thorough understanding of each muscle or muscle group and its function rather than relying on memorization alone. Improve your observational skills by analyzing the occupational performance of those around you. Developing this essential foundational knowledge will serve you well as an OT or OTA student and, more importantly, enhance your ability to promote occupational performance for your future patients.

▶**TRY IT**

What prevents a joint from moving beyond its end range (the extremes of its available motion)? In a normal, or non-injured, joint, it could be a bony block or soft tissue. For example, passively move your own elbow as far as you can into a flexed position. How does it feel? Now do the same for extension. Did you notice the difference?

End-range flexion is limited by the approximation of the muscles of the humerus and forearm and should feel springy. In contrast, extension is limited by the bony congruence, or blocking, of the humerus and ulna. Did you notice its hard end-feel?

The way a joint feels in the hands of an experienced clinician when passively moved to the end of its available range, or joint **end-feel**, also provides valuable information regarding underlying restrictions. If the joint capsule and surrounding ligaments are tight, how might the joint feel in your hands if you moved it to the end of its range? How might the end-feel be different if muscle tightness were the source of the restriction?

Capsular or ligament tightness often exhibits a firmer end-feel, while muscular tightness is springier (as muscle fibers are more extensible). A hard end-feel might indicate bone surfaces coming into contact with each other.

APPLY AND REVIEW

Review Questions

1. Which of the following describes the arrangement of a third-class lever?
   a. axis, exerted force, external force
   b. axis, external force, exerted force
   c. exerted force, axis, external force
   d. external force, axis, exerted force

2. Which word is *most* synonymous with "moment"?
   a. force
   b. synergy
   c. torque
   d. lever

3. The biomechanical concept referring to limited joint range of motion due to muscle tightness or shortening is termed
   a. active insufficiency.
   b. load to failure.
   c. yield point.
   d. passive insufficiency.

4. Which term refers to the movement of joint surfaces relative to one another?
   a. osteokinematics
   b. arthrokinematics
   c. active range of motion
   d. passive range of motion

5. Which of the following is an example of compressive force in the human body?
   a. the force between adjacent vertebrae of the spine from the weight of the body
   b. the force exerted by a tendon to move a bone
   c. the force exerted by the muscles of the trunk to stabilize the core
   d. the force of multiple muscles acting on a joint

6. Which type of bone is light and porous, typically found in the ends of large weight-bearing bones?
   a. cortical bone
   b. diaphysis
   c. compact bone
   d. cancellous bone

7. Which muscle fibers generate low force sustained over a long period, are resistant to fatigue, and make up many of the core (postural) muscles?
   a. fast-twitch muscle fibers
   b. moderate-twitch muscle fibers
   c. slow-twitch muscle fibers
   d. pennate muscle fibers

8. What type of muscle has fibers that are oblique (slanted) in relation to a central tendon and are capable of large force production?
   a. pennate muscles
   b. parallel muscles
   c. sphincter muscles
   d. Golgi tendon

9. Carrying a box with the elbows, wrists, and hands in a static (stable) position is an example of what type of muscle contraction?
   a. isotonic
   b. isometric
   c. plyometric
   d. fast-twitch

10. Flexion of the shoulder occurs *primarily* in which plane of motion?
    a. transverse
    b. frontal
    c. sagittal
    d. coronal

See Answer Key in back of book.

Notes

1. Definitions are based on the author's interpretation of American Occupational Therapy Association, *Occupational Therapy Practice Framework: Domain and Process*, 4th ed. (Bethesda, MD: AOTA Press, 2020).

2. American Occupational Therapy Association, *Occupational Therapy Practice Framework*.

3. American Occupational Therapy Association, *Occupational Therapy Practice Framework*.

4. American Occupational Therapy Association, *Occupational Therapy Practice Framework*.

5. American Occupational Therapy Association, *Occupational Therapy Practice Framework*.

6. Gary Kielhofner and Janice Posatery Burke, "A Model of Human Occupation, Part 1. Conceptual Framework and Content," *American Journal of Occupational Therapy* 34, no. 9 (September 1980): 572–81, https://doi.org/10.5014/ajot.34.9.572.

7. Roseann C. Schaaf et al., "A Frame of Reference for Sensory Integration," in *Frames of Reference for Pediatric Occupational Therapy*, 3rd ed., ed. Paula Kramer and Jim Hinojosa (Philadelphia: Lippincott Williams & Wilkins, 2010), 99–186.

8. Adapted from David Paul Greene and Susan L. Roberts, *Kinesiology: Movement in the Context of Activity*, 3rd ed. (St. Louis, MO: Elsevier, 2017), 112–15.

9. Joint descriptions are based on Andrew Biel, *Trail Guide to the Body: A Hands-On Guide to Locating Muscles, Bones, and More,* 6th ed. (Boulder, CO: Books of Discovery, 2019), 34.

10. Carol A. Oatis, *Kinesiology: The Mechanics and Pathomechanics of Human Movement*, 3rd ed. (Philadelphia: Wolters Kluwer, 2017).

Bibliography

American Occupational Therapy Association. *Occupational Therapy Practice Framework: Domain and Process*. 4th ed. Bethesda, MD: AOTA Press, 2020.

Avers, Dale, and Marybeth Brown. *Daniels and Worthingham's Muscle Testing: Techniques of Manual Examination and Performance Testing.* 10th ed. St. Louis, MO: Saunders, 2019.

Biel, Andrew. *Trail Guide to Movement: Building the Body in Motion.* 2nd ed. Boulder, CO: Books of Discovery, 2019.

Biel, Andrew. *Trail Guide to the Body: A Hands-On Guide to Locating Muscles, Bones, and More.* 6th ed. Boulder, CO: Books of Discovery, 2019.

Clarkson, Hazel M. *Joint Motion, Muscle Length, and Function Assessment: A Research-Based Practical Guide.* 2nd ed. Philadelphia: Wolters Kluwer, 2020.

Greene, David Paul, and Susan L. Roberts. *Kinesiology: Movement in the Context of Activity.* 3rd ed. St. Louis, MO: Elsevier, 2017.

Keough, Jeremy L., Susan J. Sain, and Carolyn L. Roller. *Kinesiology for the Occupational Therapy Assistant: Essential Components of Function and Movement.* 2nd ed. Thorofare, NJ: SLACK, 2017.

Kielhofner, Gary, and Janice Posatery Burke. "A Model of Human Occupation, Part 1. Conceptual Framework and Content." *American Journal of Occupational Therapy* 34, no. 9 (September 1980): 572–81. https://doi.org/10.5014/ajot.34.9.572.

Law, Mary, Barbara Cooper, Susan Strong, Debra Stewart, Patricia Rigby, and Lori Letts. "The Person-Environment-Occupation Model: A Transactive Approach to Occupational Performance." *Canadian Journal of Occupational Therapy* 63, no. 1 (April 1996): 9–23. https://doi.org/10.1177/000841749606300103.

Lundy-Ekman, Laurie. *Neuroscience: Fundamentals for Rehabilitation.* 5th ed. St. Louis, MO: Elsevier, 2018.

Oatis, Carol A. *Kinesiology: The Mechanics and Pathomechanics of Human Movement.* 3rd ed. Philadelphia: Wolters Kluwer, 2017.

Schaaf, Roseann C., Sarah A. Schoen, Susanne Smith Roley, Shelly J. Lane, Jane Koomar, and Teresa A. May-Benson. "A Frame of Reference for Sensory Integration." In *Frames of Reference for Pediatric Occupational Therapy*, 3rd ed., edited by Paula Kramer and Jim Hinojosa, 99–186. Philadelphia: Lippincott Williams & Wilkins, 2010.

Standring, Susan. *Gray's Anatomy: The Anatomical Basis of Clinical Practice, International Edition.* 41st ed. Cambridge, UK: Elsevier, 2016.

Townsend, Elizabeth A., and Helene J. Polatajko. *Enabling Occupation II: Advancing an Occupational Therapy Vision for Health, Well-Being, and Justice through Occupation.* 2nd ed. Ottawa: Canadian Association of Occupational Therapists, 2013.

CHAPTER 2

Essential Nervous System

Learning Objectives

- Demonstrate a foundational understanding of the nervous system as it relates to functional anatomy.

- Describe the organization of the peripheral nervous system, which supplies innervation for sensorimotor function.

- Explain the importance of sensorimotor function to purposeful movement and the motor performance skills that contribute to occupational performance.

Key Concepts

afferent

autonomic nervous system (ANS)

axon

axonotmesis

brachial plexus

central nervous system (CNS)

cervical plexus

cranial nerves

dendrite

dermatome

dorsal nerve root

efferent

homeostasis

lumbar plexus

motor cortex

motor nerve

motor planning area

muscle memory

neuron

neurotmesis

parasympathetic nervous system

peripheral nerve injury

peripheral nervous system (PNS)

proprioception

sacral plexus

sensorimotor system

sensory cortex

sensory nerves

somatosensation

spinal nerve

spinal tract

stereognosis

sympathetic nervous system

ventral nerve root

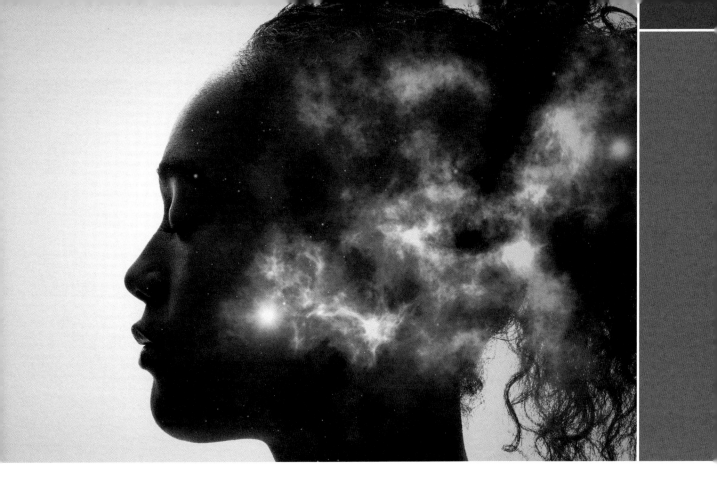

Nervous System: The Command Center

What makes us human? Is it that we move, communicate, and consciously choose how to occupy our time with meaningful activity? Is it that we think, feel, cry, and taste ice cream? Is it our social nature—friendship, a shared joke, or a first kiss? It is all of these things and more.

How do we accomplish all of this purposeful activity? We have an amazing nervous system that regulates our emotions, our sensations and perceptions, and the actions of our muscles and internal organs. This complex system works both consciously and unconsciously to regulate our body systems and facilitate occupational performance—ADLs, IADLs, rest and sleep, education, work, play, leisure, health management, and social participation.[1]

The nervous system enables us to communicate with the external world and controls our internal environment. It receives information through the senses, processes that information, and then sends motor commands that enable us to respond appropriately, such as quickly withdrawing from a painful stimulus.

All this activity is accomplished by nerve cells, or **neurons**, and the cells and connective tissue that support them. We have billions of neurons in our bodies, each consisting of a cell body with two types of extensions: axons and dendrites (**2.1**).

In general, **dendrites** are short and conduct the information received *toward* the cell body. **Axons**, or nerve fibers, are long and conduct the information *away* from the cell body.

Neurons may have a single axon (sensory unipolar) or multiple dendrites (motor multipolar) projecting from their cell body, depending on their function. The length of an axon can vary dramatically, from microscopic interneurons in the brain to peripheral nerves up to several feet in length, extending from the spinal cord to the hands or feet.

In this chapter, we explore the nervous system structures and processes primarily related to purposeful movement and the motor performance skills that contribute to occupational performance.

Peripheral Nervous System

One way of making sense of the nervous system is to subdivide it systemically. The brain and spinal cord make up the **central nervous system (CNS)**. All the remaining nerves compose the **peripheral nervous system (PNS)** (2.2).

In the PNS—the system this text primarily focuses on—each axon is wrapped in a connective tissue sheath called the **endoneurium**. Bundles of axons are then wrapped into groups, or **fascicles**, and these are surrounded by a connective tissue sheath called the **perineurium**. The fascicles are finally grouped together to form the nerves, which are also wrapped by a connective tissue sheath, the **epineurium** (2.3).

Let's take a closer look at the peripheral nerves and their contribution to sensory and motor function.

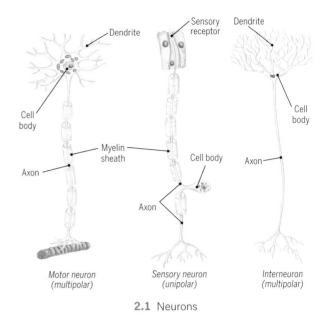

2.1 Neurons

Peripheral Nerves

The nerves of the PNS are further classified as afferent or efferent.

- **Afferent** neurons transmit sensory information toward the CNS such that the information being carried to the brain *affects* (conveys information to) the receiving end. Afferent fibers are also known as **sensory nerves**.

- **Efferent** neurons conduct motor impulses away from the CNS, typically destined for muscles. They cause an *effect* on the muscle or target tissue. Efferent nerves are also called **motor nerves**.

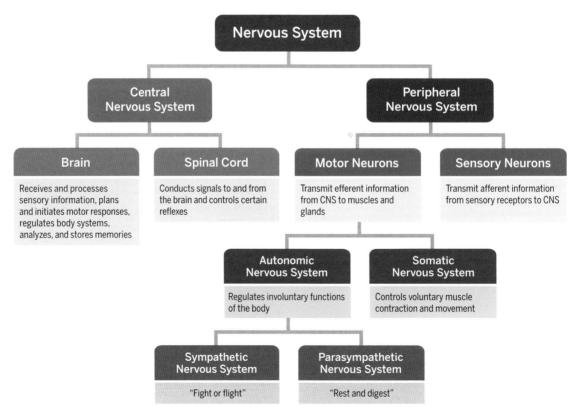

2.2 Nervous system

A nerve may contain only afferent fibers, only efferent fibers, or both, in which case it is referred to as a **mixed nerve**. The nerves of the PNS can also be classified regionally, whether they emerge directly from the skull (cranial nerves) or from the spinal cord (spinal nerves).

Cranial Nerves

Cranial nerves arise primarily from the brainstem on the inferior surface of the brain. There are twelve pairs, and each cranial nerve pair is identified by a Roman numeral (I–XII) and a descriptive name (such as olfactory or optic) that associates it with a function or location. The cranial nerves primarily innervate structures within the head and neck (**2.4**).

Entire books have been written about the cranial nerves, and while it is beyond the scope of this text to describe them in detail, **Table 2.1** gives an overview of each cranial nerve, its fiber type, and its primary function.

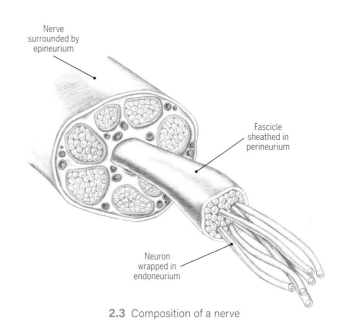

2.3 Composition of a nerve

TABLE 2.1	Overview of Cranial Nerve Function		
NUMBER	**NAME**	**SENSORY OR MOTOR**	**PRIMARY FUNCTION**
CN I	Olfactory	Sensory	Olfaction (smell)
CN II	Optic	Sensory	Vision
CN III	Oculomotor	Motor	Moving eye up, down, medially (rectus muscles); raising eyelid; constricting pupil
CN IV	Trochlear	Motor	Moving eye down and medially (superior oblique muscle)
CN V	Trigeminal	Both	Mastication (masseter, temporalis, pterygoid muscles); sensation to face and TMJ
CN VI	Abducent	Motor	Abducting the eye (lateral rectus muscle)
CN VII	Facial	Both	Facial expression; taste (sensory innervation to anterior two-thirds of tongue)
CN VIII	Vestibulocochlear	Sensory	Hearing; vestibular sense (head position relative to gravity)
CN IX	Glossopharyngeal	Both	Swallowing; taste; salivation
CN X	Vagus	Both	Visceral regulation; speech
CN XI	Spinal accessory	Motor	Scapular elevation (trapezius muscle); rotation of head (sternocleidomastoid muscle)
CN XII	Hypoglossal	Motor	Movements of tongue

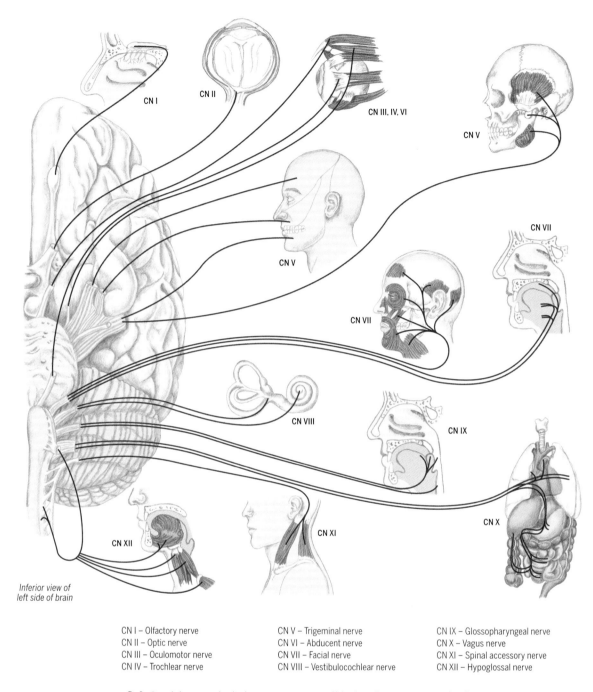

Inferior view of left side of brain

CN I – Olfactory nerve	CN V – Trigeminal nerve	CN IX – Glossopharyngeal nerve
CN II – Optic nerve	CN VI – Abducent nerve	CN X – Vagus nerve
CN III – Oculomotor nerve	CN VII – Facial nerve	CN XI – Spinal accessory nerve
CN IV – Trochlear nerve	CN VIII – Vestibulocochlear nerve	CN XII – Hypoglossal nerve

2.4 Cranial nerves include sensory nerves (*blue)* and motor nerves (*red*).

Spinal Nerves

There are thirty-one pairs of **spinal nerves** that originate at the spinal cord and connect the peripheral nerves to the central nervous system. Spinal nerve pairs are subdivided into five groups based on the five regions of the vertebral column: cervical (8), thoracic (12), lumbar (5), sacral (5), and coccygeal (1).

All except the first pair of spinal nerves exit from the vertebral column through spaces between adjacent vertebrae, or **intervertebral foramen**. The first pair exits between the first cervical vertebra (C-1, also called the atlas) and the skull. The first seven cervical nerves (C1–C7) exit *above* their respective vertebrae, while the rest of the spinal nerves (C8–L5) exit *below* their corresponding vertebrae (**2.5**).

Motor axons are located on the ventral (anterior) aspect of the spinal cord. Sensory axons are located on the dorsal (posterior) aspect. Tiny **nerve rootlets** merge

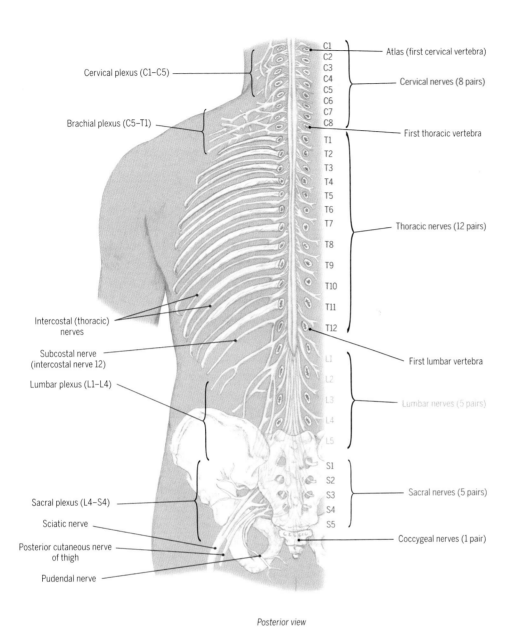

Cervical plexus (C1–C5)

Brachial plexus (C5–T1)

Intercostal (thoracic) nerves

Subcostal nerve (intercostal nerve 12)

Lumbar plexus (L1–L4)

Sacral plexus (L4–S4)

Sciatic nerve

Posterior cutaneous nerve of thigh

Pudendal nerve

C1
C2
C3
C4
C5
C6
C7
C8
T1
T2
T3
T4
T5
T6
T7
T8
T9
T10
T11
T12
L1
L2
L3
L4
L5
S1
S2
S3
S4
S5

Atlas (first cervical vertebra)

Cervical nerves (8 pairs)

First thoracic vertebra

Thoracic nerves (12 pairs)

First lumbar vertebra

Lumbar nerves (5 pairs)

Sacral nerves (5 pairs)

Coccygeal nerves (1 pair)

Posterior view

2.5 Spinal cord and spinal nerves

from the spinal cord to form **dorsal nerve roots** (sensory) and **ventral nerve roots** (motor) (**2.6**).

These dorsal and ventral nerve roots then converge, contributing both motor and sensory axons, into **dorsal rami** and **ventral rami**. The rami are the proximal portions of the peripheral nerves that provide innervation to the muscles and skin throughout the body. The dorsal rami innervate the skin and muscles of the back, and the ventral rami innervate the ventral body wall and all parts of the limbs. Therefore, only ventral rami innervate limb muscles.

Trauma or other disease processes can impair spinal nerve function, with resulting sensory and/or motor deficits depending on the site of injury. For example, based on what you have learned so far, would an injury to a dorsal nerve root result in sensory or motor loss? Nerve roots and peripheral nerves also have specific patterns of sensory and motor innervation, which are described in the next sections. Clinically, understanding these distinct patterns will help guide your assessment and intervention for patients with various peripheral nerve pathologies.

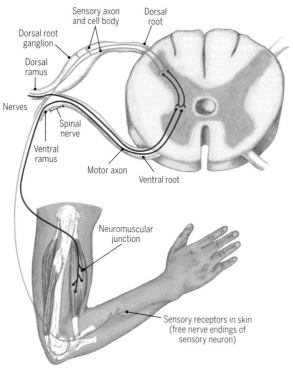

2.6 Sensorimotor function of a spinal nerve

Dermatomes

The area of skin supplied by an individual spinal nerve is called a **dermatome** (**2.7**). Generally, there is some overlap between the dermatomes of consecutive spinal nerves.

Clinically, assessment of dermatomes is useful to identify the level of a spinal cord injury (SCI) or the location of a radiculopathy (nerve root compression) at the nerve root level. For example, the loss of sensation within a single dermatome may indicate a nerve root compression between the adjacent vertebrae of the corresponding nerve root. For an individual with a complete SCI, sensation is typically impaired for all dermatomes below the level of injury, as the sensory information cannot ascend beyond the severed section of the spinal cord. Motor function is usually compromised below the level of injury as well.

What primary safety concerns would you, as a future practitioner, have for an individual with compromised sensation related to an SCI?

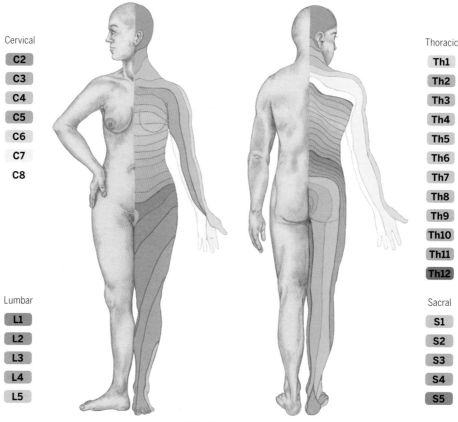

2.7 Dermatomes

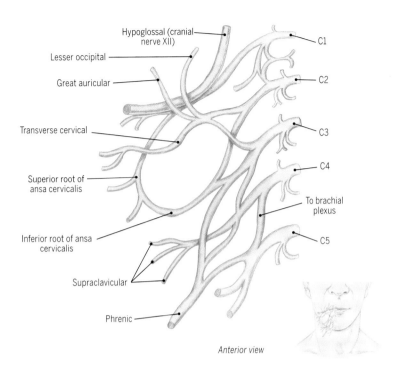

Hypoglossal (cranial nerve XII)

Lesser occipital

Great auricular

Transverse cervical

Superior root of ansa cervicalis

Inferior root of ansa cervicalis

Supraclavicular

Phrenic

C1

C2

C3

C4

To brachial plexus

C5

Anterior view

2.8 Cervical plexus

Nerve Plexuses and Peripheral Nerve Pathways

In several areas of the body, the ventral rami of spinal nerves merge to form interconnected groups of nerves known as **nerve plexuses**. There are four main spinal nerve plexuses: cervical, brachial, lumbar, and sacral.

Understanding the design of a nerve plexus and its contribution to specific peripheral nerves helps with assessment of and intervention for plexus injuries. An injury to a particular part of a nerve plexus will contribute to specific sensorimotor deficits. For example, an injury to the posterior cord of the brachial plexus will impact the radial nerve and could result in paralysis of the extensor muscles of the wrist and fingers.

The brachial plexus is of particular importance for OTs, as it gives rise to the major nerves of the upper extremity and hand, which are essential to many occupations. These nerves transmit coordinated signals for the complex gross and fine motor movements that contribute to the motor performance skills of occupational performance.

This textbook does not describe each plexus in detail, but the following sections feature a visual map of each plexus and its associated peripheral nerves. This may

serve as a reference for future clinical reasoning when you are addressing peripheral nerve injuries.

Cervical Plexus

The **cervical plexus** is formed by the anterior rami of the C1–C4 spinal nerves. The terminal nerves that emerge from this plexus innervate the diaphragm and muscles of the neck and provide sensory innervation to this region (**2.8**).

Brachial Plexus

The **brachial plexus** supplies innervation to the upper extremity through five primary terminal branches: axillary, musculocutaneous, median, radial, and ulnar (**2.9**). Collectively, these nerves provide the sensorimotor innervation to the arm and hand to support occupational performance.

This plexus begins with the ventral rami of the C5–T1 spinal nerve roots. The rami converge to form **trunks**, blending nerve fibers from different spinal levels together, before separating into **divisions**. The divisions merge again to form three distinct **cords** (lateral, posterior, and medial), which then descend to form terminal **branches** (peripheral nerves). You can use a mnemonic

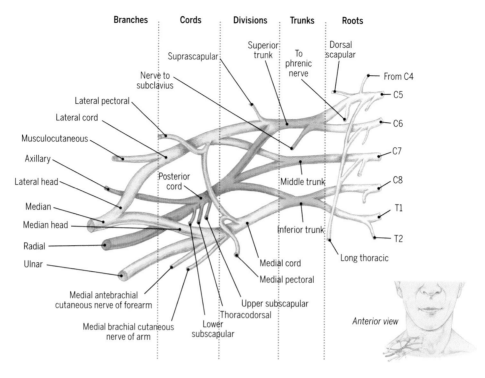

2.9 Brachial plexus

device to remember these various segments—roots, trunks, divisions, cords, branches—such as <u>R</u>ead <u>T</u>hat <u>D</u>arn <u>C</u>adaver <u>B</u>ook (how appropriate!).

The interconnections of the nerve fibers in the brachial plexus mean that individual muscles are innervated by nerves that emerge from multiple spinal levels. Practically, this arrangement creates collateral pathways for nerve signals to travel when there is damage to another area. For instance, if a nerve root or segment of a plexus is damaged, a nerve signal may still be able to get through another pathway along the plexus.

Some peripheral nerves have more collateral pathways than others. For example, the median nerve is innervated by the medial and lateral cords of the brachial plexus. However, the radial nerve receives innervation only from the posterior cord, without collateral innervation beyond this point. Injuries to various sections of the brachial plexus will have a somewhat predictable clinical presentation based on the terminal nerve impact. For example, an injury to the medial cord will lead to loss of sensorimotor innervation of the ulnar nerve, which emerges directly from this portion of the plexus.

The brachial plexus is also intimately related to the musculoskeletal anatomy of the neck and shoulder region and is susceptible to compression. Its nerve roots emerge from the anterior and middle scalene muscles of the neck before descending between the clavicle and first rib. Then the brachial plexus passes into the arm beneath the insertion of the pectoralis minor (**2.10**).

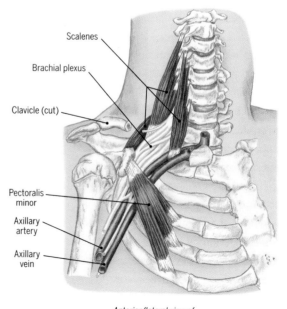

*Anterior/lateral view of
right shoulder and cervical spine*

2.10 Brachial plexus and surrounding musculoskeletal structures

▶TRY IT

The brachial plexus is complex. Drawing it out on your own may help to solidify your understanding of its various pathways and their clinical significance.

Take some time to sketch out the brachial plexus using Figure 2.9. As you form its roots, trunks, divisions, cords, and branches of individual peripheral nerves of the upper extremity, consider the impact of an injury to this delicate neural complex.

Refer to the map of the brachial plexus you have created and the motor innervation of the specific nerves of the upper extremity (2.11–2.16). Using clinical reasoning, think about the motor impairment that would occur with an injury to a specific segment of the brachial plexus. For example, what nerve would be impaired with an injury to the medial cord? What specific muscles would be affected and how would this impact occupational performance? Can you think of adaptations or modifications for someone with this type of injury and pattern of motor loss? Apply these questions to various injuries of the other components of the brachial plexus.

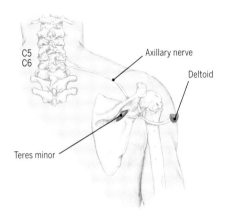

Posterior view of right shoulder

2.11 The axillary nerve (C5, C6) innervates the deltoid and teres minor, which position and stabilize the shoulder for reaching.

Tightness of these particular muscles or postural compromise may lead to compression of the brachial plexus, also known as thoracic outlet syndrome (TOS). This condition affects innervation and circulation to the upper extremity (see Chapter 5 for more detail). Traumatic injuries to the brachial plexus often involve forceful pulling of the head and neck away from the shoulder. A motorcycle accident or stretching in this area during birth (Erb's palsy) are typical causes.

As noted, there are five major terminal nerves that emerge from the brachial plexus. Figures 2.11–2.16 describe the pathway and sequential muscle innervation of each of these nerves. As you examine the nerves in detail, think about the purposeful movement that might be compromised with injury. For example, what motor loss might be present with an injury to the median nerve? How would this impact occupational performance?

The nerves that emerge from the brachial plexus are essential for motor performance skills of the upper extremity—reaching, gripping, and manipulating, as a few examples. Similarly, the lumbar and sacral plexuses innervate the muscles of the lower extremity necessary for functional mobility. Continue to think about the functional impact of injuries to these specific nerves.

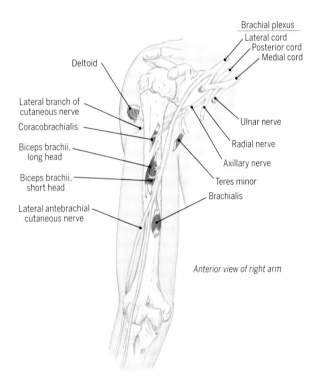

Anterior view of right arm

2.12 The relatively short musculocutaneous nerve (C5, C6, C7) innervates several shoulder and elbow flexors essential for ADL and IADL function.

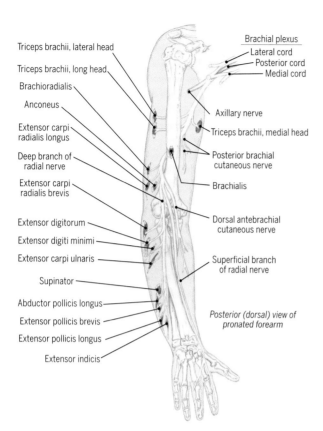

Triceps brachii, lateral head
Triceps brachii, long head
Brachioradialis
Anconeus
Extensor carpi radialis longus
Deep branch of radial nerve
Extensor carpi radialis brevis
Extensor digitorum
Extensor digiti minimi
Extensor carpi ulnaris
Supinator
Abductor pollicis longus
Extensor pollicis brevis
Extensor pollicis longus
Extensor indicis

Brachial plexus
Lateral cord
Posterior cord
Medial cord
Axillary nerve
Triceps brachii, medial head
Posterior brachial cutaneous nerve
Brachialis
Dorsal antebrachial cutaneous nerve
Superficial branch of radial nerve

Posterior (dorsal) view of pronated forearm

2.13 The radial nerve (C5–T1) innervates muscles that extend the elbow, wrist, fingers, and thumb, which are essential for object manipulation and stable grasp. Unlike the ulnar and median nerves, all of the motor innervation of the radial nerve occurs proximal to the wrist.

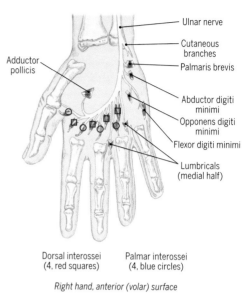

Adductor pollicis

Ulnar nerve
Cutaneous branches
Palmaris brevis
Abductor digiti minimi
Opponens digiti minimi
Flexor digiti minimi
Lumbricals (medial half)

Dorsal interossei (4, red squares)   Palmar interossei (4, blue circles)

Right hand, anterior (volar) surface

2.15 Ulnar nerve (C8–T1) in hand

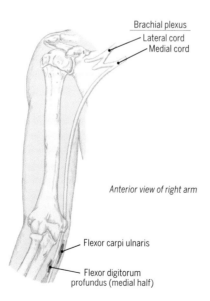

Brachial plexus
Lateral cord
Medial cord

Anterior view of right arm

Flexor carpi ulnaris
Flexor digitorum profundus (medial half)

2.14 The ulnar nerve (C8, T1) innervates two muscles near the elbow that flex the wrist and fingers. It supplies many of the small muscles within the hand (intrinsics) that are important for grip and lateral (key) pinch.

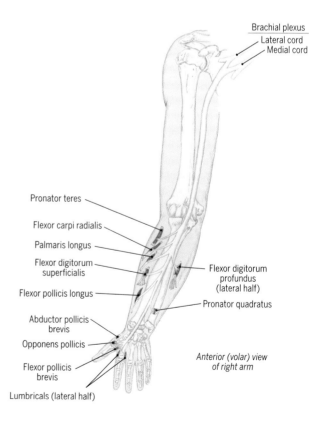

Brachial plexus
Lateral cord
Medial cord

Pronator teres
Flexor carpi radialis
Palmaris longus
Flexor digitorum superficialis
Flexor pollicis longus
Abductor pollicis brevis
Opponens pollicis
Flexor pollicis brevis
Lumbricals (lateral half)

Flexor digitorum profundus (lateral half)
Pronator quadratus

Anterior (volar) view of right arm

2.16 The median nerve (C5–T1) innervates key muscles that contribute to forearm pronation, finger flexion, and thumb motion. It also supplies valuable sensory innervation of the radial aspect of the palm and fingers to guide precise fine motor control and pinch.

CLINICAL APPLICATION
Peripheral Nerve Injuries

We have all experienced the uncomfortable pins-and-needles sensation of a hand or foot "going to sleep" from pressure or an awkward position. Prolonged pressure or tension may lead to a mild form of **peripheral nerve injury**, a direct injury to the nerve, known as neuropraxia. Neuropraxia typically resolves once the pressure on the nerve is removed, but it is also an early symptom of cumulative trauma disorders (CTDs) involving peripheral nerves. One example is carpal tunnel syndrome, which involves compression of the median nerve at the wrist (see Chapter 7).

More severe nerve injuries may involve interruption of the axons, known as an **axonotmesis**, or the entire nerve, known as a **neurotmesis**. In these cases, patients may have more severe or permanent sensory and motor loss.

Fortunately, axons can regenerate to some degree, and there are surgical procedures that include grafting or direct repair for more severe injuries.

To assess peripheral nerve function, practitioners test the strength of individual muscles along a nerve's pathway and the sensory function of the area of skin it innervates, or its sensory distribution.

Consider a specific peripheral nerve and the sensorimotor deficits associated with an injury to it:

- What motor deficit would be present with an injury to the radial nerve? How about the deep fibular (peroneal) nerve?
- What compensatory or adaptive strategies would support occupational performance for individuals with these types of injuries?

Lumbar Plexus

The **lumbar plexus** (L1–L4) innervates many of the muscles of the pelvis and thigh that stabilize the body and contribute motion and strength to the hip and knee for functional mobility (**2.17**).

Two primary motor nerves that emerge from the lumbar plexus are the femoral and obturator nerves. Their pathways and sequential motor innervation are shown in Figures **2.18** and **2.19**.

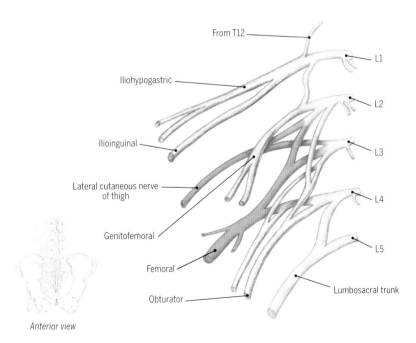

Anterior view

2.17 Lumbar plexus

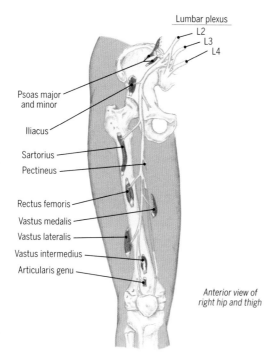

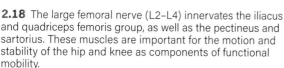

Anterior view of
right hip and thigh

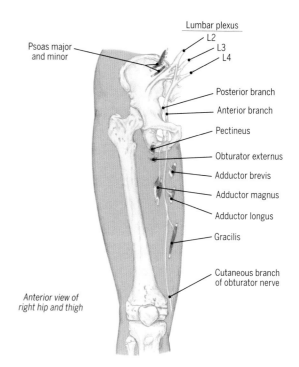

Anterior view of
right hip and thigh

2.18 The large femoral nerve (L2–L4) innervates the iliacus and quadriceps femoris group, as well as the pectineus and sartorius. These muscles are important for the motion and stability of the hip and knee as components of functional mobility.

2.19 The pathway of the obturator nerve (L2–L4) is similar to that of the femoral nerve, but the obturator nerve primarily innervates the adductors of the hip. Tightness or spasticity of this muscle group may contribute to a scissor gait pattern (see Chapter 10).

Sacral Plexus

Several nerves emerge from the **sacral plexus** and travel a short distance to innervate muscles adjacent to the plexus, such as the superior and inferior gluteal nerves (**2.20**).

Other nerves project downward through the lower limb to provide sensorimotor innervation of the posterior thigh, anterior lower leg, and foot. The pathways and sequential motor innervation of these nerves—the

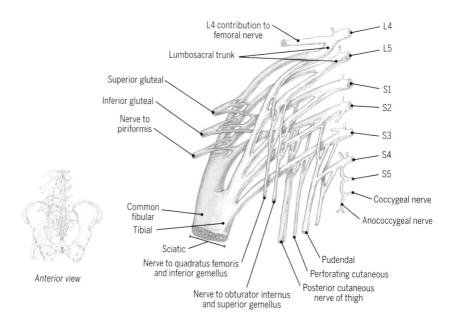

Anterior view

2.20 Sacral plexus. The terminal nerves that emerge from this plexus innervate the muscles of the pelvis and hip, the posterior thigh, the majority of the lower leg, and the entire foot.

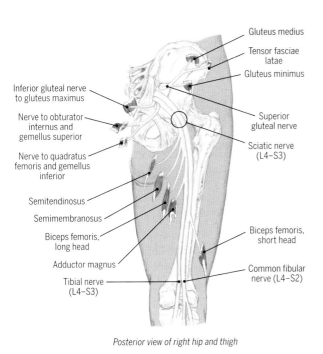

Posterior view of right hip and thigh

2.21 The largest nerve in the body, the sciatic nerve (L4–S3) divides to form two distinct nerves: the tibial and common fibular. Before these nerves separate at the knee, they innervate the hamstrings and adductor magnus.

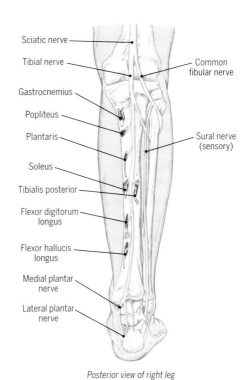

Posterior view of right leg

2.22 The tibial nerve (L4–S3) passes directly down the posterior leg to innervate the gastrocnemius and soleus, as well as the other ankle plantar flexor muscles.

sciatic, tibial, and common fibular—are shown in Figures **2.21**–**2.23**.

As you continue through this text, you will notice that many of the cadaver figures include some peripheral nerves. However, these cadaver figures often show only a portion of the entire nerve pathway. Refer back to this chapter as you identify segments of nerves on the cadaver figures for a broader perspective of the entire nerve pathway.

So far we've focused primarily on the sensorimotor function of peripheral nerves, but keep in mind that they also facilitate the autonomic functions described in the next section. As you examine the details of this system, consider how a peripheral nerve injury could affect autonomic function.

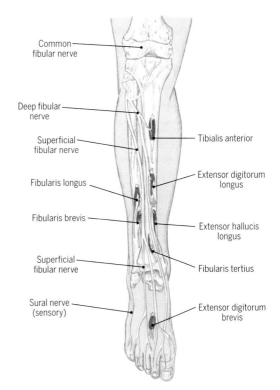

Anterior view of right leg

2.23 The common fibular nerve (L4–S2) passes around to the anterior aspect of the lower leg to innervate the ankle dorsiflexor and toe extensor muscles.

Autonomic Nervous System

As you read this book, you are making conscious, voluntary decisions—directing your gaze to the words on the page, making postural adjustments for comfort, turning (or swiping) to the next page. Many bodily processes are also occurring subconsciously—your heart is pumping, digestion is occurring, your body is maintaining a consistent temperature. These subconscious, involuntary processes are directed and regulated in large part by the **autonomic nervous system (ANS)**.

Along with the **somatic nerve** fibers that innervate striated skeletal muscle (voluntary), peripheral nerves include **visceral motor fibers** and **visceral sensory fibers**. These nerve fibers transmit motor and sensory signals, respectively, to and from the body's organs (viscera). Functionally, they provide pathways for the ANS to monitor and regulate the activity of various organs to maintain **homeostasis**, or equilibrium within the systems of the body.

The ANS is categorized into two subsystems—sympathetic and parasympathetic. These systems typically have opposing functions and effects throughout the body.

Activity in the **sympathetic nervous system** typically involves expending energy within the body. The overall function of the sympathetic nervous system is described as "fight or flight," which refers to the body processes required when it's time to take action, such as when playing a sport or responding to a perceived threat. The **parasympathetic nervous system**, in contrast, works to conserve energy, or "rest and digest," when the situation does not demand expending high energy, as when sleeping. Although the detailed anatomy and processes of the autonomic nervous system are beyond the scope of this text, Figure **2.24** is a quick reference for these systems.

In clinical practice, it is important to be able to explain the general functions of the nervous system in a way that is easy to understand.

- How would you describe the general functions of the sympathetic nervous system in your own words?
- How would you describe the general functions of the parasympathetic nervous system in your own words?

Now that we understand the peripheral nerve pathways and how information is transmitted throughout the body, let's briefly examine the central nervous system and its role in purposeful movement.

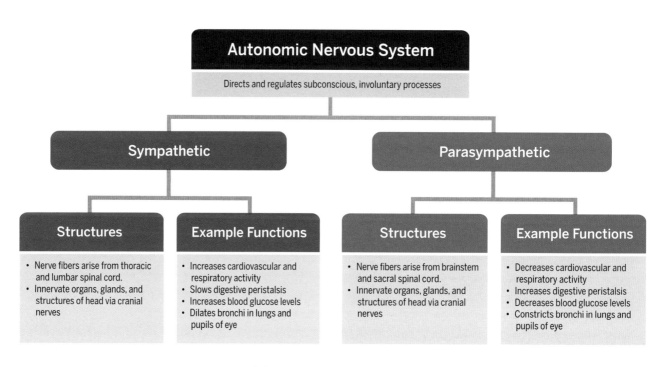

2.24 Autonomic nervous system

Central Nervous System

While the peripheral nervous system supplies the wiring (innervation) of the body, the central nervous system (CNS), made up of the brain and spinal cord, serves as its control center. Moving, thinking, learning, choosing, feeling, and more are all directed by specific interconnected functional areas of the brain. To help you better understand the motor skills that support occupational performance, the following is a general overview of the brain structures related to purposeful movement.

Sensorimotor System

With your eyes closed, turn a page (or swipe) to the next page in this textbook and then turn the page back (**2.25**). How were you able to accomplish this simple task without seeing the book? The sensory receptors in your fingertips were able to guide your brain to send the appropriate purposeful motor signals. This is a simple example of the **sensorimotor system**, or sensorimotor loop, in action.

Sensory input guides motor output. You will hear this concept in some form throughout your OT education. Basically, it means that the brain requires accurate sensory information to produce any type of purposeful movement.

When you turned the page with your eyes closed, you used your fingers to feel the edge of the page (or screen), telling the brain where to place the fingertips. The forearm then cooperated, pronating (rotating) to flip the page. How did your muscles know how to do this?

Repeating an act over and over creates **muscle memory**, allowing seemingly subconscious motor commands to be sent to accomplish familiar tasks. Think about typing, tying your shoes, or buttoning a shirt. After so many repetitions, the sensorimotor process becomes nearly automated. Often, therapists working with individuals after neurological injuries like a stroke emphasize high-repetition activities to reinforce these functional sensorimotor pathways.

Let's talk about the structures of the nervous system required for sensorimotor function. **Somatosensation**, or tactile sensation, describes the sensation received from the skin, limbs, and joints.

Sensory receptors in the joints and skin provide detailed, specific information about the location and quality of sensation. In the joints, **proprioceptors** send

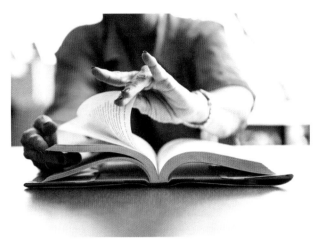

2.25 Sensory input guides motor output, such as when using touch to turn the page of a book.

information about the body's position and movement, or **proprioception**. Sensory receptors in the skin, including **mechanoreceptors** and **thermoreceptors**, send signals to the brain about light touch, pressure, or changes in temperature.

Sensory information travels through the peripheral nerves of the body. For example, touch the tip of your index finger to your thumb. The sensation you felt was transmitted to the brain by the median nerve.

The brain creates associations between sensory input and various objects, allowing you to identify an object based on sensory input alone, or **stereognosis**. Think about putting your hand in your pocket to retrieve a quarter from a group of coins. Your fingers search out the largest coin with a rough outer edge. You might even feel the smooth outline of George Washington's profile on one side and the coarse imprint of an eagle on the other, discerning a quarter from among the other coins by its distinct sensory characteristics.

Each part of the body has a peripheral nerve dedicated to **cutaneous** (skin) **sensation**. The sensory input then passes into the spinal cord via the dorsal nerve root. Once in the spinal cord, sensory information ascends to the brain via different **spinal tracts**, which are bundles of axons dedicated to a particular type of sensory input.

For example, pain or coarse touch travels up the **spinothalamic** (anterolateral) **tracts** in the anterior part of the spinal cord, while other somatosensation like light touch and proprioception travels through the **dorsal column tracts** in the posterior part of the spinal cord. The **corticospinal tracts** are primary motor tracts,

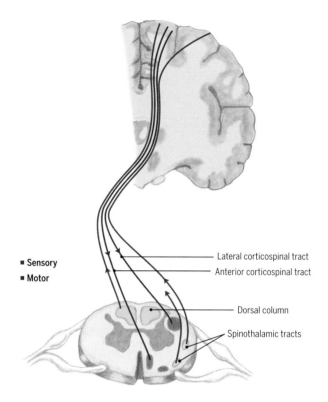

- ■ Sensory
- ■ Motor

— Lateral corticospinal tract
— Anterior corticospinal tract

— Dorsal column

— Spinothalamic tracts

2.26 Major sensory and motor tracts within the spinal cord

transmitting motor commands from the brain to the muscles of the body (**2.26**). There are many other tracts that transmit other types of information to and from the brain and body, but these are a few of the primary tracts related to voluntary sensorimotor function.

Once the sensory information reaches the brain, it is routed to various structures for processing and use in decision-making and motor movement. For example, the **vestibular system**, **cerebellum**, and **basal ganglia** use sensory information to make unconscious, involuntary adjustments to posture, body position, and coordinated motor activity.

Recall that sensory input guides purposeful movement of the body. The CNS and PNS demonstrate a continuous real-time process to guide body movement to meet environmental and functional demands (**2.27**). Conscious sensory information is received and processed by the **sensory cortex** of the **parietal lobe**. The **primary sensory cortex** provides simple sensory interpretation, like sharp, cold, or soft, while the **secondary sensory cortex** and **association cortex** interpret its meaning, associating the feeling with stored memories of similar sensory input for object identification.

Primary sensory cortex	Secondary sensory cortex	Association cortex	Motor planning areas	Primary motor cortex
Perceives and discriminates sensory information (location, quality, intensity)	Recognizes specific sensation (object, environment, or person)	Connects sensory perception to prior memory, interprets meaning of sensation, and facilitates goal-directed planning and use of sensation	Plans specific movements, sequence, and timing	Executes planned motor response via efferent commands from cortex

2.27 Overview of sensorimotor process

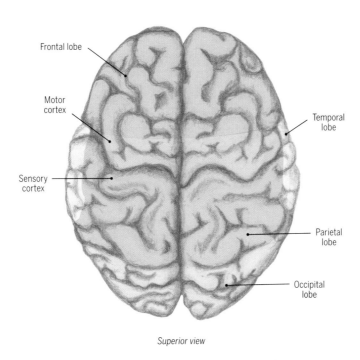

Superior view

2.28 Lobes, sensory cortex, and motor cortex of the brain

Recall a sensation such as having someone put ice down the back of your shirt or cutting your finger. The brain learns quickly, associating these unique sensations with a prank or something more dangerous.

Once the sensation is perceived and interpreted, the information is used to plan purposeful movements by the **motor planning areas** of the **frontal lobe**. This is the reason the sensory cortex and motor cortex are adjacent to one another anatomically, facilitating the continuous interaction of sensory input and motor output (**2.28**).

After movements are planned, the motor commands are sent by the primary **motor cortex** through motor tracts (corticospinal) in the spinal cord to the muscles involved in the specific motion via the peripheral nerves. These motor signals are modified by various structures in the brain, like the basal ganglia and cerebellum, which regulate the signals to produce fluid, coordinated motion.

Take a moment to review what you've just learned about the sensorimotor system. Then answer the following question: How would you describe the sensorimotor loop to a patient who sustained a stroke with a partial loss of sensation and movement on one side of their body (hemiparesis)?

As you continue your study of occupation-based anatomy, consider how sensory input guides motor output. Think about how a loss of sensation, muscle paralysis, or impaired coordination impacts sensorimotor function. This will give you an idea of the potential impact of certain pathologies, like a stroke or SCI, on your future patients and how you might rehabilitate or compensate for these deficits.

Review Questions

1. What is the term for the area of skin innervated primarily by a single spinal nerve root?
   a. a myotome
   b. peripheral innervation
   c. a dermatome
   d. cutaneous sensation

2. What term describes the ability to sense the position of the joints and body in space?
   a. tactile sensation
   b. cutaneous sensation
   c. stereognosis
   d. proprioception

3. Reaching deep into a coat pocket to retrieve a small key, among other objects, without the aid of vision requires which of the following types of functional sensation?
   a. proprioception
   b. stereognosis
   c. somatosensation
   d. touch localization

4. Which of the following ADL tasks would be *most* difficult with sensory loss of the median nerve? (Think about the median nerve's sensory contribution to the hand and fingers.)
   a. buttoning the top button of a shirt
   b. putting on a pair of pants
   c. buckling a belt
   d. washing your hands

5. The autonomic nervous system is responsible for all of the following *except*
   a. regulation of metabolism.
   b. coordinating motor movements of the body.
   c. increasing or decreasing cardiovascular activity.
   d. initiating a fight-or-flight response.

6. What structure describes interconnected nerve pathways that supply sensorimotor innervation to the upper extremity?
   a. lumbar plexus
   b. cervical plexus
   c. brachial plexus
   d. sacral plexus

7. All *but* which of the following are part of the central nervous system (CNS)?
   a. spinal nerve roots
   b. brain
   c. spinal cord
   d. brainstem

8. A radial nerve impairment may result in which of the following?
   a. loss of active finger flexion
   b. loss of active wrist and finger extension
   c. intrinsic hand muscle weakness
   d. loss of thumb adduction

9. Which of the following terms refers to a bundle of axons transmitting a similar type of information within the spinal cord?
   a. peripheral nerve
   b. cranial nerve
   c. dorsal root ganglion
   d. tract

10. Which of the following statements regarding cranial nerves is *not* true?
    a. They emerge from the brainstem.
    b. They innervate structures *only* within the head.
    c. They are located in the central nervous system but function similar to peripheral nerves.
    d. They are arranged in twelve pairs.

See Answer Key in back of book.

Notes

1. American Occupational Therapy Association, *Occupational Therapy Practice Framework: Domain and Process*, 4th ed. (Bethesda, MD: AOTA Press, 2020).

Bibliography

American Occupational Therapy Association. *Occupational Therapy Practice Framework: Domain and Process*. 4th ed. Bethesda, MD: AOTA Press, 2020.

Biel, Andrew. *Trail Guide to Movement: Building the Body in Motion*. 2nd ed. Boulder, CO: Books of Discovery, 2019.

Biel, Andrew. *Trail Guide to the Body: A Hands-On Guide to Locating Muscles, Bones, and More*. 6th ed. Boulder, CO: Books of Discovery, 2019.

Keough, Jeremy L., Susan J. Sain, and Carolyn L. Roller. *Kinesiology for the Occupational Therapy Assistant: Essential Components of Function and Movement*. 2nd ed. Thorofare, NJ: SLACK, 2017.

Lundy-Ekman, Laurie. *Neuroscience: Fundamentals for Rehabilitation*. 5th ed. St. Louis, MO: Elsevier, 2018.

Oatis, Carol A. *Kinesiology: The Mechanics and Pathomechanics of Human Movement*. 3rd ed. Philadelphia: Wolters Kluwer, 2017.

Standring, Susan. *Gray's Anatomy: The Anatomical Basis of Clinical Practice, International Edition*. 41st ed. Cambridge, UK: Elsevier, 2016.

PART II

Spine—The Core of Purposeful Movement

CHAPTER 3

Spine

Learning Objectives

- Describe the bones, joints, and muscles contributing to purposeful movement of the spine.

- Identify the primary purposeful movements of the spine within the context of occupational performance.

- Explain the importance of trunk control to occupational performance.

- Begin to develop clinical reasoning to identify limitations of the spine that may affect occupational performance.

Key Concepts

adaptive equipment (AE)

axial skeleton

cerebral palsy (CP)

cervical spine

co-contraction

core

dermatome

differential diagnosis

fusion

intra-abdominal pressure

laminectomy

low back pain (LBP)

lumbar spine

myotome

primary curve

radiculopathy

secondary curve

spinal cord injury (SCI)

stagger stance

thoracic spine

trunk

vertebral (spinal) column

weight-shifting

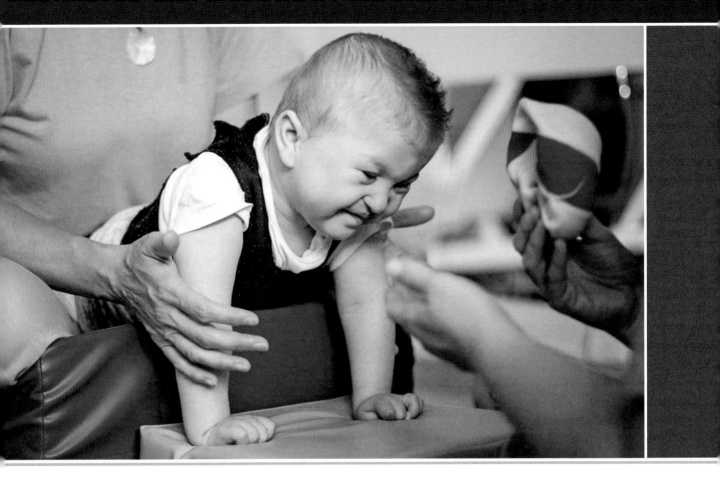

 # Occupational Profile: Max Carter

MAX CARTER is a twenty-month-old boy who has been diagnosed with cerebral palsy. Like many children with cerebral palsy, Max has abnormal muscle tone—mild spasticity, or increased muscle tightness, throughout his body. This pattern creates an imbalance of forces between the agonist and antagonist muscles, limiting his trunk control and purposeful use of his arms and legs.

He lives with his parents and older brother and has been receiving in-home occupational therapy services as part of an early intervention program. Max's cognitive and language skills are similar to those of other children his age. His primary limitations are related to motor performance skills needed for his daily activities and occupations.

Specifically, he is unable to sit independently and can only mobilize throughout his home by belly crawling (on his stomach) with assistance. He is able to hold his head up when he's held in a sitting position or lying on his stomach (prone). He will also reach for and grasp small objects but has difficulty using objects for a particular purpose. For example, he is not able to use a spoon to feed himself. Like all children, Max's primary occupation at this age is play. He especially enjoys finger painting with his brother.

The family is seeking OT services to address his functional mobility, use of his arms and legs, and participation in self-feeding and dressing. As we discuss the related anatomy of the trunk, consider these questions:

- Pediatric occupational therapy practitioners address many areas of development—cognitive, gross motor, fine motor, and socioemotional, to name a few. How might Max's abnormal muscle tone and limited trunk control impact these areas of development?
- What effect might his limited trunk control have on his ability to participate in play, self-feeding, and dressing in his home environment?

Note: Pediatrics is a very complex area of occupational therapy practice. This case study introduces some basic concepts regarding the importance of trunk control to develop and function. It is not intended to represent a comprehensive approach to pediatrics.

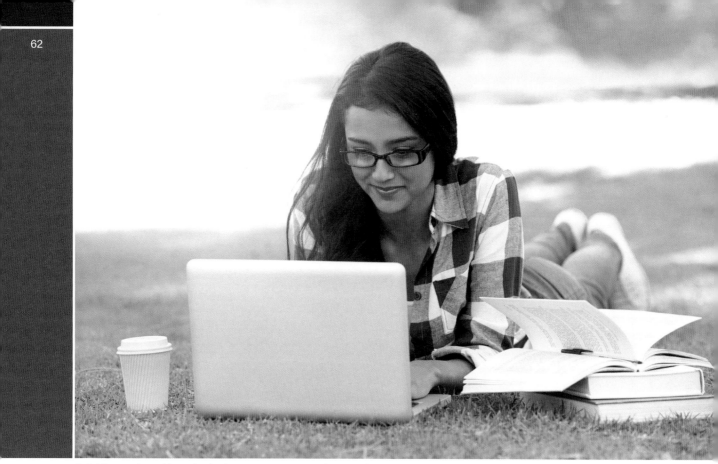

3.1 The trunk positions the body to support occupational performance.

Spine: A Central Scaffold

How are you sitting as you read this book? Are you sitting up? Lying on your back or stomach? Slouching in a recliner, trying to stay awake to cram for an early exam tomorrow morning? In whatever posture you find yourself, the core—or trunk—of your body is the central scaffold for maintaining or transitioning to these various positions (**3.1**). The muscles that form the core surround the axial skeleton and often demonstrate **co-contraction**, or simultaneous activation of agonist and antagonist muscles, contributing to static and dynamic stability for occupational performance.

Look up the motor performance skills in the *Occupational Therapy Practice Framework*, fourth edition (OTPF-4). Notice that "positioning the body" (aligns, positions, stabilizes) precedes motor performance skills involving the arms and legs (reaches, moves, walks).[1] This intentional sequence reflects a key principle of practice: purposeful use of the extremities depends on a stable trunk to support movement.

Before we begin our discussion of this region, it is important to clarify some terms. The chapter is titled "**Spine**," as it covers the entire neck and back. However, the term **trunk** is also used to describe the body's

core region—the back, abdomen, thorax (chest), and pelvis—from which the head, arms, and legs project. The terms *trunk* and *core* are used somewhat interchangeably, though trunk is the more formal and accepted clinical term. **Vertebral (spinal) column** is used to describe all of the vertebrae that form the skeletal structure of the spine.

As motion of the human body is grounded in its trunk, postural imbalance or instability may affect function of the arms and legs. For this reason, clinicians commonly assess an individual's motor skills from proximal (trunk) to distal (extremities), ensuring a stable foundation for purposeful movement.

This chapter describes the skeletal structures, joints, and muscles that form, stabilize, and move the spine. You will find opportunities to apply occupational and clinical perspectives to the spine and trunk through text activities ("Try It"), discussion (from safe lifting and transfer techniques to spinal injuries and adaptive equipment), and digital resources for practicing palpation.

Along the way, we will discuss Max. Imagine that you have the opportunity to work alongside his occupational therapist during a session in Max's home. In contrast to working in clinical settings, working in the home provides an opportunity to assess and support occupational performance within the individual's typical environment, often in collaboration with family members or a caregiver.

Osteology: Bones of the Spine

The **axial skeleton** of the human body includes the vertebral column, ribs, and sternum, as well as the skull (presented in Chapter 4). As a skeletal scaffold, the axial skeleton provides central attachment sites for the large muscle groups that control the trunk, proximal extremities, neck, and head (3.2). The heart and lungs are protected by the rib cage and sealed below by the diaphragm, creating an airtight compartment that supports cardiovascular function, breathing, and the ability to speak.

As you work through the detailed information for each bone, use the digital resources with this textbook to guide your identification and palpation of the bony landmarks that are accessible beneath the skin. Knowledge of these anatomical features, many of which are attachment sites for muscles, will also help your understanding of muscle function and movement.

Let's examine these skeletal structures as a foundation for the functional anatomy of the trunk.

Vertebral (Spinal) Column

The vertebral (spinal) column is composed of five distinct regions of vertebrae: **cervical** (7), **thoracic** (12), **lumbar** (5), **sacral** (5), and **coccygeal** (4). The vertebrae of the cervical, thoracic, and lumbar segments move independently but also in concert, while the sacral and coccygeal vertebrae are fused.

The vertebrae within each segment vary in size and shape, contributing to the natural curvature of the spine (3.3). An anatomical S is formed with an anterior curve (lordosis) of the cervical spine, posterior (kyphosis) thoracic curve, lumbar lordosis, and sacral kyphosis. These alternating curves function similar to a coiled spring, absorbing the considerable compressive forces imposed on the spine with upright function (sitting or standing). When a compressive load is introduced to the spine, such as when carrying a backpack, the curvatures increase. Once the load is removed, they recoil to their original shape.

While individual vertebrae vary to some degree in size and shape, each is made up of a vertebral body and vertebral arch. The **vertebral body** is the main portion of the vertebra, made up largely of cancellous (spongy) bone to absorb compressive forces within the spine. The **vertebral arch** is formed by the **pedicles** and

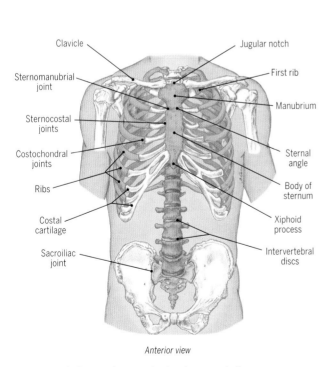

Anterior view

3.2 Anterior vertebral column and rib cage

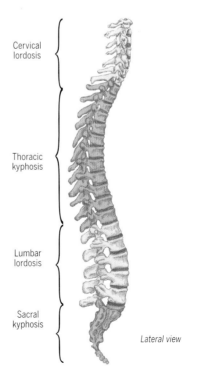

Lateral view

3.3 Vertebral column

MAX CARTER | At birth, the entire vertebral column demonstrates a single kyphotic curvature (concave anteriorly), known as its **primary curve. Secondary curves** in the form of lordosis (concave posteriorly) develop in the cervical and lumbar spine as a child learns to extend the head and neck, sit, stand, and walk. The primary kyphotic curve is maintained in the thoracic and sacral regions.

While observing Max, you notice during his in-home therapy session that he has some head and neck control but still cannot sit without support and does not attempt to walk.

- How might these limitations affect the formation of the secondary curves of his spine?
- What general recommendations might an OT make for infants to encourage the development of these functional curves?

laminae and serves as a bony base for the processes that project from the vertebra (**3.4**).

The vertebral arch forms an opening posterior to the vertebral body known as the **vertebral foramen**. All of the vertebral foramen align vertically within the vertebral column, creating a protected bony canal for the spinal cord to transmit signals between the brain and peripheral nerves of the body.

An additional opening exists between adjacent vertebrae called the **intervertebral foramen**. This provides a passage for the spinal nerves as they emerge from various levels of the spinal cord.

Adjacent vertebral bodies are separated by an **intervertebral disc**, which acts as a stabilizer and shock absorber while allowing some movement to occur between vertebrae. The intervertebral disc consists of a fibrous outer ring called the **annulus fibrosus** surrounding a gel-like inner core called the **nucleus pulposus**. We'll look more closely at these discs when we discuss joints (see **3.22**).

Bony Landmarks of the Vertebral Column

Each vertebra has seven distinct processes, or bony extensions, that serve as articular (joint) surfaces as well as attachments for muscles and ligaments.

The **spinous process** projects dorsally and inferiorly, while dual **transverse processes** extend laterally from each side of the vertebra (**3.5**). The spinous process is easily palpable in the center of the back and is a surface landmark to identify various segments of the spinal cord. With the neck flexed, the C-7 spinous process is typically the most prominent, helping to delineate the cervical and thoracic vertebrae.

There are two **superior facets** and two **inferior facets** on each side of the vertebra. They feature flat, smooth articular surfaces, forming joints between adjacent vertebrae. The thoracic vertebrae have additional **costal facets** that supply articular surfaces for the ribs (**3.6**).

CLINICAL APPLICATION
Radiculopathy

Vertebral fractures, osteoarthritis, or thinning of the intervertebral disc may result in a narrowing of the intervertebral foramen, which might lead to compression of the nerve root. This condition is known as a **radiculopathy**, or nerve root compression. It may result in sensorimotor deficits of the dermatome (area of skin) or muscles innervated by that particular spinal nerve (see Chapter 2).

Clinically, sensory and motor testing may help you identify the location of a spinal nerve compression or differentiate the symptoms from a peripheral nerve issue. For example, what area of sensory loss would you anticipate with a radiculopathy at the C-6 level? How would this be different from a compression of the median nerve at the wrist (carpal tunnel syndrome)? Differentiating symptoms of various diagnoses, or **differential diagnosis**, is an important part of clinical reasoning.

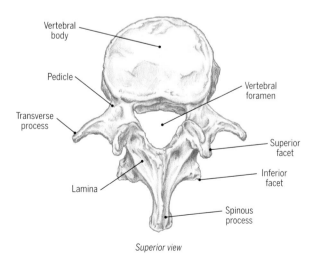

Superior view

3.4 Vertebra

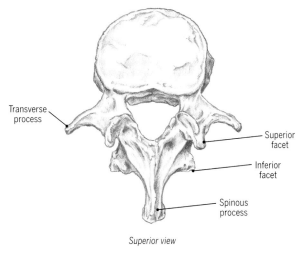

Superior view

3.5 Processes and facets of vertebrae

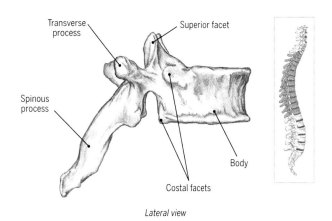

Lateral view

3.6 Costal facets of thoracic vertebrae

Cervical Vertebrae

The seven cervical vertebrae make up the **cervical spine**. The first (C-1) and second (C-2) cervical vertebrae form the **upper cervical spine**. They are uniquely designed to be the interface between the skull and spinal column (**3.7**).

The **atlas** (C-1) is formed by anterior and posterior arches, which connect to create a large vertebral foramen. The foramen serves as the superior entrance for the spinal cord into the vertebral column. Its anterior arch has facets—smooth concave surfaces—on which

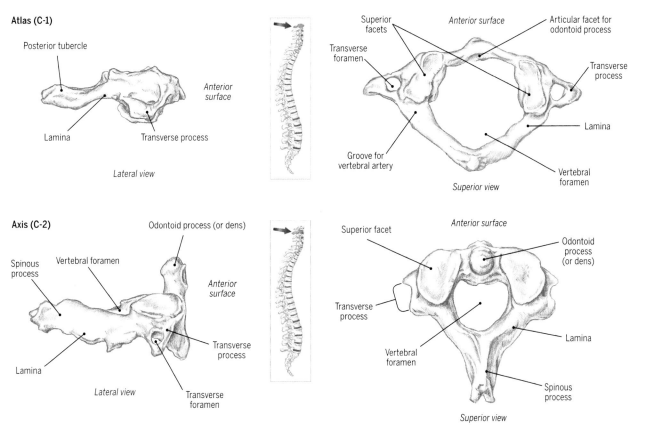

3.7 Atlas and axis

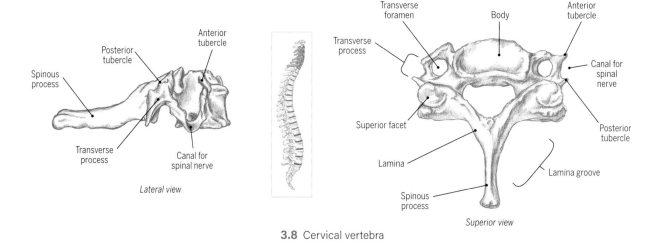

3.8 Cervical vertebra

the skull rests, similar to the mythical Atlas holding the weight of Earth on his shoulders.

The **axis** (C-2) allows for rotation of the skull on the spinal column. It has a unique superior projection called the **odontoid process**, or **dens**, which projects upward through the foramen of the atlas. The odontoid process serves as a vertical pivot for rotation of the head, supported on the atlas. The atlas and axis provide approximately half of the rotation available in the head and neck.

The remaining cervical vertebrae (C-3–C-7) make up the **lower cervical spine** and are relatively consistent in shape and size. Their spinous and transverse processes supply levers for motion of the head and neck (**3.8**).

The cervical spine is the most mobile segment of the spinal column, with the lower cervical column complementing the motions of the atlas and axis. The transverse processes of the cervical vertebrae (except C-1) each have a **transverse foramen** through which the vertebral artery and vein ascend, supplying blood to the brain (**3.8**, **3.9**).

The **nuchal ligament** is a unique structure of the cervical spine that extends inferiorly from the **external occipital protuberance** of the skull (**3.10**).

Animals that walk on all fours, such as sheep and cattle, have a similar ligament that supports the weight of the head against gravity. In animals, this ligamentous structure is referred to as a "paddywhack" and is sold as a dog treat (think of the nursery rhyme line "With a knick-knack, paddywhack, give a dog a bone"). In humans, this finlike nuchal ligament is an important attachment site for the **trapezius** and **splenius capitis** muscles.

▶TRY IT

To identify the end of the cervical spine and the beginning of the thoracic spine, you can easily palpate the C-7 spinous process (**3.10**). It is often the most prominent vertebra.

Palpate the occiput at the base of your skull, and then slowly run your fingers down the middle of your spine while maintaining gentle pressure. You will start to feel large bony protrusions. These are the spinous processes of the cervical vertebrae.

Keep moving your fingers inferiorly until you feel the largest spinous process. This should be C-7. If you extend your neck, the spinous process above (C-6) should disappear while the C-7 spinous process remains because it is less mobile. These are often important landmarks to delineate in order to assess the mobility of the cervical spine. Additionally, the spinous process inferior to C-7 marks the beginning of the thoracic spine, described in the next section.

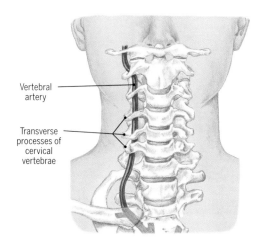

3.9 Cervical spine and vertebral artery

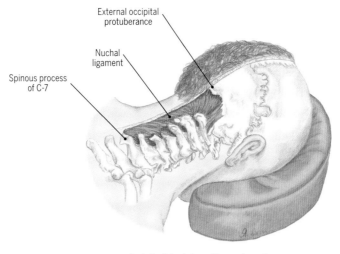

*Posterior/lateral view with muscles and
tissue removed from right side*

3.10 Nuchal ligament and external occipital protuberance

Thoracic Vertebrae

The twelve thoracic vertebrae form the **thoracic spine**, spanning the central part of the vertebral column and providing the posterior attachment for the ribs (**3.11**). They are slightly thicker posteriorly and thinner anteriorly, contributing to the kyphotic (posterior) curvature of the thoracic spine. The vertebral bodies are progressively larger moving toward the lumbar spine, enhancing the weight-bearing surface of the lower vertebrae, which absorb more compressive force.

Costal facets on the vertebral body and transverse processes serve as attachments for the head and tubercle of each rib. Because the ribs project laterally around the trunk and are close together, side bending of the thoracic spine is limited.

Sternum

The **sternum** is a flat vertical bone aligned with the vertebral column in the sagittal plane that supplies anterior structural support for the rib cage (**3.12**). It is made up of the manubrium, body, and xiphoid process, with articular surfaces for the ribs forming **sternocostal joints**.

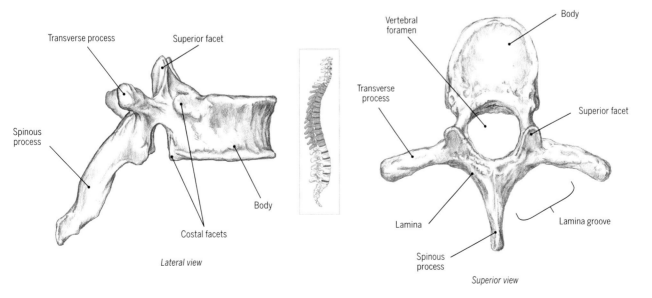

Lateral view   *Superior view*

3.11 Thoracic vertebra

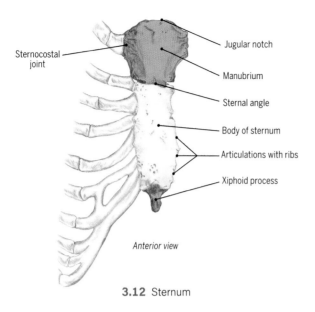

Jugular notch

Sternocostal joint

Manubrium

Sternal angle

Body of sternum

Articulations with ribs

Xiphoid process

Anterior view

3.12 Sternum

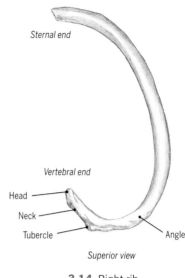

Sternal end

Vertebral end

Head

Neck

Tubercle

Angle

Superior view

3.14 Right rib

Ribs

The **rib cage** is formed by twelve pairs of ribs resembling bucket handles. The ribs are held to the skeleton by the vertebrae and sternum, with the rounded handles wrapping around the upper trunk (**3.13**, **3.14**).

The first seven ribs are referred to as **true ribs**. These ribs have direct links to the sternum via **costal cartilage**. Ribs eight through ten are called **false ribs** because they converge with a common costal cartilage connection to the sternum. The final two ribs are termed **floating ribs**. These have no bony connection to the anterior sternum and are joined to the skeleton only by the vertebrae.

The rib cage gives structure to the core of the body and essential protection to the vital organs within. The **diaphragm** serves as a muscular seal to the inferior rib cage, controlling the volume of the thoracic cavity for respiration and speech. When the diaphragm contracts, the **thoracic (chest) cavity** expands, bringing air into the lungs. Relaxation of the diaphragm decreases the volume of the thoracic cavity, expelling air from the lungs.

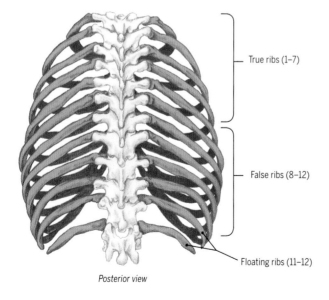

True ribs (1–7)

False ribs (8–12)

Floating ribs (11–12)

Posterior view

3.13 Rib cage

CLINICAL APPLICATION
Rib Fractures

Individual or multiple rib fractures can result from traumatic injuries like motor vehicle accidents (MVAs) or falls. Because the ribs are held in place by the intercostal muscles, mild rib fractures are often nondisplaced (the bones remain connected) and will heal on their own in approximately six weeks if protected from further injury.

Severe displaced fractures can also damage the lungs. The sharp fractured end of a rib may puncture a lung, causing leakage of air (pneumothorax). An injury of this nature is potentially life-threatening and requires surgery to address the compromised lung and stabilize the ribs.

How might a rib fracture temporarily impair trunk mobility or respiration (breathing)?

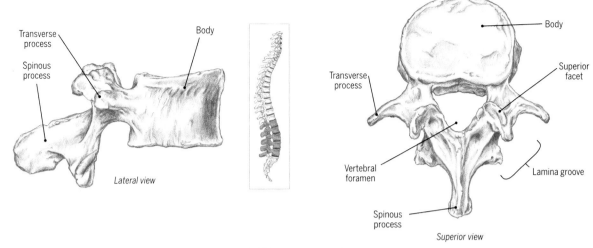

Transverse process

Body

Spinous process

Lateral view

Body

Transverse process

Superior facet

Vertebral foramen

Spinous process

Lamina groove

Superior view

3.15 Lumbar vertebra

Lumbar Vertebrae

The five lumbar vertebrae that form the **lumbar spine** are the largest and least mobile of the vertebral column, providing a stable base of support for the upper body. In contrast to the thoracic vertebrae, they are thicker anteriorly, which collectively creates lordosis at this level of the spinal column (**3.15**).

The lumbar vertebrae are supported posteriorly by a thick fascial membrane called the **thoracolumbar fascia (TLF)**, which limits shear force between the vertebrae with bending and lifting (**3.16**).

Sacrum

The **sacrum** is a triangular bone located beneath the fifth lumbar vertebra, forming the posterior pelvic wall (**3.17**). It has five connected segments that fuse in adulthood. **Foramina**, or openings, on its anterior and posterior surfaces create passageways for spinal nerves.

The **sacral alae**, located on the lateral aspects of the superior sacrum, provide the articular surfaces for the pelvis. The **coccyx**, or tailbone, is the terminal segment of the vertebral column, formed by three to five small vertebrae.

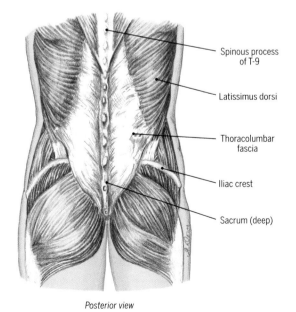

Spinous process of T-9

Latissimus dorsi

Thoracolumbar fascia

Iliac crest

Sacrum (deep)

Posterior view

3.16 Lower thorax and pelvis

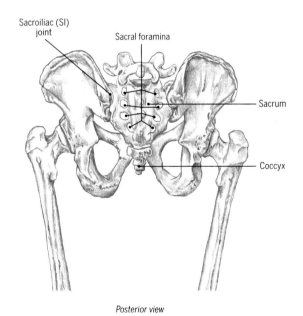

Sacroiliac (SI) joint

Sacral foramina

Sacrum

Coccyx

Posterior view

3.17 Sacrum

MAX CARTER | As you continue working with Max in his home environment, you notice the OT supports him in some different positions.

In sitting, Max's trunk remains flexed forward, and he places his hands on the floor for support. But when the OT supports him at his hips and trunk, he sits more upright and begins to reach forward, exploring the environment with his hands. You hold out his favorite small toy while the OT supports him in sitting, and he reaches out to hold it with both hands for several seconds before releasing it.

The OT helps Max transition into a prone position supported on a wedge brought from the clinic. With help, Max is able to prop up through his arms with his elbows and wrists extended (see photo). The OT continues to support his trunk while you hold out the small toy in front of him.

Max seems uncomfortable at first, but slowly he begins to raise his head. He reaches out with one hand for the toy and holds it for a few seconds.

The OT then works with Max while he is lying on his back (supine). He seems most content in this position. With a big smile, he reaches for small objects with both hands at midline (the center of his body). During the session, you also notice that Max can follow simple verbal instructions.

- How might this activity be graded up or down to increase or decrease the level of difficulty for Max?
- Why do you think the OT is working with Max in different positions? How might this address abnormal muscle tone and trunk control?
- Why do you think Max seems to have more head and neck control, as well as improved hand function, with his trunk stabilized?
- A child's primary occupation is play. What other play-based interventions could you recommend for Max in a supported seated, prone, side lying, or supine position?

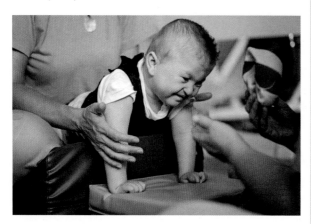

Now that we have discussed the bones that supply the skeletal structure of the spine, let's examine the unique joints that contribute to trunk motion.

Joints

Similar to links in a chain, the spinal vertebrae move relative to one another, contributing to global movements of the entire chain (spine) (**3.18**). The sum of motion between individual vertebrae produces the gross movements of the trunk required for functional activity—flexion, extension, side bending, and rotation.

In an upright position—sitting, standing, or walking/running—the spine is functioning in a closed-chain pattern. Adjacent vertebrae are compressed together under the weight of gravity, increasing the interdependence of their movement. The vertebrae demonstrate more mobility with open-chain functional positions and reduced compressive forces, such as when the body is horizontal while sleeping.

An injury or loss of mobility in an individual vertebra or portion of the vertebral column will affect the other interconnected links. A neutral spine, with its three natural curves present and supported, is most conducive to

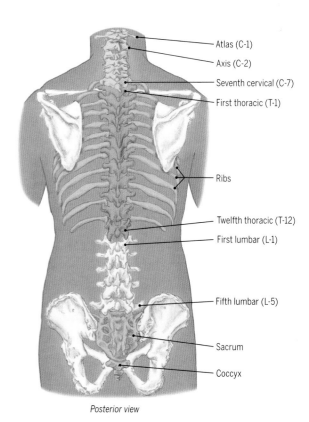

Atlas (C-1)
Axis (C-2)
Seventh cervical (C-7)
First thoracic (T-1)
Ribs
Twelfth thoracic (T-12)
First lumbar (L-1)
Fifth lumbar (L-5)
Sacrum
Coccyx

Posterior view

3.18 Spinal vertebrae

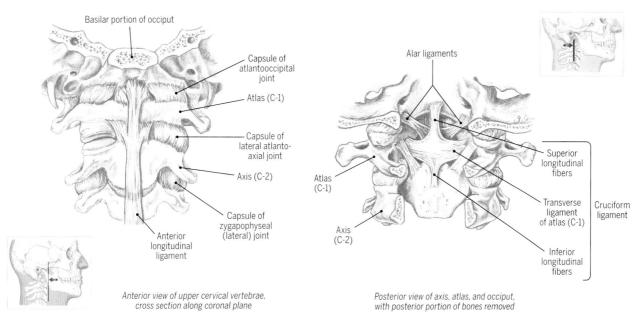

Anterior view of upper cervical vertebrae,
cross section along coronal plane

Posterior view of axis, atlas, and occiput,
with posterior portion of bones removed

3.19 Atlantooccipital joint

optimal occupational performance. It is from this position that the body is most stable and designed to move. Dysfunction of the skeletal elements of the spine often leads to muscle fatigue, postural imbalance, and pain.

Atlantooccipital Joint

The **atlantooccipital (AO) joint** is the interface between the skull and vertebral column (**3.19**). It consists of the convex occipital condyles articulating with the concave superior facets of the atlas (C-1). This joint is supported by articular synovial capsules, as well as the

anterior and **posterior atlantooccipital membranes**. Sometimes referred to as the "yes joint," it provides the initial movement for flexion and extension of the head.

Atlantoaxial Joint

The **atlantoaxial (AA) joint**, in contrast, is referred to as the "no joint" because it supplies much of the rotation of the head (**3.20**). The most mobile portion of this joint is formed by the odontoid process, which extends vertically through the **anterior arch** and is supported by the **transverse ligament** of the atlas,

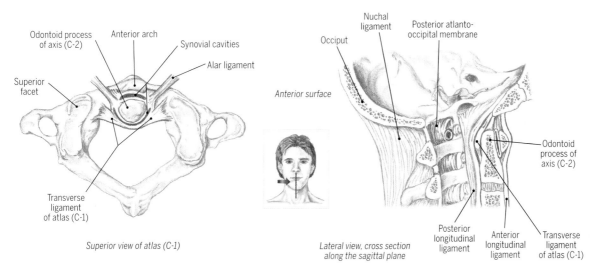

Superior view of atlas (C-1)

Anterior surface

Lateral view, cross section
along the sagittal plane

3.20 Atlantoaxial joint

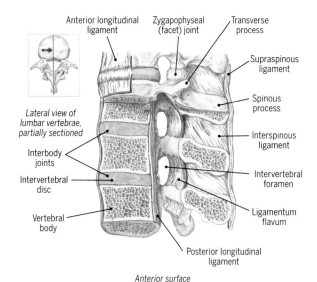

Lateral view of lumbar vertebrae, partially sectioned

Anterior surface

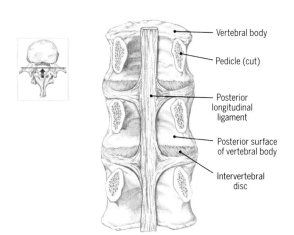

Posterior view of vertebral bodies

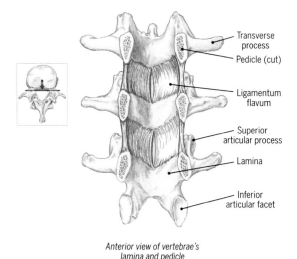

Anterior view of vertebrae's lamina and pedicle

3.21 Intervertebral joints

serving as a pivot for rotation. There are also two synovial facet joints, one on either side of the vertebra, that are further stabilized by the **anterior** and **posterior atlantoaxial membranes**.

Intervertebral Joints

There are three distinct articulations between adjacent vertebrae in the spinal column: one interbody joint and two zygapophyseal (facet) joints (**3.21**). Motion of the intervertebral joints varies between each region of the spinal column, contributing to the delicate balance of core stability and mobility required for function. As mentioned earlier, mobility varies depending on the functional purpose of the specific region of the spine.

The cervical spine is the most mobile region, allowing broad movement of the head and neck, which enhances the visual field for occupations like driving. The vertebrae of the lumbar spine are less mobile, supplying the stability needed in the lower core for the compressive forces associated with functional mobility or lifting.

The primary ligaments that support the intervertebral joints are the **anterior longitudinal ligament (ALL)**, **posterior longitudinal ligament (PLL)**, and **ligamentum flavum** (**3.21**). The longitudinal ligaments are thick membranes that span the volar and dorsal aspects of the vertebral bodies, stabilizing and preventing excessive glide (shear) between vertebrae. The ligamentum flavum provides stability between segments, connecting at the laminae of adjacent vertebrae. Other supporting ligaments include the zygapophyseal joint capsule and the **intertransverse** and **interspinous ligaments**, which connect the processes of the vertebrae.

Interbody Joints

The **interbody joints** consist of adjacent vertebral bodies vertically aligned, with the intervertebral disc acting as a cushion between the two weight-bearing surfaces (**3.21**).

Similar to a waterbed conforming to the weight of a body, the nucleus pulposus within the disc displaces to accommodate movement between adjacent vertebrae to contribute to collective motion of the entire spine. The annulus fibrosis—the thick fibrocartilage barrier around the disc—limits the amount of displacement and stabilizes the disc, similar to the rubber covering of a tire. This arrangement allows the interbody joints to individually flex, extend, laterally flex, and rotate, contributing to these same gross movements of the trunk (**3.22**).

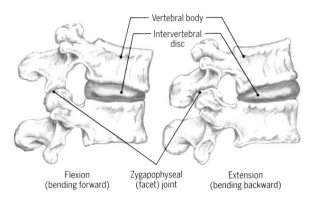

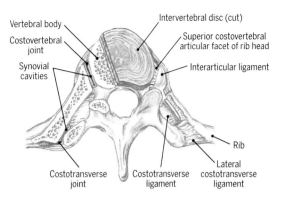

Flexion (bending forward)   Zygapophyseal (facet) joint   Extension (bending backward)

Superior view of thoracic vertebra, left side of illustration cut in cross section

3.22 The nucleus pulposus within the intervertebral disc displaces to facilitate movement between adjacent vertebrae.

Zygapophyseal (Facet) Joints

The **zygapophyseal (facet) joints** are formed by the superior and inferior facets of adjacent joints on either side of the vertebrae (**3.22**). True synovial joints, they are surrounded by joint capsules and allow a small amount of motion between the vertebrae.

The alignment of the zygapophyseal joints varies within the spinal column and limits certain motions. For example, in the cervical spine, the facets are aligned near the frontal plane, allowing for rotation, flexion, and extension while limiting translation. In contrast, the facets in the lumbar spine are aligned near the transverse plane (medial and lateral), limiting rotation and promoting stability in the lower vertebrae.

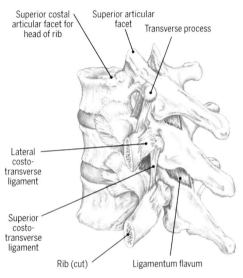

Lateral/posterior view

Costal Joints

Costal joints are the connections between the ribs and skeleton and are found at the sternum and thoracic vertebrae (**3.23**). There are two articulations between the posterior ribs and thoracic vertebrae: the **costovertebral** and **costotransverse joints**, which connect at the vertebral body and transverse process, respectively. Anteriorly, the **sternoclavicular (SC) joints** are the connection between the ribs and sternum (described in Chapter 5).

The costal joints demonstrate variable amounts of gliding and rotation, allowing the ribs to elevate and depress with respiration. As mentioned, the ribs resemble bucket handles with anterior and posterior connections to the skeleton. Symmetrical movement of individual ribs requires cooperative motion of the costal joints.

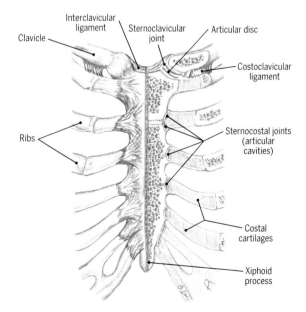

Anterior view, right side of illustration shown in coronal cross section

3.23 Costal joints

Given what you now know about the segments of the spine, answer the following questions:

- Why do you think radiculopathy is most common in the cervical and lumbar spine?
- Why do you think painful conditions of the spine are most often focused in the lumbar area?
- Why are compression fractures in the older adult population most prevalent in the thoracic spine?

 MAX CARTER | Let's think about Max again. How would the lack of development of the secondary curves of his spine (cervical and lumbar lordosis) impact the alignment and function of the vertebral joints in these regions?

Now that you have an understanding of the skeletal components and articulations of the spinal column, let's discuss the muscles that contribute to stability and movement of the trunk.

Musculature and Movement

The muscles that act on the spine form the muscular core of the body and serve to position, align, and stabilize the trunk for occupational performance (**3.24**, **3.25**). These muscles feature a blend of slow- and fast-twitch fibers and are nearly continuously active in some capacity.

The spinal muscles surround and support the vertical spinal column, similar to how the guylines of a tent or

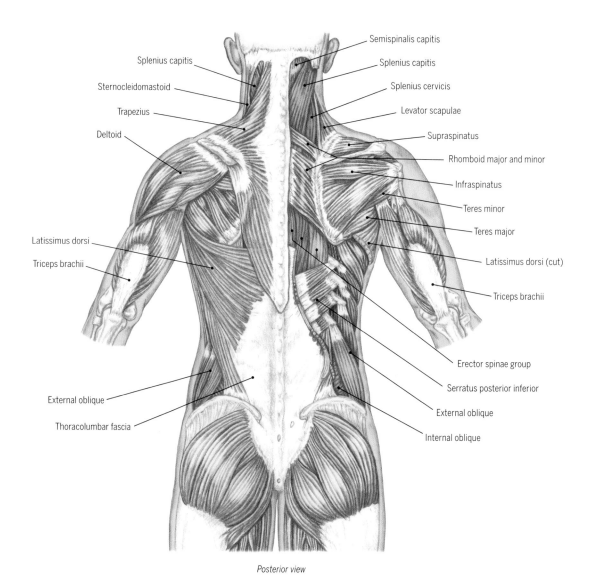

Semispinalis capitis
Splenius capitis
Sternocleidomastoid
Trapezius
Deltoid
Latissimus dorsi
Triceps brachii
External oblique
Thoracolumbar fascia

Semispinalis capitis
Splenius capitis
Splenius cervicis
Levator scapulae
Supraspinatus
Rhomboid major and minor
Infraspinatus
Teres minor
Teres major
Latissimus dorsi (cut)
Triceps brachii
Erector spinae group
Serratus posterior inferior
External oblique
Internal oblique

Posterior view

3.24 Superficial muscles of the back. The deltoid, trapezius, and latissimus dorsi are removed on the right side.

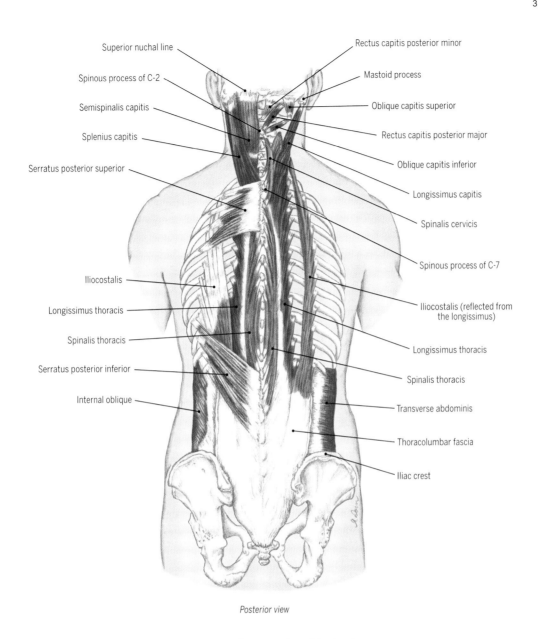

Superior nuchal line

Spinous process of C-2

Semispinalis capitis

Splenius capitis

Serratus posterior superior

Iliocostalis

Longissimus thoracis

Spinalis thoracis

Serratus posterior inferior

Internal oblique

Rectus capitis posterior minor

Mastoid process

Oblique capitis superior

Rectus capitis posterior major

Oblique capitis inferior

Longissimus capitis

Spinalis cervicis

Spinous process of C-7

Iliocostalis (reflected from the longissimus)

Longissimus thoracis

Spinalis thoracis

Transverse abdominis

Thoracolumbar fascia

Iliac crest

Posterior view

3.25 Intermediate muscles of the back

cell tower support a central pole by exerting force in opposing directions (**3.26**). The agonist and antagonist muscle groups often act simultaneously, referred to as co-contraction, exerting force in different directions to stabilize or act as synergists for purposeful movement. For example, when standing upright in a relatively static position, perhaps at a wedding or similar event, the slow-twitch fibers of the erector spinae and abdominal muscles generate opposing low-amplitude forces. These counterbalancing forces contribute to isometric contractions, stabilizing the spine in the neutral vertical position. Functional flexion and extension of the trunk, as when picking up a child, illustrate synergy between these muscle groups. The erector spinae eccentrically contract with abdominal shortening to facilitate trunk flexion. Returning the trunk to neutral reverses this pattern: the erector spinae concentrically contract as the abdominals elongate.

Many superficial core muscles are long and broad, spanning and applying force to the entire spine with numerous attachments to the vertebrae and ribs. These muscles are often paired, extending from the lower vertebrae and pelvis in symmetrical patterns. Some deeper muscles are small and attach only to adjacent vertebrae, enhancing the core stability needed for various functional postures.

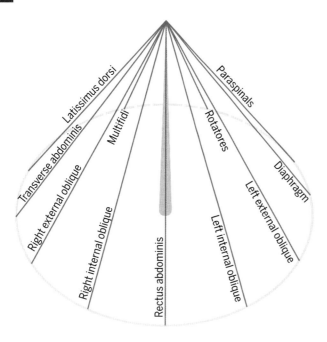

3.26 The core muscles are similar to the guylines of a cell tower or tent, balancing the forces that keep the trunk upright.

The muscles of this region also make contributions beyond movement. The abdominal and spinal muscles, for example, form a muscular wall that surrounds and protects the digestive system. An entrance to this vital center, in the form of the esophagus and trachea (windpipe), allows life-sustaining air and nutrients to enter. The muscles of the pelvic floor and its openings supply an exit for waste (see Chapter 8).

In the next sections, we'll explore the muscles of the core, grouped by region and depth relative to the spinal column. As you examine these muscles, consider their antagonists and how the opposing forces may facilitate stability or movement of the trunk.

Posterior Musculature

Collectively, the muscles of the posterior spine act to extend, rotate, and laterally flex the trunk and neck. Along with the anterior muscles, they contribute significantly to balanced stability of the trunk.

These muscles are active for static and dynamic positioning and movement of the trunk, such as when standing at a mirror to complete your morning hygiene routine or watering the lawn with a garden hose. They also return the trunk to a neutral position after flexing forward, such as after bending forward to tie your shoes.

Erector Spinae Group

Iliocostalis

Longissimus

Spinalis

The **erector spinae—iliocostalis**, **longissimus**, and **spinalis** (from lateral to medial)—are the most superficial muscles on the posterior spine, spanning from the lower vertebral column and pelvis to the base of the skull (**3.27**).

The muscles are secured inferiorly to the pelvis, lumbar spine, and thoracolumbar fascia, providing an anchor to exert force for extension of the trunk. The muscle fibers ascend the spine in symmetrical vertical pairs, balancing the forces that act upon the vertebrae and rib cage.

Fibers are subdivided as they ascend, splitting away from the main muscle like branches of a tree (**3.28– 3.30**). They are named according to the region of the spine they act upon. For example, the **longissimus capitis** extends the skull (capitis), while the **longissimus cervicis** extends the neck (cervicis) (**3.29**).

The erector spinae bring the core of the body back to neutral (extension) after flexing for activities like picking up a toddler or putting on socks. They also cooperate with the abdominals for static standing, such as when standing at a sink to wash dishes.

ERECTOR SPINAE GROUP	
Purposeful Activity	
P	**Maintaining an upright position for ADLs/IADLs**
A	*Unilaterally:* **Laterally flex** vertebral column to the same side *Bilaterally:* **Extend** the vertebral column
O	Common tendon (thoracolumbar fascia) that attaches to the posterior surface of sacrum, iliac crest, and spinous processes of the lumbar and last two thoracic vertebrae
I	Various attachments at the posterior ribs, spinous and transverse processes of thoracic and cervical vertebrae, and mastoid process of temporal bone
N	Spinal

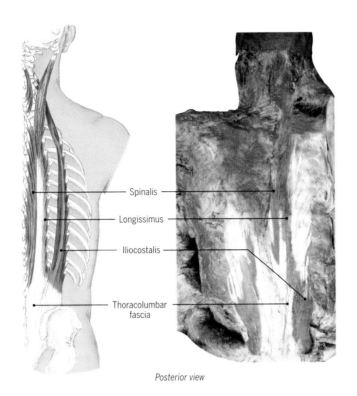

Spinalis

Longissimus

Iliocostalis

Thoracolumbar
fascia

Posterior view

3.27 Erector spinae group

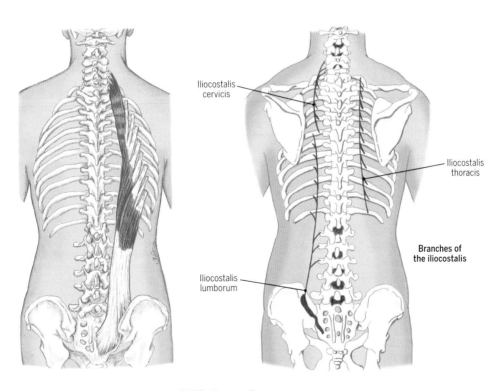

Iliocostalis
cervicis

Iliocostalis
thoracis

**Branches of
the iliocostalis**

Iliocostalis
lumborum

3.28 Iliocostalis

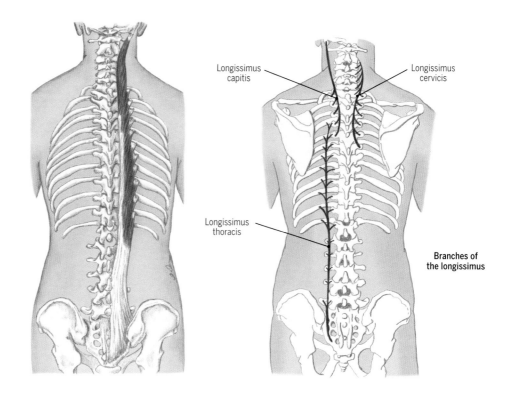

3.29 Longissimus

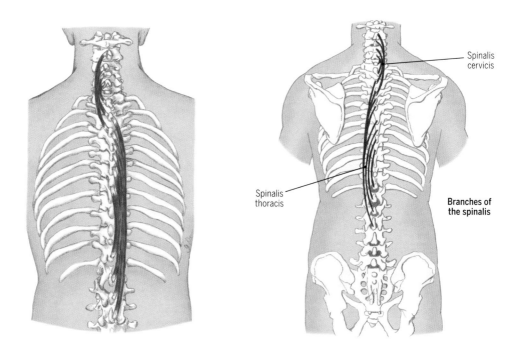

3.30 Spinalis

Transversospinalis Group

Multifidi

Rotatores

Semispinalis capitis

The muscles of the transversospinalis group—**multifidi**, **rotatores**, and **semispinalis**—lie deep to the erector spinae and connect individual vertebrae (**3.31**).

Their fibers are short and narrow, often connecting the spinous and transverse processes of adjacent vertebrae. As the erector spinae exert force across various regions of the spine, the transversospinalis muscles act similarly on individual vertebrae, enhancing the force and stability of trunk extension and rotation.

The most inferior multifidi are anchored to the sacrum, and the rest originate on the transverse vertebral processes (**3.32**). These muscle fibers span two to four vertebrae and insert on the spinous processes.

The rotatores have the same vertebral attachments, but they span only one or two vertebrae. The multifidi and rotatores provide deep postural support between adjacent vertebrae to align or stabilize the trunk for occupational performance in activities such as tai chi or yoga.

The semispinalis capitis originates on the transverse processes of C-4 to T-5, attaching to the skull to extend the head (**3.33**).

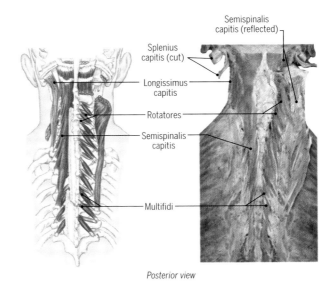

Posterior view

3.31 Transversospinalis group

MULTIFIDI AND ROTATORES
Purposeful Activity
P Tai chi or yoga (deep postural stability)
A *Unilaterally:* Rotate the vertebral column to the opposite side
Bilaterally: Extend the vertebral column
O Multifidi: Sacrum and transverse processes of lumbar through cervical vertebrae
Rotatores: Transverse processes of lumbar through cervical vertebrae
I Spinous processes of lumbar vertebrae through second cervical vertebra
(Multifidi span two to four vertebrae; rotatores span one to two vertebrae)
N Spinal

SEMISPINALIS CAPITIS
Purposeful Activity
P Using a computer workstation, looking overhead
A Extend the vertebral column and head
O Transverse processes of C-4 to T-5
I Between the superior and inferior nuchal lines of the occiput
N Cervical

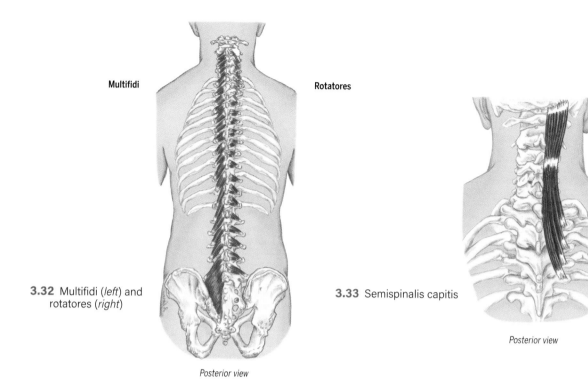

3.32 Multifidi (*left*) and rotatores (*right*)

Posterior view

3.33 Semispinalis capitis

Posterior view

Splenii

Splenius capitis
Splenius cervicis

The **splenius capitis** and **splenius cervicis** lie deep to the trapezius on the upper back and neck (**3.34**).

These muscles have similar oblique pathways. They extend from the spinous processes of the upper back (C-7–T-6) to the cervical transverse processes (cervicis;

C-1–C-3) and mastoid process (capitis) of the skull. Their actions contribute to rotation, lateral flexion, and extension of the head and neck—important for gathering visual input as you navigate your surrounding environment.

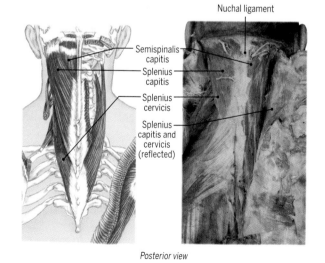

Nuchal ligament

Semispinalis capitis
Splenius capitis
Splenius cervicis
Splenius capitis and cervicis (reflected)

Posterior view

3.34 Splenii

SPLENIUS CAPITIS AND CERVICIS	
Purposeful Activity	
P	Social interaction, driving
A	*Unilaterally:* **Rotate** the head and neck to the same side **Laterally flex** the head and neck to the same side *Bilaterally:* **Extend** the head and neck
O	Capitis: Inferior one-half of ligamentum nuchae and spinous processes of C-7 to T-4 Cervicis: Spinous processes of T-3 to T-6
I	Capitis: Mastoid process and lateral portion of superior nuchal line Cervicis: Transverse processes of C-1 to C-3
N	Cervical

Suboccipitals

Rectus capitis posterior major
Rectus capitis posterior minor
Oblique capitis superior
Oblique capitis inferior

The **suboccipitals** are four paired muscles, the deepest of the neck, that lie at the base of the posterior skull (occiput) (**3.35**). These muscles stabilize and contribute to small, precise movements of the head. They are active as you turn your head in small increments to scan the text on this page, for instance. Crossing the atlas, axis, and occiput, they also promote positional stability at the vertebral level.

The fibers of the **rectus capitis posterior major** and **minor** span the posterior atlas and axis to the nuchal line of the occiput, supplying force for extension and rotation of the head. The **oblique capitis superior** originates at the transverse process of C-1 and inserts into the nuchal line, contributing to lateral flexion and extension. Spanning the spinous process of C-2 to the transverse process of C-1, the **oblique capitis inferior** contributes to rotation of the atlantoaxial joint.

SUBOCCIPITALS	
Purposeful Activity	
P	Scanning a computer monitor, reading a book
A	Rectus capitis posterior major, rectus capitis posterior minor, and oblique capitis superior: **Rock** and **tilt** the head back into extension
	Rectus capitis posterior major and oblique capitis inferior: **Rotate** the head to the same side
	Oblique capitis superior: **Laterally flex** the head to the same side
N	Suboccipital

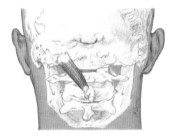

Rectus capitis
posterior major

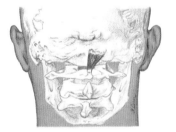

Rectus capitis
posterior minor

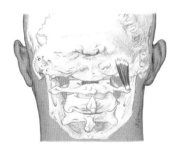

Oblique capitis
superior

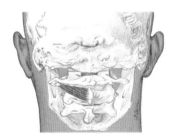

Oblique capitis
inferior

Posterior views

3.35 Suboccipitals

Quadratus Lumborum

The **quadratus lumborum** is an important contractile link between the pelvis and lower back, acting to stabilize the lower back, elevate the pelvis, or flex the trunk laterally (**3.36**). This muscle is active whenever elevating one side of the hip, as when climbing a ladder.

QUADRATUS LUMBORUM	
Purposeful Activity	
P	**Lifting, walking**

A	*Unilaterally:* **Laterally tilt** (elevate) the pelvis **Laterally flex** the vertebral column to the same side Assist to **extend** the vertebral column *Bilaterally:* **Fix** the last rib during forced inhalation and exhalation
O	Posterior iliac crest
I	Last rib and transverse processes of first through fourth lumbar vertebrae
N	Lumbar plexus T12, L1 to L3

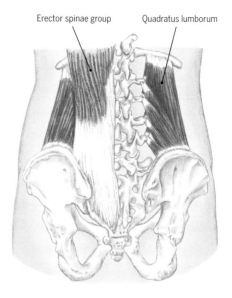

Posterior view, erector spinae group removed on right side

3.36 Quadratus lumborum

Intertransversarii and Interspinales Muscles

The **intertransversarii** attach to adjacent transverse processes in the lumbar and cervical regions, stabilizing and contributing to lateral flexion between the vertebrae (**3.37**).

The **interspinales** similarly connect adjacent spinous processes of the lumbar and cervical vertebrae, contributing to trunk extension (**3.38**).

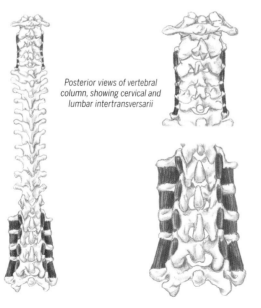

Posterior views of vertebral column, showing cervical and lumbar intertransversarii

3.37 Intertransversarii

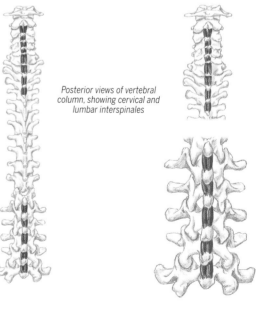

Posterior views of vertebral column, showing cervical and lumbar interspinales

3.38 Interspinales

Serratus Posterior Superior and Inferior

The **serratus posterior superior** and **inferior** lie at opposite ends of the spinal column (**3.39**). The superior fibers extend from the spinous processes of the upper vertebrae (C-7–T-3). The inferior fibers originate from the lower vertebrae (T-12–L-3) and attach to adjacent ribs. The main function of these muscles is to elevate (superior) and depress (inferior) the ribs during respiration.

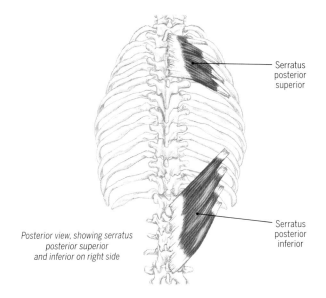

Posterior view, showing serratus posterior superior and inferior on right side

3.39 Serratus posterior superior and inferior

Anterior Musculature

Counterbalancing the posterior muscles, the muscles of the anterior spine stabilize, flex, rotate, and laterally flex the trunk and neck. These muscles also form a continuous muscle layer around the abdomen as a protective barrier for the viscera.

Sternocleidomastoid

The **sternocleidomastoid (SCM)** is a large superficial muscle that is visible when turning the head to the side (**3.40**). It has two heads—**sternal** and **clavicular**—and

its fibers follow an oblique pathway to insert at the mastoid process of the temporal bone.

As it traverses the cervical spine and inserts on the skull, the SCM is capable of contralateral rotation and lateral flexion of both the head and neck, which, as with the splenii, is helpful when visually scanning your environment. When acting bilaterally, the SCM also contributes to flexion of the neck and elevation of the rib cage for deep respiration.

STERNOCLEIDOMASTOID	
Purposeful Activity	
P	Watching an athletic event, socializing, driving
A	*Unilaterally*: Laterally **flex** the head and neck to the same side; **Rotate** the head and neck to the opposite side. *Bilaterally:* **Flex** the neck; Assist to **elevate** the rib cage during inhalation
O	Sternal head: Top of manubrium; Clavicular head: Medial one-third of the clavicle
I	Mastoid process of temporal bone and the lateral portion of superior nuchal line of occiput
N	Spinal accessory (XI) nerve, C2 and C3

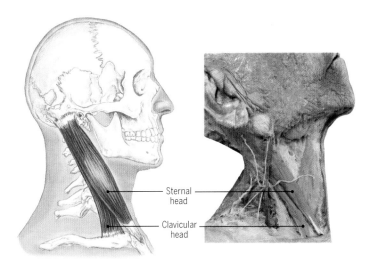

Lateral view

3.40 Sternocleidomastoid

Scalenes

Anterior
Middle
Posterior

The **anterior**, **middle**, and **posterior scalene** muscles are positioned on the lateral aspect of each side of the cervical spine (**3.41**).

As a group, the scalenes contribute primarily to lateral flexion (unilateral action) and flexion (bilateral action) of the cervical spine. They also help elevate the first and second ribs for deep respiration. Note that the brachial plexus and the subclavian artery pass between the anterior and middle scalene muscles (**3.42**).

Scalene tightness can compress these neurovascular structures, which may cause pain, numbness, and tingling in the upper extremity. This condition is known as **thoracic outlet syndrome (TOS)** and is described further in Chapter 5.

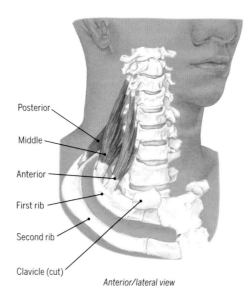

Posterior
Middle
Anterior
First rib
Second rib
Clavicle (cut)

Anterior/lateral view

3.41 Scalenes

ANTERIOR SCALENE
Purposeful Activity

P Driving, deep breathing with exertion (running, cycling)

A *Unilaterally:*
With the ribs fixed, **laterally flex** the head and neck to the same side
Rotate head and neck to the opposite side

Bilaterally:
Elevate the ribs during inhalation
Flex the head and neck

O Transverse processes of third through sixth cervical vertebrae (anterior tubercles)

I First rib

N C3 to C8

MIDDLE SCALENE
Purposeful Activity

P Driving, deep breathing with exertion (running, cycling)

A *Unilaterally:*
With the ribs fixed, **laterally flex** the head and neck to the same side
Rotate head and neck to the opposite side

Bilaterally:
Elevate the ribs during inhalation

O Transverse processes of second through seventh cervical vertebrae (posterior tubercles)

I First rib

N C3 to C8

POSTERIOR SCALENE
Purposeful Activity

P **Driving, deep breathing with exertion (running, cycling)**

A *Unilaterally:*
With the ribs fixed, **laterally flex** the head and neck to the same side
Rotate head and neck to the opposite side

Bilaterally:
Elevate the ribs during inhalation

O Transverse processes of sixth and seventh cervical vertebrae (posterior tubercles)

I Second rib

N C3 to C8

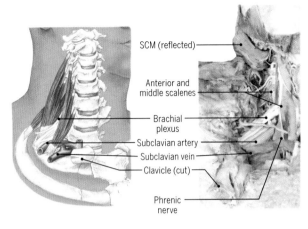

Anterior view

3.42 Brachial plexus, subclavian artery, and subclavian vein

Abdominal Muscles

The **abdominal wall** serves as the anterior musculature support for the trunk and as a counterbalance to the erector spinae (**3.43**). Additionally, the abdominals serve as a muscular shield, protecting the viscera of the lower abdomen that lie outside the rib cage.

On the surface, these muscles may seem isolated to the vertical row of "abs" overlying the stomach. But this muscle group forms a circumferential muscular girdle spanning the ribs, pelvis, and thoracolumbar fascia. The muscles overlap with varied fiber direction for balanced postural stability and trunk motion.

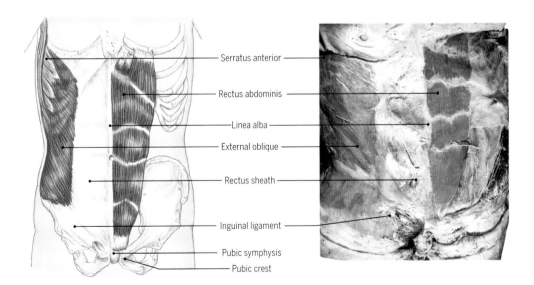

Anterior view

3.43 Abdominal wall

Rectus abdominis

Rectus abdominis is the central muscle of the abdominal wall, with vertical fibers extending from the pubic crest to ribs five through seven and the xiphoid process (**3.43**). The muscles are encased within the **rectus sheath** and segmented by **tendinous intersections**, forming the boundaries of the often-coveted six-pack abs.

Functionally, this muscle acts to flex the trunk, bringing the rib cage toward the pelvis or bringing the inferior pelvis toward the rib cage, known as **posterior pelvic tilt**. Contraction of the rectus abdominis also increases **intra-abdominal pressure**, which stabilizes the lumbar spine for lifting and facilitates respiration, childbirth, and defecation.

RECTUS ABDOMINIS	
Purposeful Activity	
P	**Lower body dressing, bed mobility (supine to sit)**
A	**Flex** the vertebral column **Tilt** pelvis posteriorly
O	Pubic crest, pubic symphysis
I	Cartilage of fifth, sixth, and seventh ribs and xiphoid process
N	Ventral rami of T5 to T12

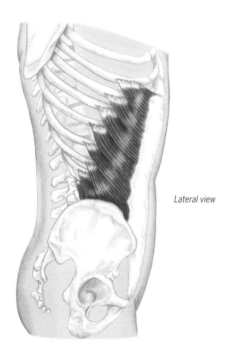

Lateral view

3.44 External oblique

External oblique

The **external oblique** muscles slant inferiorly and medially from the ribs toward the iliac crest and rectus sheath of the rectus abdominis (**3.44**). To conceptualize the pathway of this muscle, put your hands in the front pockets of your pants but leave your thumbs sticking out. Your fingers will now point in the direction of the muscle fibers of the external oblique.

Its association with the rectus abdominis, via the rectus sheath, allows the external oblique to enhance the actions of trunk flexion and abdominal compression. The oblique muscle's fiber orientation also contributes to ipsilateral flexion and contralateral rotation of the trunk, such as when playing a racket sport.

EXTERNAL OBLIQUE		
Purposeful Activity		
P	**Bed mobility, lifting (increasing intra-abdominal pressure to stabilize lumbar spine)**	
A	*Unilaterally:* **Laterally flex** vertebral column to the same side **Rotate** vertebral column to the opposite side *Bilaterally:* **Flex** the vertebral column **Compress** abdominal contents	
O	External surfaces of fifth to twelfth ribs	
I	Anterior part of the iliac crest, rectus sheath to linea alba	
N	Ventral rami of T5 to T12	

MAX CARTER | The erector spinae and abdominal muscle groups contribute a counterbalance of respective extension and flexion forces to maintain the trunk in an upright neutral position.

As you continue to observe Max in his home environment, you notice that his trunk is often in a flexed position. What effect do you think this has on his erector spinae and abdominal muscles? How might this affect his musculoskeletal development and occupational performance?

Internal oblique

The **internal oblique** lies just deep to the external oblique (**3.45**), but its fibers slant in the opposite direction, upward to the ribs from the thoracolumbar fascia and iliac crest. The internal oblique works in synergy with the external oblique for trunk flexion and lateral flexion. In contrast, it also rotates the trunk to the same side with force exerted from its posterior fibers anchored to the thoracolumbar fascia.

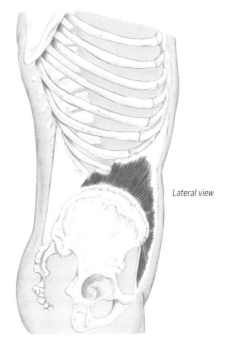

Lateral view

3.45 Internal oblique

INTERNAL OBLIQUE	
Purposeful Activity	
P	**Bed mobility, playing a racket sport (trunk rotation), lifting (increasing intra-abdominal pressure to stabilize lumbar spine)**
A	*Unilaterally:* **Laterally flex** vertebral column to the same side **Rotate** vertebral column to the same side *Bilaterally:* **Flex** the vertebral column **Compress** abdominal contents
O	Lateral inguinal ligament, iliac crest, and thoracolumbar fascia
I	Internal surface of lower three ribs, rectus sheath to linea alba
N	Ventral rami of T7 to T12, L1, iliohypogastric, and ilioinguinal

Transverse abdominis

Fibers of the **transverse abdominis** are mainly horizontal, wrapping the abdomen like a corset or lower back support (**3.46**).

Extending from the iliac crest, thoracolumbar fascia, and lower six ribs to the rectus sheath, the transverse abdominis is able to pull back on the abdominal wall, increasing pressure and stabilizing the pelvis and spine. This stabilization helps with activities such as lifting, for example.

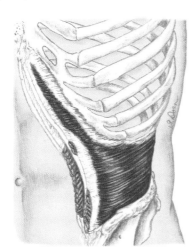

Anterior view, both obliques reflected

3.46 Transverse abdominis

TRANSVERSE ABDOMINIS	
Purposeful Activity	
P	**Carrying a child or pet (increasing intra-abdominal pressure to stabilize lumbar spine)**
A	**Compress** abdominal contents
O	Lateral inguinal ligament, iliac crest, thoracolumbar fascia, and internal surface of lower six ribs
I	Rectus sheath to linea alba
N	Ventral rami of T7 to T12, L1, iliohypogastric, and ilioinguinal

Diaphragm

The **diaphragm** is a broad muscular membrane that forms the floor of the **thoracic cavity**, the area inside the rib cage (**3.47**). Its fibers converge from the lower six ribs, upper lumbar vertebrae, and xiphoid process to a **central tendon**, controlling the volume of the thoracic cavity as it contracts and relaxes (**3.48**).

As the diaphragm contracts, it moves downward, increasing volume and allowing air to fill the expanding lungs. Relaxation has the opposite effect, with the diaphragm elevating and forcing air out of the lungs. **Diaphragmatic breathing**, or deep breathing, is used by vocalists to optimize air intake, producing forceful, sustained notes.

DIAPHRAGM	
Purposeful Activity	
P	**Singing, playing a trumpet (deep breathing)**
A	Draw down the central tendon of the diaphragm Increase the volume of the thoracic cavity during inhalation
O	Costal attachment: Inner surface of lower six ribs Lumbar attachment: Upper two or three lumbar vertebrae Sternal attachment: Inner part of xiphoid process
I	Central tendon
N	Phrenic C3 to C5

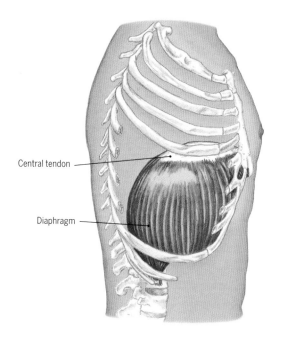

Lateral view

3.47 Diaphragm, shown in position of exhalation

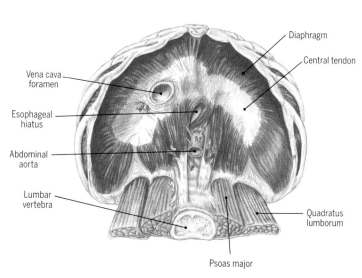

Inferior view

3.48 Diaphragm

Intercostals

As the name implies, the **intercostals** lie between adjacent ribs in two layers—external and internal fibers that run perpendicular to one another (**3.49**). These muscles assist with elevating and depressing the ribs with deep breathing, as when singing or after a long run.

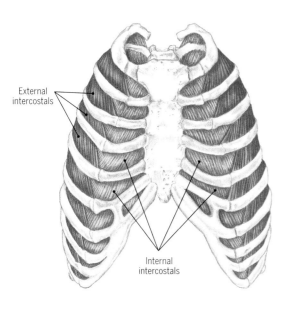

3.49 Intercostals

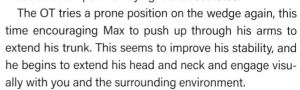

INTERCOSTALS		
Purposeful Activity		

P Singing, playing the trumpet (deep breathing)

A External intercostals: **Draw the ribs superiorly** (increasing the space of the thoracic cavity) to assist with **inhalation**
Internal intercostals: **Draw the ribs inferiorly** (decreasing the space of the thoracic cavity) to assist with **exhalation**

O Inferior border of the rib above

I Superior border of the rib below

N Thoracic

Now that you have an understanding of the muscles of the spine, let's discuss their contribution to stability and movement.

MAX CARTER | The treatment session with Max continues and you notice several distinct patterns of increased muscle tone. It seems that his flexor muscles are most affected, and he has difficulty extending not only his trunk but also his elbows, hands, and knees. His abdominal muscles seem particularly tight and restricted.

The OT tries a prone position on the wedge again, this time encouraging Max to push up through his arms to extend his trunk. This seems to improve his stability, and he begins to extend his head and neck and engage visually with you and the surrounding environment.

After a few minutes in the prone position, the OT transitions Max back to a seated position, and he is able to sit for several seconds with less support. His mother is very pleased and asks what changed. Take a moment to reflect on what you've just learned about the musculature of this region, and apply it to these questions:

- Abdominal muscle tightness affects the position of the pelvis. What specific impact would tightness of the rectus abdominis have on pelvic position?
- Why do you think lying in a prone position with trunk extension on the wedge improved Max's ability to sit upright with less support?

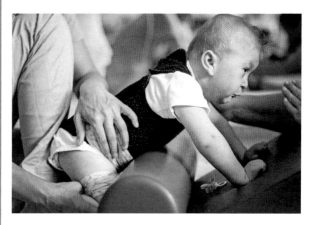

Purposeful Movement of the Spine

Remember that movement of the entire spine is the sum of motion of adjacent vertebrae in the cervical, thoracic, and lumbar segments of the spine. Adjacent vertebrae move a small amount relative to one another, similar to links in a chain, collectively flexing, extending, or rotating the neck (cervical spine) or trunk (thoracolumbar spine).

When the body is in an upright position (sitting, standing, walking), the spine functions in a closed kinetic chain, its segments functionally "fused" through the compressive force of gravity. A loss of mobility between individual vertebrae or in a vertebral region (like the lumbar spine) has an impact on the entire vertebral column, specifically when functioning in this closed-chain pattern, as when carrying a heavy load.

Take some time to review the performance skills outlined in the OTPF-4 and consider the role of the cervical spine. Its contribution extends beyond motor performance skills.[2] The neck positions, aligns, and stabilizes the head for self-feeding, swallowing, and scanning the visual environment. It turns toward, looks at, and along with facial expression conveys nonverbal communication and emotion. Limitations in cervical spine mobility may significantly impair occupations like driving or community mobility, which require an expansive and shifting visual field.

Gross movement of the thoracolumbar (thoracic and lumbar) spine positions, aligns, and stabilizes the entire body for occupational performance. Because motion of the trunk involves all of the vertebrae, many muscles—both superficial and deep—contribute to core movement. The muscles work in synergy to produce motion and counterbalance one another to supply stable motion or static stability for function.

The next sections illustrate the movements of the cervical and thoracolumbar spine.

Cervical Spine (Neck)

Figures **3.50–3.53** feature muscles that contribute to purposeful movement of the cervical spine, with prime movers listed first. Asterisks indicate muscles not shown.

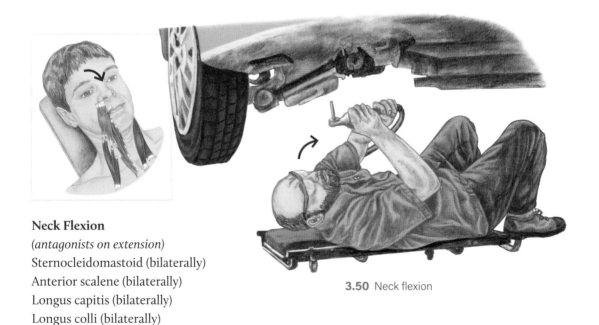

Neck Flexion

(*antagonists on extension*)
Sternocleidomastoid (bilaterally)
Anterior scalene (bilaterally)
Longus capitis (bilaterally)
Longus colli (bilaterally)

3.50 Neck flexion

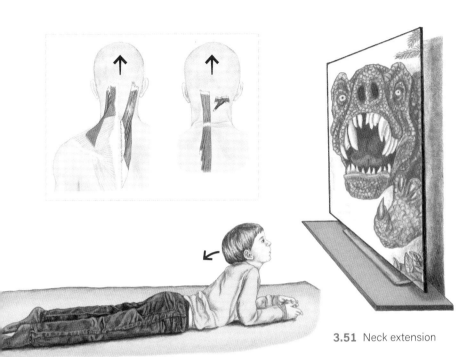

Neck Extension
(antagonists on flexion)
Trapezius (upper fibers, bilaterally)
Levator scapulae (bilaterally)
Splenius capitis (bilaterally)
Splenius cervicis (bilaterally)
Rectus capitis posterior major
Rectus capitis posterior minor
Oblique capitis superior
Semispinalis capitis
Longissimus capitis (assists)*
Longissimus cervicis (assists)*
Iliocostalis cervicis (assists)*
Multifidi (bilaterally)*
Rotatores (bilaterally)*
Intertransversarii (bilaterally)*
Interspinalis*

3.51 Neck extension

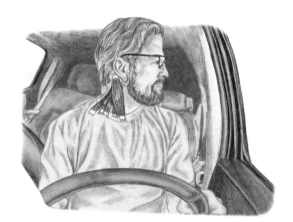
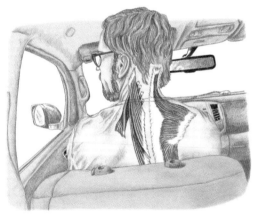

3.52 Neck rotation

Ipsilateral Neck Rotation
(unilaterally to the same side)
Levator scapulae
Splenius capitis
Splenius cervicis
Rectus capitis posterior major*
Oblique capitis inferior*
Longus colli*
Longus capitis*
Longissimus capitis (assists)*
Longissimus cervicis (assists)*
Iliocostalis cervicis (assists)*

Contralateral Neck Rotation
(unilaterally to the opposite side)
Trapezius (upper fibers)
Sternocleidomastoid
Anterior scalene
Middle scalene
Posterior scalene
Multifidi*
Rotatores*

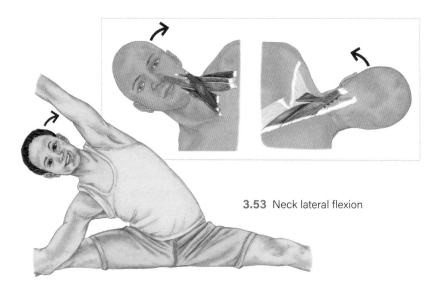

3.53 Neck lateral flexion

Neck Lateral Flexion
(unilaterally to the same side)
Trapezius (upper fibers)
Levator scapulae
Sternocleidomastoid
Anterior scalene (with ribs fixed)
Middle scalene (with ribs fixed)
Posterior scalene (with ribs fixed)
Splenius capitis
Splenius cervicis
Longus capitis
Longus colli
Longissimus capitis (assists)*
Longissimus cervicis (assists)*
Iliocostalis cervicis (assists)*
Oblique capitis superior*
Intertransversarii*

Thoracolumbar Spine (Trunk)

Figures **3.54–3.59** feature muscles that contribute to purposeful movement of the thoracolumbar spine and rib cage, with prime movers listed first. Asterisks indicate muscles not shown.

Trunk Flexion
(antagonists on extension)
Rectus abdominis
External oblique (bilaterally)
Internal oblique (bilaterally)*
Psoas major (with the insertion fixed)*
Iliacus (with the insertion fixed)*

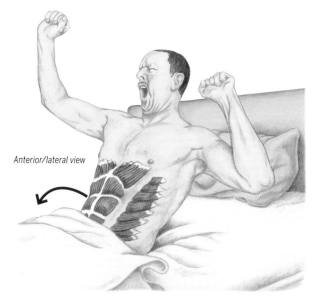

Anterior/lateral view

3.54 Trunk flexion

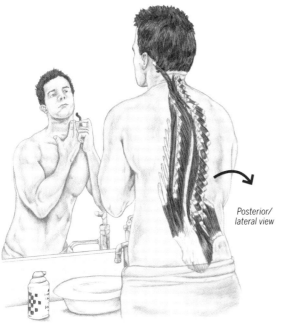

Trunk Extension
(antagonists on flexion)
Longissimus (bilaterally)
Iliocostalis (bilaterally)
Multifidi (bilaterally)
Rotatores (bilaterally)*
Semispinalis capitis
Spinalis (bilaterally)
Quadratus lumborum (assists)
Interspinalis*
Intertransversarii (bilaterally)*
Latissimus dorsi (assists when arm is fixed)*

Posterior/lateral view

3.55 Trunk extension

3.56 Trunk rotation

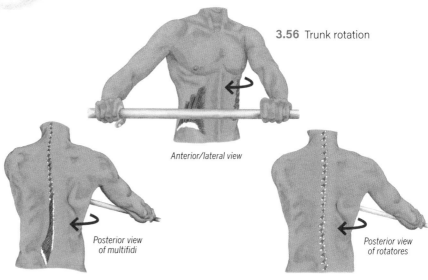

Trunk Rotation
(all unilaterally)
External oblique (to the opposite side)
Internal oblique (to the same side)
Multifidi (to the opposite side)
Rotatores (to the opposite side)

Anterior/lateral view

Posterior view of multifidi

Posterior view of rotatores

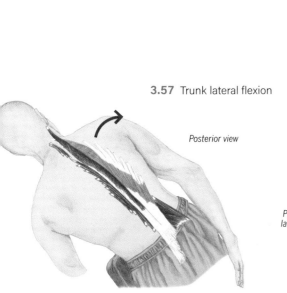

3.57 Trunk lateral flexion

Posterior view

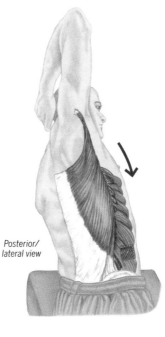

Posterior/lateral view

Trunk Lateral Flexion
(unilaterally to the same side)
Iliocostalis
External oblique
Internal oblique
Longissimus
Quadratus lumborum
Psoas major (assists)*
Intertransversarii*
Spinalis
Latissimus dorsi (assists)

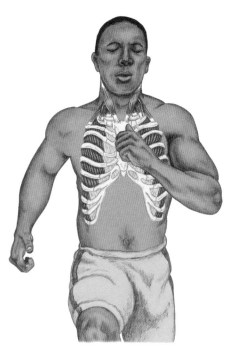

Rib Cage Elevation/Expansion (involved with inhalation)

(antagonists on depression)

Anterior scalene (bilaterally)
Middle scalene (bilaterally)
Posterior scalene (bilaterally)
Sternocleidomastoid (assists)
External intercostals (assists)
Serratus posterior superior*
Pectoralis major (all fibers may assist
    if arm is fixed)*
Pectoralis minor (if scapula is fixed)*
Serratus anterior (if scapula is fixed)*
Subclavius (first rib)*

3.58 Rib cage elevation/expansion

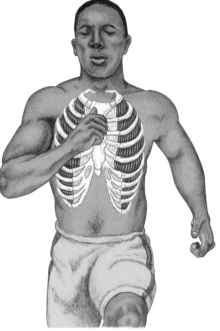

Rib Cage Depression/Collapse (involved with exhalation)

(antagonists on elevation)

Internal intercostals (assists)
Serratus posterior inferior*

3.59 Rib cage depression/collapse

 OT Guide to Goniometry & MMT: Trunk and Neck

Now that you have examined the muscles of the trunk and neck and conceptualized their contribution to occupational performance, let's consider the assessment of movement and strength for this region of the body.

To assess mobility of the trunk and neck, practitioners often visually examine symmetry of movement and overall flexibility as a starting point, or screening, for deficits. For example, instructing a patient to look as far as they can over their right and then left shoulder may help to identify a gross deficit in neck rotation. The same technique may work to generally assess lateral flexion. Additionally, the distance from the fingertips to the floor with trunk flexion or lateral flexion, maintaining the hips and knees in neutral, provides an approximate measure of the flexibility of the thoracolumbar spine.

The neck, or cervical spine, is the most mobile part of the spinal column, and there are goniometric techniques to more precisely measure movement in this portion of the spine. The *OT Guide to Goniometry & MMT* eTextbook describes these techniques in detail, along with MMT assessment. With a partner, practice assessing general mobility of the neck by visual observation. Then, practice goniometry and MMT as a more precise method of assessment for each movement. Describe the muscles that contribute force for each motion, as well as the importance of the movement for occupational performance. Consider: How do these movements affect the visual field, facilitate social interaction, or support feeding and swallowing? How would deficits in movement or strength impact the performance of these occupations?

Maintaining the balance of forces acting on the spine by its surrounding muscles will support the neutral position of the spine emphasized throughout this chapter. Think about the broad impact of muscular imbalance:

- How would the trunk be positioned with tightness and shortening of the abdominal muscles and with elongation of the erector spinae group?
- What effect would this position have on an individual's occupational performance?
- How could this imbalance be prevented in a developing child or an adult worker?

Occupational and Clinical Perspectives

Now that you have an understanding of the bones, joints, and muscles that contribute to trunk control, let's examine this region of the body through the lens of occupation and clinical reasoning. The following sections further integrate the functional anatomy of this region into occupational performance as well as several common pathologies you may encounter as a practitioner.

Core Stability and Occupational Performance

We have seen how, functionally, the spine serves as the central skeletal scaffolding of the body that supports purposeful movement of the extremities. You may hear this principle expressed in different ways, but "proximal stability before distal mobility" is a common adage within occupational therapy, emphasizing the need for a stable proximal core to maximize function of the distal extremities.

The ability to voluntarily position and stabilize the body's core, or **trunk control**, is also an essential motor component of occupational performance. An infant needs trunk control to develop the ability to crawl, an industrial worker needs trunk control for safe lifting, and trunk control and stability are essential components of safe functional mobility for older adults. Trunk control also plays a significant role in sitting and standing balance, both static (such as sitting still and paying attention in an important meeting) and dynamic (such as driving).

Regardless of the population, trunk balance and control are important for safe, optimal occupational performance.

Some neurological conditions may also contribute to **hypertonia**, increased muscle tone, or **hypotonia**, decreased tone throughout the body. Individuals with

▶**TRY IT**

Let your trunk slouch back in your chair with no muscle support like a "wet noodle." Then try to reach forward and use your hands.

It's not easy, is it? Without trunk support, we expend significant energy and attention just trying to stabilize the trunk, which limits purposeful use of the arms and legs.

In some cases, an individual's trunk strength and stability may be improved through various interventions to support occupational performance. For example, using a mirror for visual feedback to improve postural alignment might facilitate improved trunk stability for ADL performance. In other cases, core instability or dysfunction may be more permanent due to a neurological pathology like cerebral palsy.

How would your approach and interventions be different depending on whether or not muscle strength and control could be improved? What are some specific adaptive or compensatory strategies for long-term or permanent loss of trunk control?

these conditions may benefit from more adaptive or compensatory strategies, such as adding external supports to maintain upright posture in a wheelchair to improve function.

Patient Transfers and Safe Lifting

The spine is uniquely designed to absorb compressive forces in an upright, vertical position, as the weight of the body and ground reaction forces converge on the vertebrae. However, forces applied to a flexed spine generate shear forces, or surfaces moving against one another in opposite directions, between vertebrae. Shear forces increase the likelihood of injury.

You have likely heard a common guiding principle of safe lifting, "Lift with your legs, not your back." The legs are designed to generate large forces from a flexed position, as when standing up from a low commode; the spine is not. Keeping the back straight (extended) allows the vertebrae to function as they were designed: aligned vertically to absorb compressive forces (**3.60**).

A **stagger stance**, with one foot slightly in front of the other and the hips and knees somewhat flexed, has several benefits when lifting or performing IADLs like vacuuming or sweeping a floor (**3.61**).

The stagger stance position maintains a more neutral pelvis and reduces the strain on the spine by allowing

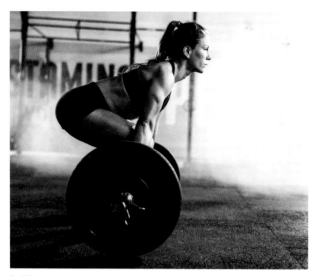

3.60 Forces through the spine when lifting. What impact do shear forces have on the vertebrae of the spine? How can shear forces be minimized when lifting or completing a patient transfer?

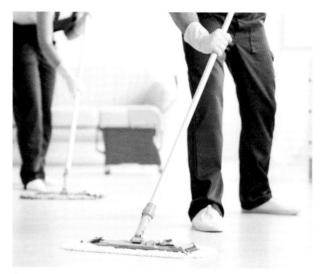

3.61 Stagger stance. What are the benefits of this functional stance when sweeping or mopping?

functional **weight-shifting**, moving the weight of the body from one leg to the other. Weight-shifting facilitates purposeful movement of the body, such as when advancing a vacuum or mop, generating motion from the strong muscles of the legs rather than from the spine, which remains in a neutral position. A staggered stance with weight-shifting is often an appropriate strategy for any type of lifting, carrying, or moving of objects, as well as patient transfers.

Body mechanics are particularly important for OTs and OTAs who frequently complete and educate others on patient transfers (**3.62**). Working with patients on safe transfers from one functional surface to another,

such as from a hospital bed to a bedside commode (BSC), is a common part of practice in many clinical settings.

The transfer technique will vary based on the level of assistance the patient requires and the environment, as well as the relative sizes of the patient and clinician. Specific transfer techniques are described in Chapter 10 in relation to functional mobility.

Many IADLs and work occupations involve some form of materials handling or lifting. Consistent use of proper body mechanics and lifting technique may prevent back injuries, promoting employee health and productivity. General recommendations for safe lifting include a stagger stance, bending the legs, keeping the

▶TRY IT

To better understand and appreciate the benefits of using a stagger stance when completing IADLs or lifting, locate a vacuum or broom. Hold onto the item and keep your feet together beneath your body with your hips and knees straight. In this position, try to vacuum or sweep.

Did you notice the movement and engagement of the muscles in your core? How is your balance?

Now stagger your feet with one in front of the other, flex your hips and knees, and try again. Shift your weight from the back leg to the front leg, keeping your trunk in a neutral position.

Did you notice the difference in which muscle groups were engaged and in your overall stability? This concept applies to safe lifting, ADL/IADL training, and patient transfers.

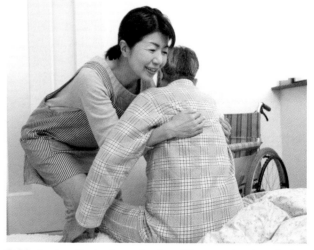

3.62 Analyze the body mechanics of the caregiver transferring this individual. Do you have any recommendations?

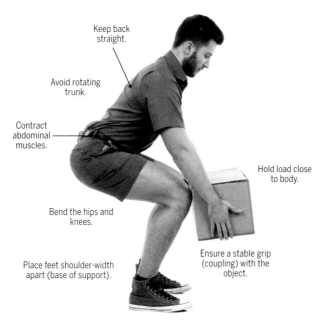

Keep back straight.

Avoid rotating trunk.

Contract abdominal muscles.

Bend the hips and knees.

Place feet shoulder-width apart (base of support).

Hold load close to body.

Ensure a stable grip (coupling) with the object.

3.63 Safe lifting. How do these common lifting recommendations promote safety and protect the back?

back straight, holding the load close to the body, and avoiding rotation of the trunk (**3.63**). Contracting the abdominal muscles increases intra-abdominal pressure, which stabilizes the lumbar spine, and is recommended during a lift (**3.64**).[3]

Because the lumbar spine absorbs most of the compressive force with lifting, it is important to maintain stability in this area—but not too much. If the spine is too rigid, it will not absorb the inevitable forces of flexion, extension, and torsion (twisting) associated with body movements,

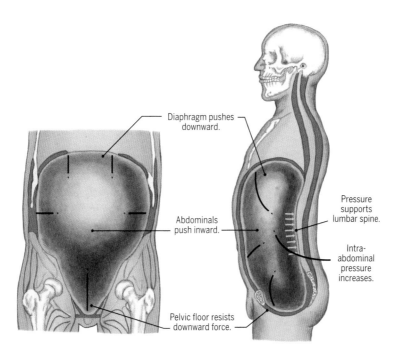

Diaphragm pushes downward.

Pressure supports lumbar spine.

Abdominals push inward.

Intra-abdominal pressure increases.

Pelvic floor resists downward force.

3.64 Intra-abdominal pressure. How can the abdominal muscles stabilize the lumbar spine when lifting?

increasing the chance of injury. A balance of stability and mobility is required and largely depends on the person and occupation.

For example, when working with a ballerina, a practitioner might emphasize flexibility to achieve the graceful extremes of posture required. However, when working with a factory worker whose job involves repetitive lifting, stability might be the priority.

Now that we have reviewed some strategies to promote a neutral spine and prevent injury, what specific strategies might you recommend to the following individuals?

- an adult worker who primarily stocks shelves at a grocery store
- an older adult who enjoys landscaping and gardening
- an adult who enjoys weight lifting as a primary leisure and health management occupation

We often consider the position and movement of the trunk when an individual is standing upright, walking, or lifting. But it is also important to consider the position and support of the spine when the body is horizontal, as when resting on a couch or sleeping in a bed, described in the next section.

Rest and Sleep

Have you ever fallen asleep on the floor or a couch and woken up with stiffness and pain (**3.65**)? In what position do you typically sleep—on your back (supine), on your stomach (prone), or lying on your side (side lying)?

Regardless of your preferred position, supporting the neutral position and natural curvature of your spine—keeping the head, shoulders, and hips aligned—during rest and sleep is just as important as for daily upright function.

Sleeping on your back is often the recommended position. However, this may strain the lumbar spine as its curvature (lordosis) is unsupported on a flat surface. A bolster or other support under the back of your knees will flex the hips slightly and reduce the strain. This strategy may also make your patients more comfortable when they are lying supine on a plinth in the clinic. A pillow for the head should support the lordosis of the cervical spine, aligning the ears and shoulders.

Sleeping on your stomach is not ideal, though it may be habitual and preferred for some individuals (**3.66**). Placing a pillow under the pelvis and stomach may prevent excessive lordosis or extension of the low back to support a more neutral spine. This position typically involves rotation of the neck to facilitate breathing, so using no pillow or a small pillow may prevent excessive rotation. Sleepers should avoid positioning their arms overhead, to prevent straining their shoulders.

When sleeping on your side, placing a pillow between your knees or under your waist may help to keep the pelvis in a neutral position, preventing lateral flexion or rotation of the spine. You might need a larger pillow for your head to keep the cervical spine neutral relative to the trunk.

Unlike some IADLs or leisure occupations, rest and sleep are universal. Quality rest is essential to the physical, cognitive, and emotional aspects of occupational performance. Many factors contribute to a good night's rest, but the position and support of a neutral spine are among the most important.

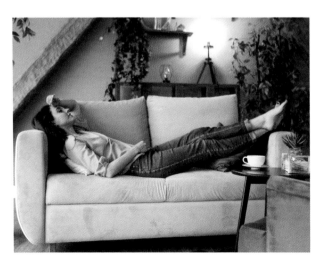

3.65 Sleep and spinal alignment. How would sleeping in this position affect the spine?

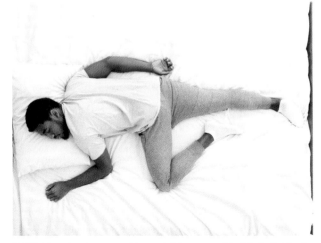

3.66 Sleeping in prone. How might you modify this individual's sleep position to promote a neutral spine?

Abnormal Muscle Tone

There are many neurological diagnoses that relate to muscle tone in the body. Two common conditions are cerebral palsy and hemiparesis.

Cerebral palsy (CP) typically involves abnormal muscle tone, which often affects core strength, function, and development, even when cognition is intact. For example, a child with low muscle tone may not be able to sit upright, limiting arm function and preventing developmental milestones like self-feeding or dressing. Postural supports may enhance proximal stability to improve the purposeful use and development of the arms and hands (**3.67**). For children with high muscle tone, like Max in the case study, practitioners often use play-based interventions in different positions (like prone, supine, or high-kneeling), stretching, or orthotics to decrease muscle tightness.

A stroke or traumatic brain injury (TBI) may also lead to abnormal muscle tone, weakness, or complete paralysis of the muscles of the trunk, often on one side of the body. This unilateral weakness, or **hemiparesis**, contributes to significant musculoskeletal imbalance of the trunk. Impairment of the sensory systems of the body—visual, vestibular, or somatosensory—may also affect an individual's ability to maintain an upright position. Depending on the severity of the brain injury,

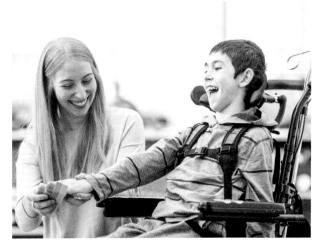

3.67 Wheelchair positioning. How do the physical supports on this wheelchair contribute to the child's hand function for occupational performance?

sensorimotor control and core strength may or may not return. Interventions that focus on postural control and symmetry of the body, such as working in front of a mirror, may help to restore postural balance and function.

Spinal Injuries

Improper lifting, traumatic injury, or age-related changes may lead to a herniated or slipped disc, an injury to the intervertebral disc between the vertebrae (**3.68**).

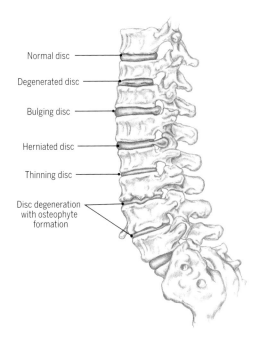

Normal disc

Degenerated disc

Bulging disc

Herniated disc

Thinning disc

Disc degeneration with osteophyte formation

3.68 Examples of disc problems. How might degeneration of the spinal vertebrae contribute to compression of a spinal nerve root (radiculopathy)? What symptoms would you expect?

A herniated disc can cause compression of a nerve root within the intervertebral foramen, or radiculopathy. Over time the compression may impact the spinal nerve's specific sensory pathway, or **dermatome**, or the muscles it innervates, its **myotome**. In certain cases, this compression may exert pressure on the adjacent spinal cord, leading to paralysis or loss of sensation.

The vertebrae and intervertebral discs are also subject to traumatic injury or degeneration over time, which can decrease the tight spaces (foramen) between the vertebrae. Aging and postural compromise affect the alignment and strength of these structures, changing the dynamics of load-bearing through the spine. As a result, older adults are more susceptible to stress fractures or arthritic changes that may cause significant pain and functional limitations.

Conservative management of vertebral injuries may include efforts to stabilize the spine as well as prevention of further injury. **Fusion** of adjacent vertebrae and **laminectomy**, removal of the lamina, are common surgical procedures for addressing back pain associated with vertebral instability.

A **spinal cord injury (SCI)**, in broad terms, is an injury to the spinal cord that blocks the transmission of neurological signals from the brain and body, resulting in functional impairment. An SCI is often the result of high-impact trauma, such as a motor vehicle accident (MVA) or diving injury. The injury may be complete, with the entire cord severed, or partial, preserving some connection between the brain and body. Sensory and motor function is generally lost below the level of injury, with higher-level injuries causing more functional impairment. For example, an injury in the cervical spine will impact the arms, legs, and trunk (quadriplegia), while an injury in the lumbar spine will affect only the legs (paraplegia). SCIs are complex, and it is far beyond the scope of this text to describe them in detail. The diagnosis is mentioned here because it relates to this region of the body and practitioners commonly encounter individuals with SCIs in rehabilitation.

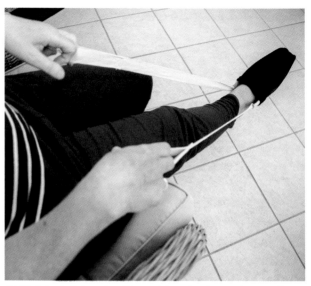

3.69 Adapted dressing. How might adaptive equipment like a sock aid decrease stress on the spine for lower body dressing?

Adaptive Equipment

Many ADLs involve trunk flexion, such as lower extremity dressing, including donning or doffing pants, socks, and shoes. Spinal flexion may be limited after surgery or related to **low back pain (LBP)**. Specialized **adaptive equipment (AE)** supports these occupations while limiting trunk flexion.

A **reacher** serves as an extension of the upper extremity for object manipulation or guiding pants onto the lower legs, limiting demands on the trunk. A **sock aid** also provides an alternative method to don socks without flexing the trunk (**3.69**).

Individuals with poor trunk control may also benefit from adaptive seating and mobility services. A customized seating system offers additional support to the trunk with cushions, backrests, lateral supports, and headrests catered to individual needs. Backrests and cushions can be custom designed with contours to support spinal postures associated with kyphosis or scoliosis.

Specialty chairs may also tilt or recline, providing gravity-assisted trunk extension and the ability to change positions frequently to safely distribute pressure (**3.70**). A supported upright posture in a custom seating system enhances mobility as well as breathing, self-feeding, engaging with family and friends, and overall quality of life.

As you continue to study the regions and functional anatomy of the body, consider the role of the trunk in supporting (or inhibiting) purposeful movement of the entire person. Interventions to improve trunk control and stability, whether rehabilitative, compensatory, or adaptive, often significantly enhance a patient's engagement and participation in occupation.

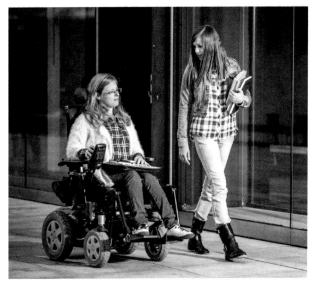

3.70 Power mobility. How might this power wheelchair facilitate engagement in occupation beyond mobility?

APPLY AND REVIEW

Max Carter

The OT has worked with Max for nearly an hour, including grading the activity up by having Max attempt to crawl up the incline of the wedge (see photo). Max is exhausted and has fallen asleep in his mother's arms. His tone seems to have relaxed, and his trunk is in a more neutral position. His mother is encouraged by the OT session today, particularly with Max's ability to sit upright for a few seconds with less support to engage in play with his toys. She asks what else they can do at home to improve his function.

Working with a child involves working with a family or caregiver, and fortunately, Max's family is very engaged and supportive.

- Provide Max's mother with some safe play-based activities that Max can complete at home to promote his trunk control and function.
- What are some strategies you can recommend to support Max's participation in other ADLs, such as dressing, self-feeding, and bathing?

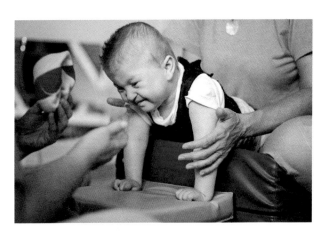

- What everyday items could the family safely use in place of the wedge to continue similar activities throughout the week?

Review Questions

1. Which of the following muscles is the *primary* flexor of the trunk?
   a. rectus abdominis
   b. external oblique
   c. erector spinae
   d. quadratus lumborum

2. What structures form a closed kinetic chain that resembles a bucket handle?
   a. clavicle and first rib
   b. lumbar vertebrae and sacrum
   c. thoracic vertebrae, ribs, and sternum
   d. cervical spine and clavicle

3. Contraction of the diaphragm has what effect on the volume of the thoracic cavity?
   a. decreased volume
   b. neutral volume
   c. stabilized volume
   d. increased volume

4. What vertebral region supports the majority of the compressive load of the spine?
   a. cervical
   b. lumbar
   c. thoracic
   d. coccyx

5. Maintaining a neutral spine and lifting with the legs reduces what type of force between adjacent vertebrae?
   a. compression
   b. distraction
   c. shear (translation)
   d. concentric

6. What type of stance supports occupational performance by facilitating weight-shifting and maintaining a neutral pelvis?
   a. straight leg
   b. neutral
   c. parallel
   d. stagger

7. The medial and lateral orientation of the _____ joints limits rotation and enhances stability in the lumbar spine.
   a. zygapophyseal (facet)
   b. laminar
   c. interbody
   d. atlantoaxial

8. What structure provides a flexible cushion between adjacent vertebrae, absorbing axial compression and allowing for some motion?
   a. transverse process
   b. thoracolumbar fascia
   c. intervertebral disc
   d. synovial capsule

9. Contraction of the abdominal muscles while lifting increases _____, which helps to stabilize the lumbar spine.
   a. thoracic cavity volume
   b. intra-abdominal pressure
   c. cervical mobility
   d. low back pain

10. What portion of the vertebral column is the most mobile and facilitates occupational performance by greatly increasing the visual field?
    a. lumbar spine
    b. sacral spine
    c. thoracic spine
    d. cervical spine

See Answer Key in back of book.

Notes

1. American Occupational Therapy Association, *Occupational Therapy Practice Framework: Domain and Process*, 4th ed. (Bethesda, MD: AOTA Press, 2020).

2. American Occupational Therapy Association, *Occupational Therapy Practice Framework*.

3. Karen Jacobs, *Ergonomics for Therapists*, 3rd ed. (St. Louis, MO: Mosby Elsevier, 2008).

Bibliography

American Occupational Therapy Association. *Occupational Therapy Practice Framework: Domain and Process*. 4th ed. Bethesda, MD: AOTA Press, 2020.

Biel, Andrew. *Trail Guide to Movement: Building the Body in Motion*. 2nd ed. Boulder, CO: Books of Discovery, 2019.

Biel, Andrew. *Trail Guide to the Body: A Hands-On Guide to Locating Muscles, Bones, and More*. 6th ed. Boulder, CO: Books of Discovery, 2019.

Clarkson, Hazel M. *Joint Motion, Muscle Length, and Function Assessment: A Research-Based Practical Guide*. 2nd ed. Philadelphia: Wolters Kluwer, 2020.

Greene, David Paul, and Susan L. Roberts. *Kinesiology: Movement in the Context of Activity*. 3rd ed. St. Louis, MO: Elsevier, 2017.

Jacobs, Karen. *Ergonomics for Therapists*. 3rd ed. St. Louis, MO: Mosby Elsevier, 2008.

Keough, Jeremy L., Susan J. Sain, and Carolyn L. Roller. *Kinesiology for the Occupational Therapy Assistant: Essential Components of Function and Movement*. 2nd ed. Thorofare, NJ: SLACK, 2017.

Oatis, Carol A. *Kinesiology: The Mechanics and Pathomechanics of Human Movement*. 3rd ed. Philadelphia: Wolters Kluwer, 2017.

Pendleton, Heidi McHugh, and Winifred Schultz-Krohn. *Pedretti's Occupational Therapy: Practice Skills for Physical Dysfunction*. 8th ed. St. Louis, MO: Elsevier, 2017.

CHAPTER 4

Head and Neck

Learning Objectives

- Describe the bones, structures, and muscles contributing to facial expression, speech, swallowing, and eye movement.

- Explain the role of the head and face in nonverbal communication (facial expression), speech, swallowing, and eye movement.

- Begin to develop clinical reasoning to identify limitations of the head and neck that may affect occupational performance.

Key Concepts

aphasia

aspiration

Bell's palsy

deglutition

diplopia

dysarthria

dysphagia

esophageal phase

hard palate

homonymous hemianopsia

modified barium swallow study

optokinetic reflex

oral preparatory phase

oral transit phase

paranasal sinuses

pharyngeal phase

phonemes

swallowing

therapeutic use of self

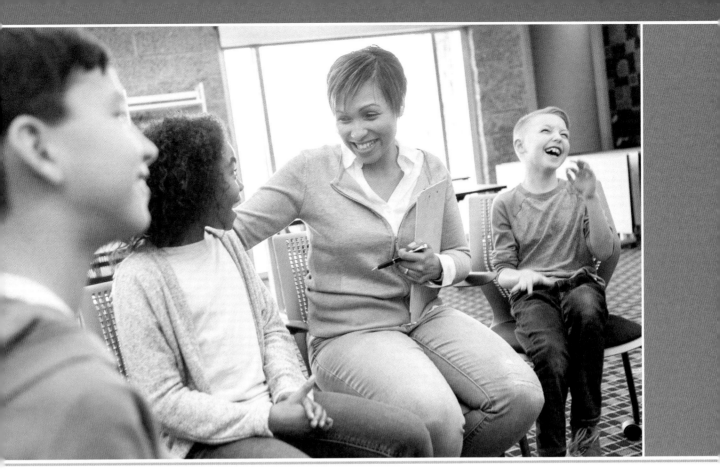

Occupational Profile: Charity Rose

CHARITY ROSE is a social worker who works in a large metropolitan school system. Recently married, she and her spouse, Shane, have just bought a new home. They enjoy cooking together, traveling, and spending time with their family and friends.

While driving home from work yesterday, Charity felt some weakness on the side of her face. When she looked in the mirror, she noticed the left side of her face was drooping. Concerned that she might be having a stroke, she drove herself to the emergency room.

Oddly, she did not notice any weakness or loss of sensation in her arms or legs and had no issues with her vision or cognition. Think about Charity's symptoms and answer the following questions:

- Do you think Charity's symptoms are consistent with a stroke?
- Are her symptoms consistent with any other type of neurological diagnosis (refer to Chapter 2)?

Keep Charity in mind as we discuss the functional anatomy of the head and neck.

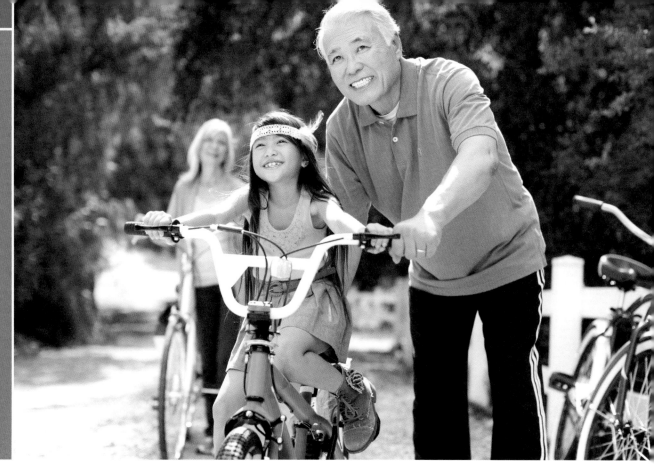

4.1 The head and neck contain functional pathways that are essential to occupational performance.

Head and Neck: Functional Pathways

The head and face are essential to occupational performance, contributing to motor, processing, and social interaction skills (**4.1**). Close your eyes and think about an occupation you enjoy. What does it look and sound like? What does it feel like? Does it have an aroma? The sensory pathways of the head and processing ability of the brain make this memory possible, enhancing the meaning of purposeful activity.

Motion of the cervical spine, coupled with movements of the eye, allows for more than 180° of real-time visual input for safe driving or navigating a run through an urban area. Verbal communication involves the mouth, tongue, and lips forming the syllables of language or song. The ears receive auditory input, which is interpreted by the brain as language, a signal of danger, or a familiar tune from the airwaves passing through. Powerful nonverbal messages ("If looks could kill...") are also conveyed by the muscles of facial expression, communicating joy, fear, or anger.

The tongue and nose perceive complementary sensations of taste and smell, allowing us to savor our favorite dish or appreciate the complexities of a fine wine. How-ever, the brain must process, interpret, and record this sensory input to have meaningful interaction, memories, or an appropriate motor response.

This chapter presents the unique structures of the head and face that facilitate these essential functions. Clinical perspectives are imbedded in the chapter along with a case study to emphasize the importance of the functional anatomy of the head and face to future practice. Consider the functional roles of the structures described in the next section. Several of these structures serve multiple roles in different systems of the body, and their dysfunction often has a broad impact on occupational performance.

Osteology: Bones of the Head and Neck

The skull serves as a bony cavity to protect the brain and its continuous processes—vital organ regulation, sensorimotor function, hormonal regulation, and cognition, to name a few. The mandible and hyoid bone are skeletal components that give structure to the functions of speech, eating, and swallowing. Use the digital palpation resources with this book to identify the various surface anatomy landmarks described for each bone.

Skull

The **head** refers to the skull and all the structures on its surface and within, whereas the **skull** consists solely of the bones of the **cranium** and **mandible**. The skull is composed of interconnected bones, similar to pieces of a three-dimensional puzzle (**4.2**, **4.3**). The bones form two distinct portions: the rounded top of the skull, called the neurocranium, and the facial bones, or viscerocranium. These are joined by **sutures**, or **synarthrodial joints**.

The **neurocranium** is divided into a roof and a base. Its roof, or **calvarium**, is formed by the superior portions of the **frontal**, **occipital**, and two **parietal** bones. The base is formed by parts of the frontal (2), occipital, and **temporal** (2) bones, as well as the **ethmoid** and **sphenoid** bones.

The **viscerocranium**, the skeleton of the face, comprises fourteen distinct bones: **zygomatic** (2), **lacrimal** (2), **nasal** (2), **inferior nasal concha** (2), **maxilla** (2),

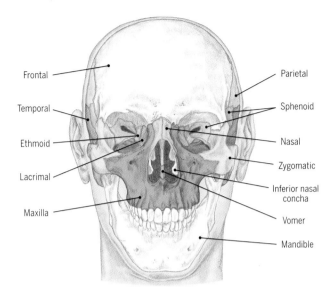

Facial bones (14)	
Inferior nasal concha (2)	Nasal (2)
Lacrimal (2)	Palatine (2)
Mandible	Vomer
Maxilla (2)	Zygomatic (2)

4.3 Anterior view of the skull

palatine (2), **vomer**, and mandible. These bones provide the skeletal structure for the skin and muscles of the face and form cavities for the eyes, nose, and mouth.

Bony Landmarks of the Skull

As the skull lies just beneath the skin, it is easily palpable, and many bony landmarks can be clearly identified (**4.4**, **4.5**).

At the base of the posterior skull, the rounded occipital bone can be palpated by gliding the fingers upward from the neck. The **external occipital protuberance** is the most posterior point of the occiput, palpable at the midline of the bone.

Moving laterally around the skull, the **mastoid process** projects outward just behind the ear, providing an anatomical attachment for the sternocleidomastoid muscle to rotate the head. Anterior to the opening of the ear is the **zygomatic arch**, a bony ridge composed of parts of the zygomatic and maxillary bones that forms the superior skeletal border of the cheek.

The **alveolar process**, a thickened ridge of bone on the inferior border of the maxilla, contains **dental alveoli**, or tooth sockets, for the upper teeth. The palatine process of the maxilla spans this horseshoe-shaped ridge,

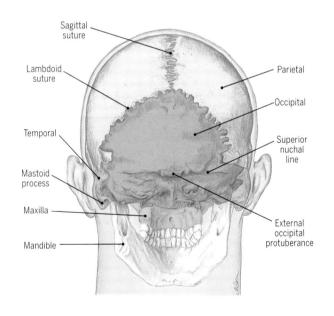

Cranial bones (8)	
Ethmoid	Parietal (2)
Frontal	Sphenoid
Occipital	Temporal (2)

4.2 Posterior view of the skull

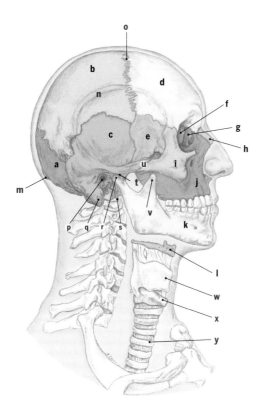

a. Occiput
b. Parietal
c. Temporal
d. Frontal
e. Sphenoid
f. Ethmoid
g. Lacrimal
h. Nasal
i. Zygomatic
j. Maxilla
k. Mandible
l. Hyoid
m. External occipital protuberance
n. Temporal lines of parietal bones
o. Coronal suture
p. External auditory meatus
q. Mastoid process
r. Condyle of the mandible
s. Styloid process of the temporal bone
t. Temporomandibular joint
u. Zygomatic arch
v. Coronoid process
w. Thyroid cartilage
x. Cricoid cartilage
y. Trachea

Black letters indicate bones; **red** letters indicate bony landmarks or other structures.

4.4 Lateral view of the skull

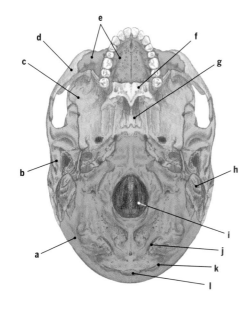

a. Occiput
b. Temporal
c. Sphenoid
d. Zygomatic
e. Maxilla
f. Palatine
g. Vomer
h. Mastoid process
i. Foramen magnum
j. Inferior nuchal line
k. Superior nuchal line
l. External occipital protuberance

Black letters indicate bones; **red** letters indicate bony landmarks or other structures.

4.5 Inferior view of the skull

forming the anterior two-thirds of the **hard palate**, or bony roof of the mouth, with the **horizontal plate** of the palatine bone making up the posterior third (**4.6**).

The bony superior rim of the **orbit**, or eye socket, is palpable beneath the eyebrow and around the periphery of the eyelids. The **optic canal** is the opening posterior to the orbit, and the optic nerve and ophthalmic artery pass through here (**4.7**).

The nasal bones lie centrally between the orbits, creating the bony foundation for the cartilage of the nose. The ethmoid bone forms the roof of the nasal cavity and is lined by the **cribriform plate**, which has many small openings called **olfactory foramina**. The olfactory foramina are passageways for the branches of the **olfactory nerve** to enter the nasal cavity, transmitting smell sensations to the brain.

Several other significant openings in the skull are important passageways for sensory input and motor output, blood vessels, and nerves:

- **foramen magnum**—in the occipital bone for the spinal cord and vertebral arteries
- **external auditory meatus** (ear canal)—for the passage of sound to the eardrum
- **supraorbital foramen**—in the frontal bone for the supraorbital vein, artery, and nerve (branch of trigeminal nerve)
- **infraorbital foramen**—in the maxilla for the infraorbital nerve
- **foramen rotundum**—in the sphenoid bone for the maxillary nerve

CLINICAL APPLICATION
Cleft Lip and Cleft Palate

In utero, a baby's lips begin to form between the fourth and seventh weeks of pregnancy. The palate forms between the sixth and ninth weeks. The tissues that form the lips and palate grow toward the center of the face. Sometimes, however, they fail to completely join.

A **cleft lip** indicates a gap, or split, in the upper lip. A **cleft palate** describes an opening in the hard or soft palate in the roof of the oral cavity. These conditions vary in severity and may affect only the upper lip, partial palate, or both the upper lip and entire palate.

These birth defects impair the function of the nasal and oral cavities, impacting the development of feeding, swallowing, and language skills. Early surgical repair, often involving tissue grafting, is generally successful in restoring closure of the lip and palate to facilitate development of these skills.[1] How would successful surgical closure of the lips and palate contribute to these functional skills?

- **stylomastoid foramen**—in the temporal bone for the facial nerve
- **foramen ovale**—in the sphenoid bone for the mandibular nerve
- **mental foramen**—in the mandible for the mental nerve

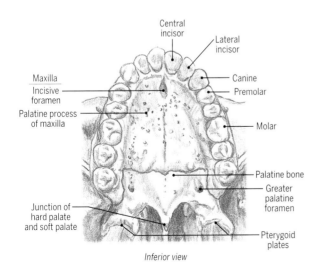

4.6 Hard palate

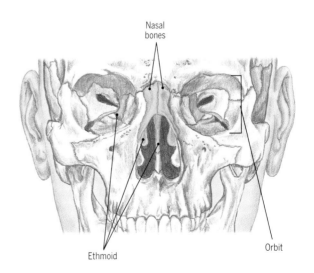

4.7 Nasal bones

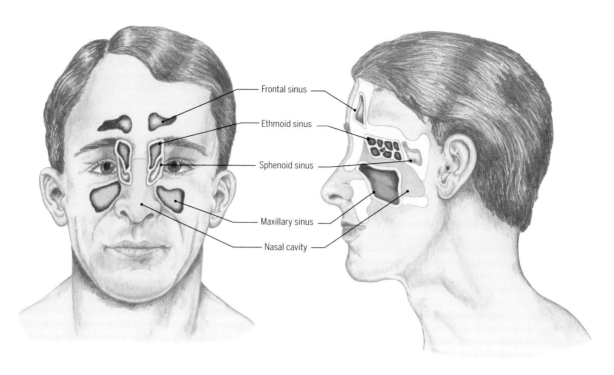

4.8 Paranasal sinuses

Paranasal Sinuses

The **paranasal sinuses** are hollow, air-filled spaces within the skull that decrease the weight of the skull and contribute to vocal quality. The paranasal sinuses are paired and positioned adjacent to the nasal cavity (maxillary), posterior to the eyebrow (frontal), between the orbits (ethmoid), and posterior to the ethmoid sinuses (sphenoid) (**4.8**).

Mandible

The U-shaped **mandible**, or jawbone, supports the lower teeth and serves as the mobile skeletal floor of the mouth (**4.9**). The **mandibular condyle** and **coronoid process** project upward from the ramus of the mandible, separated by the mandibular notch. The mandibular body extends anteriorly and contains sockets (alveoli) for the sixteen teeth of the lower jaw.

Bony Landmarks of the Mandible

The **body** of the mandible refers to the flat surface of the bone beneath the teeth (**4.9**). The **base** is its sharp inferior edge, or jawline. The **submandibular fossa** is located on the interior aspect of the mandible and forms

a small depression on which the submandibular gland rests. The mandibular condyle emerges just anterior to the ear. When opening the jaw, it moves along the zygomatic arch.

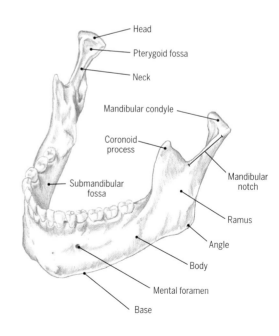

4.9 Bones and bony landmarks of the mandible

Hyoid and Larynx

The **hyoid bone** is also a U-shaped bone that serves as an attachment point for many muscles involved in speech and swallowing (**4.10**, **4.11**).

Suspended in the upper neck, the hyoid is an attachment site for the muscles of the tongue above and muscles of the **larynx** (voice box) below (**4.12**). The larynx is formed by six distinct cartilages, three of which are paired—**arytenoid**, **corniculate**, and **cuneiform**—and three of which are unpaired—**thyroid**, **cricoid**, and **epiglottic**.

Along with the trachea and larynx, many other delicate vascular structures and glands are positioned adjacent to or pass through the bones of the head and neck. Clinically, it is important to understand the specific locations of these structures. For example, the carotid artery is a site of blockage related to stroke, and lymph nodes in the axilla and neck may be removed to address certain types of cancer.

The **common carotid arteries** ascend and divide into internal and external branches, supplying blood to the

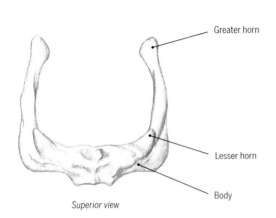

Greater horn

Lesser horn

Body

Superior view

4.10 Hyoid bone

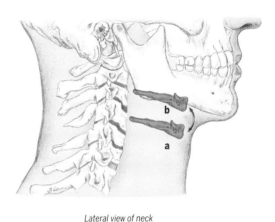

b

a

Lateral view of neck

4.11 The hyoid bone at rest (*a*) and during swallowing (*b*)

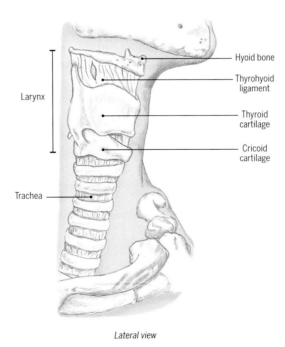

Larynx

Trachea

Hyoid bone

Thyrohyoid ligament

Thyroid cartilage

Cricoid cartilage

Lateral view

4.12 Neck

brain (internal), neck (external), and face (external) (**4.13**). The **internal jugular vein** runs along with the common carotid artery, and the **external jugular vein** runs superficial to the sternocleidomastoid muscle (**4.14**).

Additionally, the salivary gland, thyroid gland, and many lymph nodes lie beneath the jaw and around the neck (**4.15**).

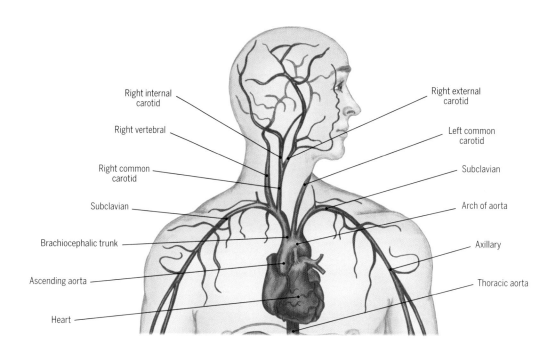

4.13 Arteries of the upper body

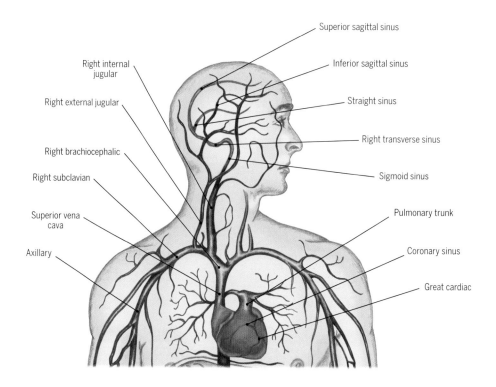

4.14 Veins of the upper body

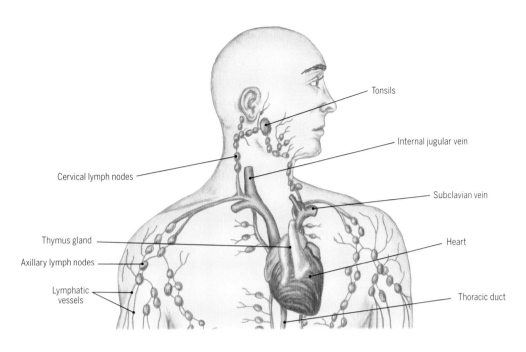

4.15 Lymphatic system of the upper body

Oral Cavity and Pharynx

The oral cavity and pharynx provide a two-way functional anatomical pathway for speaking, eating, and breathing. The **oral cavity** describes the space from the mouth to the **soft palate**, including the gums, lining of the cheeks, floor of the mouth, and anterior two-thirds of the tongue (**4.16**).

The oral cavity is a vital passageway serving as the beginning of the **alimentary (digestive) tract** and **upper respiratory tract** for inhalation (along with the nose). The oral cavity and nose are also exits for deoxygenated air exhaled from the lungs during respiration. Additionally, the oral and nasal cavities serve as acoustic chambers, shaping exhaled air into the syllables (**phonemes**) of words spoken or sung.

Moving posteriorly, we find the **pharynx**, a functional channel shared by the digestive and respiratory systems that leads to the esophagus and larynx. Anatomically, the pharynx is divided into three distinct segments: the **nasopharynx** is the portion posterior to the nasal cavity, the **oropharynx** lies behind the oral cavity, and the **laryngopharynx** spans the area between the hyoid bone and esophagus.

Functionally, the pharynx is a pathway for food to reach the esophagus and for air to reach the larynx. The pharynx is formed by two layers of muscles that facilitate swallow-

ing: an inner longitudinal layer containing the **stylopharyngeus**, **salpingopharyngeus**, and **palatopharyngeus**, and an outer circular layer made up of the **inferior, middle**, and **superior constrictor** muscles.

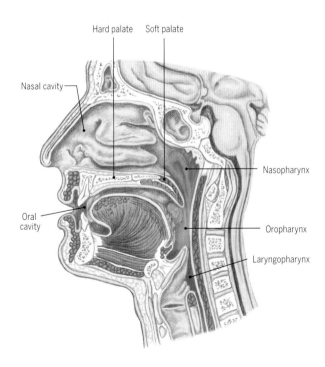

4.16 Oral cavity and pharynx

Joints

We typically associate the joints of the body with movement. However, some joints are designed to stabilize adjacent bones, as is the case with many of the bones of the skull. The following sections describe the stabilizing joints of the skull as well as the temporomandibular joint and its articulation with the jaw to facilitate speech, eating, and swallowing.

Sutures of the Skull

Unlike the synovial joints of the limbs, the bones of the skull are held together by sutures, which are classified as **synarthroses**, or unmoving joints (**4.17**).

The sutures are held together by dense fibrous tissue called **Sharpey's fibers**. The sutures of an infant's skull are flexible, allowing the skull to expand as the brain grows. With age, the sutures ossify and become more rigid.

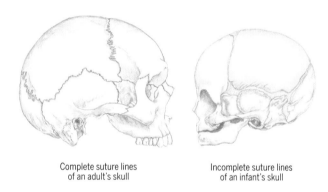

Complete suture lines
of an adult's skull

Incomplete suture lines
of an infant's skull

4.17 Sutures of the skull

CHARITY ROSE | Charity's temporomandibular joint does not seem to be impaired. She is able to move her jaw through its full range of motion and to forcefully clench her teeth. However, she is having difficulty closing her lips together to seal her mouth on the left side. She first noticed this when attempting to drink water out of a straw while waiting in the emergency room.

As we discuss the muscles of the head and face, keep these deficits in mind. See if you can identify the specific muscles that are impaired.

Temporomandibular Joint

The **temporomandibular joints (TMJs)**, positioned on each side of the jaw, are synovial joints (**4.18**). These joints operate in tandem for symmetrical, functional motion of the mandible, including elevation, depression, lateral deviation, protraction, and retraction.

The TMJs are vital for many occupations—eating, hygiene, singing, or playing an instrument, to name a few. These joints move an estimated two to three thousand times per day.

To allow motion and reduce friction between the articular surfaces—the mandibular condyle and articular fossa—each TMJ is equipped with an **articular disc** that moves with the condyles as the jaw opens and closes (**4.19**).

Ligament support of the TMJs includes a joint capsule as well as the **stylomandibular**, **sphenomandibular**, and **temporomandibular ligaments**, enhancing stability between the skull and mandible (**4.18**, **4.19**).

Musculature, Function, and Movement

Most muscles of the face, unlike muscles of the limbs, move the surrounding soft tissue instead of the joints. Facial expression, opening and closing the eyes or mouth,

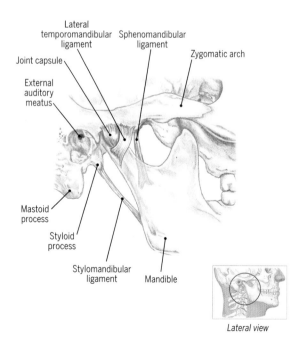

Lateral
temporomandibular
ligament

Sphenomandibular
ligament

Zygomatic arch

Joint capsule

External
auditory
meatus

Mastoid
process

Styloid
process

Stylomandibular
ligament

Mandible

Lateral view

4.18 Lateral skull and mandible

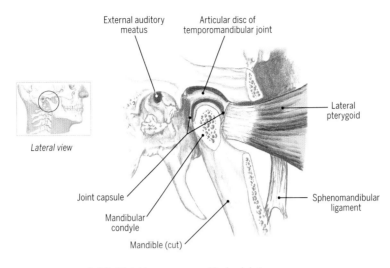

External auditory meatus

Articular disc of temporomandibular joint

Lateral pterygoid

Lateral view

Joint capsule

Sphenomandibular ligament

Mandibular condyle

Mandible (cut)

4.19 Right temporomandibular joint

and blowing a kiss are examples of functional soft tissue movements of the face. Other muscles are involved with chewing, swallowing, or verbal communication—actions that include movement of the TMJ and structures of the throat.

The muscles that move the head and neck, outside of the TMJ, are covered in Chapter 3. The following sections present the other muscles of the head and neck (**4.20**, **4.21**) in functional groups for an occupation-based perspective focusing on purposeful activity.

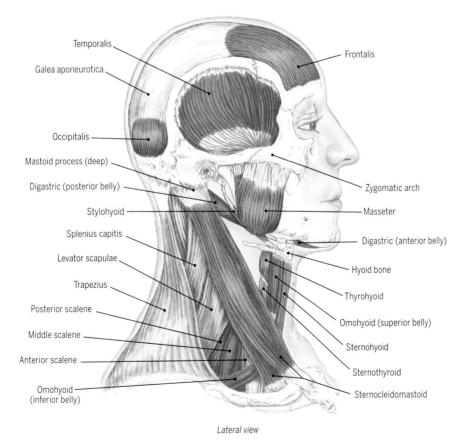

Temporalis

Galea aponeurotica

Frontalis

Occipitalis

Mastoid process (deep)

Digastric (posterior belly)

Stylohyoid

Zygomatic arch

Splenius capitis

Masseter

Levator scapulae

Digastric (anterior belly)

Trapezius

Hyoid bone

Posterior scalene

Thyrohyoid

Middle scalene

Omohyoid (superior belly)

Anterior scalene

Sternohyoid

Omohyoid (inferior belly)

Sternothyroid

Sternocleidomastoid

Lateral view

4.20 Muscles of the head and neck

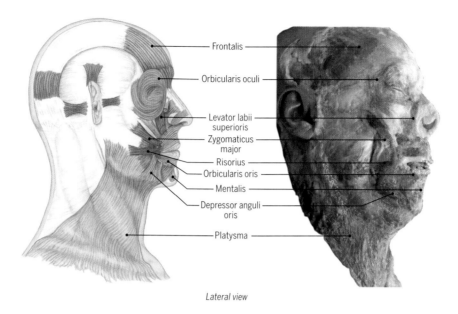

Lateral view

4.21 Superficial muscles of the head and neck

Muscles of Facial Expression

The muscles of facial expression are classified as **integumentary muscles** and attach to the underlying fascia and skin of the face (**4.22**).

Because of this unique arrangement, their attachment sites are not described in detail here. Rather, their positions and orientations are presented in each figure in a functional context.

As the primary functional purpose of these facial muscles is to express emotion, they are known as **mimetic** muscles. The muscles are typically superficial, just beneath the skin, and their attachment sites become more visible with specific expressions. For example, when smiling, the corners of the mouth elevate, revealing the pathway of the zygomaticus major.

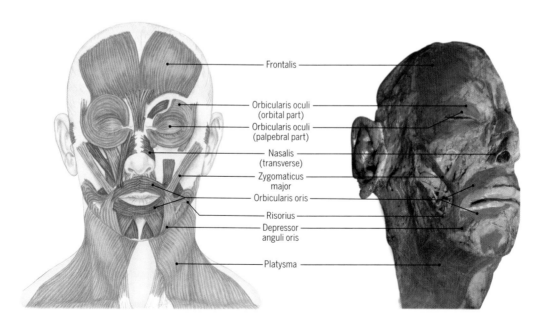

Anterior view

4.22 Muscles of facial expression

Figures **4.23–4.40** present the muscles that act on the mouth, nose, eyes, or scalp, in subgroups.

Muscles of the Mouth

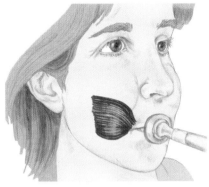

Buccinator
- Contracts the cheeks to narrow the mouth
- Directs a **bolus** (mass of chewed food) and prevents food particles from falling between the teeth and gums
- Engages when blowing up a balloon or playing the trumpet

4.23 Buccinator

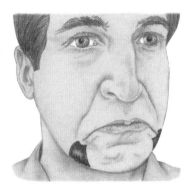

4.24 Depressor anguli oris

Depressor anguli oris
- Depresses and pulls corners of the mouth inferior and lateral
- Expresses sadness

Depressor labii inferioris
- Depresses, protrudes, and pulls the lips laterally
- Exposes the lower teeth for brushing and flossing

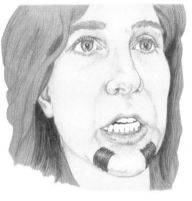

4.25 Depressor labii inferioris

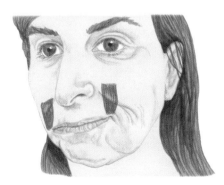

4.26 Levator anguli oris

Levator anguli oris
- Elevates the angles of the mouth
- With bilateral contraction, expresses a warm smile
- With unilateral contraction, may express a self-confident smirk

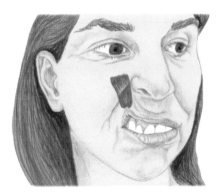

4.27 Levator labii superioris

Levator labii superioris
- Elevates and protrudes the upper lip
- Exposes the upper teeth for brushing or flossing
- Expresses a contemptuous snarl

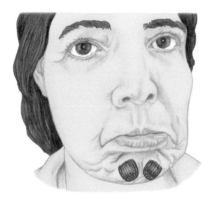

4.28 Mentalis

Mentalis

- Elevates the medial skin of the chin
- Protrudes the lower lip
- Expresses significant sadness

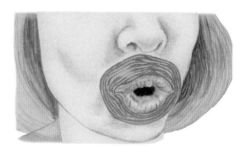

4.29 Orbicularis oris

Orbicularis oris

- Closes and shapes the lips
- Contours to the mouthpiece of an instrument
- Allows for drinking from a straw or removing food from spoon
- Seals mouth for swallowing
- Puckers up for a kiss

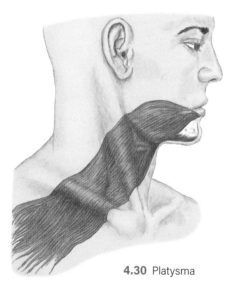

4.30 Platysma

Platysma

- Depresses the jaw and corners of the mouth
- Tightens the fascia of the neck
- Expresses rage or terror

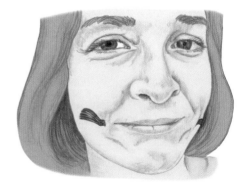

4.31 Risorius

Risorius

- Retracts the corners of the mouth
- May express a fake smile

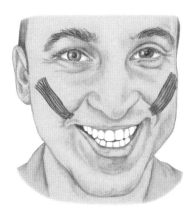

Zygomaticus major
- Elevates and pulls corners of the mouth laterally
- Contracts with the orbicularis oculi to express authentic joy in the form of a smile or laughter

Zygomaticus minor
- Elevates and protrudes the upper lip
- Puffs out the superior cheeks
- Expresses a genuine smile or a skeptical grimace

4.32 Zygomaticus major

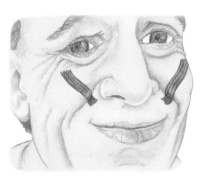

4.33 Zygomaticus minor

Muscles of the Nose

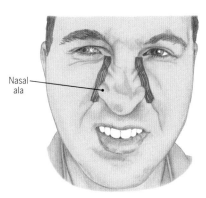

Nasal ala

Levator labii superioris alaeque nasi
- Flares the nostrils
- Expresses disgust

4.34 Levator labii superioris alaeque nasi

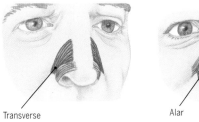

Transverse

Alar

4.35 Nasalis

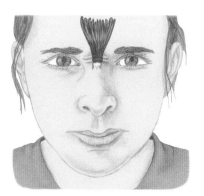

4.36 Procerus

Nasalis
- Constricts the nostrils (transverse fibers)
- Flares the nostrils (alar fibers)
- Controls circumference of nostrils to regulate airflow through nose

Procerus
- Pulls skin between eyebrows down
- Expresses concentration

Muscles of the Eyes

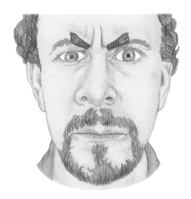

4.37 Corrugator supercilii

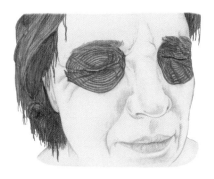

4.38 Orbicularis oculi

Corrugator supercilii
- Depresses and pulls the eyebrow medially
- Expresses concern or confusion

Orbicularis oculi
- Involuntarily closes the eyelid such as when blinking or sleeping (palpebral fibers)
- Forcefully closes the eye such as when squinting or expressing pain (orbital fibers)

Muscles of the Scalp

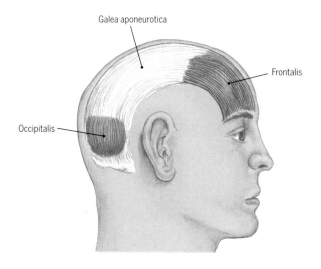

4.39 Occipitofrontalis (frontalis and occipitalis)

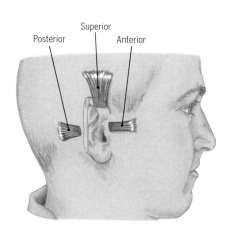

4.40 Auricularis (anterior, superior, posterior)

Occipitofrontalis (frontalis and occipitalis)
- Elevates both eyebrows to express surprise
- Elevates one eyebrow to express skepticism

Auricularis (anterior, superior, posterior)
- Wiggles the ears (for those who can activate these muscles—can you?)

Muscles of Mastication and Speech

Masseter

Temporalis

Medial and lateral pterygoids

Muscles that control the mouth and tongue produce the forces involved with mastication (chewing and grinding) and the syllables (phonemes) of speech. Several of these muscles act directly on the TMJ to open and close the jaw, and others control the tongue.

The masseter, temporalis, medial pterygoid, and lateral pterygoid (**4.41–4.44**) are the primary muscles of mastication. Other muscles in this functional group control the tongue, which is active for both speech production and the oral phase of digestion (deglutition). Compared to the muscles of facial expression, the muscles of mastication and speech have better-defined attachments to the bones of the face and mandible.

Masseter

- Generates biting force up to 150 pounds
- Elevates and protrudes the mandible for speech and chewing

CHARITY ROSE | Charity was evaluated by a physician in the emergency room who administered a few formal cognitive and physical exams. The physician noted equal range of motion (ROM) and strength throughout Charity's extremities as well as normal cognition and orientation.

She then asked Charity to smile, raise her eyebrows, whistle, and puff out her cheeks. These tasks were hard to complete as it seemed the left side of her face would not cooperate. Charity also noticed she could swallow fine. Her tongue seemed to work normally for speaking, but her words were somewhat muddled.

Magnetic resonance imaging (MRI) of her brain revealed no evidence of a stroke or other brain injury.

- What do the findings of Charity's exam suggest? Does this information help to identify a specific diagnosis?
- Which muscles of the face appear to be impacted? Why do you think only these muscles are affected?
- Refer to Charity's occupational profile at the beginning of the chapter. How might her symptoms hinder her occupational performance? Consider her ADLs and IADLs as well as her roles as a social worker and spouse.

MASSETER	
Purposeful Activity	
P	Eating, playing the trumpet
A	**Elevate** the mandible (TMJ) May assist to **protract** the mandible (TMJ)
O	Zygomatic arch
I	Angle and ramus of mandible
N	Trigeminal (V) nerve (mandibular division)

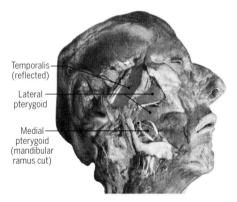

Temporalis (reflected)
Lateral pterygoid
Medial pterygoid (mandibular ramus cut)

4.41 Masseter

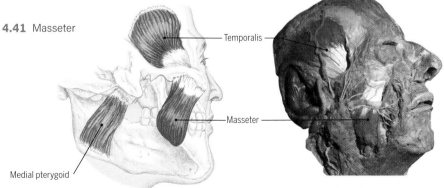

Temporalis
Masseter
Medial pterygoid

Lateral view

Temporalis

- Elevates and retracts the mandible for speech and chewing

TEMPORALIS	
Purposeful Activity	
P	**Eating, verbal communication**
A	**Elevate** the mandible (TMJ) **Retract** the mandible (TMJ)
O	Temporal fossa and fascia
I	Coronoid process and anterior edge of ramus of the mandible
N	Trigeminal (V) nerve (mandibular division)

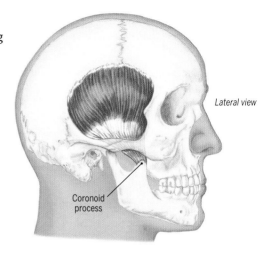

Lateral view

Coronoid process

4.42 Temporalis

Medial and Lateral Pterygoids

- Protrudes mandible
- Laterally and medially deviates mandible to grind food

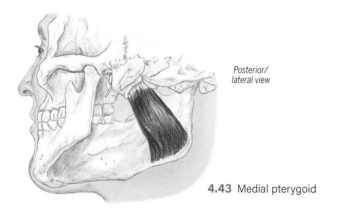

Posterior/ lateral view

4.43 Medial pterygoid

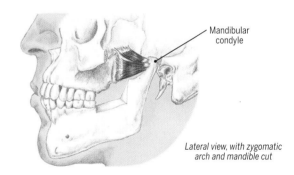

Mandibular condyle

Lateral view, with zygomatic arch and mandible cut

4.44 Lateral pterygoid

MEDIAL PTERYGOID	
Purposeful Activity	
P	**Eating (grinding food)**
A	*Unilaterally:* **Laterally deviate** the mandible to the opposite side *Bilaterally:* **Elevate** the mandible **Protract** the mandible
O	Medial surface of lateral pterygoid plate of sphenoid bone and tuberosity of maxilla
I	Medial surface of ramus of the mandible
N	Trigeminal (V)

LATERAL PTERYGOID	
Purposeful Activity	
P	**Eating (grinding food)**
A	*Unilaterally:* **Laterally deviate** the mandible to the opposite side *Bilaterally:* **Protract** the mandible
O	Superior head: Infratemporal surface and crest of greater wing of sphenoid bone Inferior head: Lateral surface of lateral pterygoid plate of sphenoid bone
I	Articular disc and capsule of TMJ, neck of mandible
N	Trigeminal (V)

Muscles of Swallowing

Suprahyoids (strap muscles)
Infrahyoids (strap muscles)
Extrinsic muscles of the tongue
Intrinsic muscles of the tongue

Swallowing is a complex mechanism that involves both voluntary and involuntary muscle function to propel food from the mouth to the esophagus. Figures **4.45–4.50** illustrate the muscles primarily involved with swallowing. They form the floor of the mouth and act on the tongue and larynx. The specific phases of swallowing are described later in this chapter.

Suprahyoids (Strap Muscles)

Geniohyoid
Mylohyoid
Stylohyoid
Digastric

Geniohyoid, mylohyoid, and stylohyoid
- Form the muscular floor of the mouth beneath the tongue
- Elevate the hyoid and larynx for swallowing
- Depress the mandible

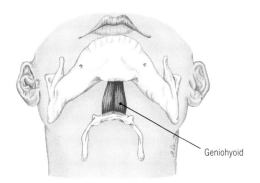

Anterior/inferior view

4.45 Geniohyoid

GENIOHYOID, MYLOHYOID, AND STYLOHYOID	
Purposeful Activity	
P	**Verbal communication, singing, swallowing**
A	**Elevate** hyoid and tongue **Depress** mandible (TMJ)
O	Geniohyoid, mylohyoid: Underside of mandible Stylohyoid: Styloid process
I	Hyoid bone
N	Geniohyoid: C1 and C2 Mylohyoid: Trigeminal (V) Stylohyoid: Facial (VII)

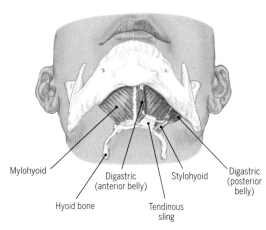

Anterior/inferior view

4.46 Mylohyoid and stylohyoid. Geniohyoid is deep to mylohyoid.

Digastric

- Spans the mastoid process and inferior border of mandible
- Attaches to the hyoid via tendinous sling
- Depresses the mandible (hyoid fixed)
- Elevates the hyoid (mandible fixed)

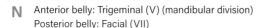

DIGASTRIC	
Purposeful Activity	
P	Swallowing, verbal communication
A	With hyoid bone fixed, **depress** the mandible (TMJ) With mandible fixed, **elevate** the hyoid bone **Retract** the mandible (TMJ)
O	Mastoid process (deep to sternocleidomastoid and splenius capitis)
I	Inferior border of the mandible
N	Anterior belly: Trigeminal (V) (mandibular division) Posterior belly: Facial (VII)

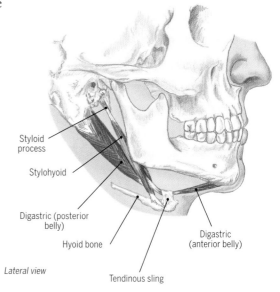

Styloid process

Stylohyoid

Digastric (posterior belly)

Hyoid bone

Digastric (anterior belly)

Lateral view

Tendinous sling

4.47 Digastric

Infrahyoids (Strap Muscles)

Sternohyoid
Sternothyroid
Thyrohyoid
Omohyoid

- Depress the hyoid (antagonists to suprahyoids) during swallowing and speech

INFRAHYOIDS	
Purposeful Activity	
P	Swallowing, verbal communication
A	**Depress** the hyoid bone and thyroid cartilage
O	Sternohyoid and sternothyroid: Top of manubrium Thyrohyoid: Thyroid cartilage Omohyoid: Superior border of the scapula
I	Sternohyoid, thyrohyoid, and omohyoid: Hyoid bone Sternothyroid: Thyroid cartilage
N	Sternohyoid, sternothyroid, and omohyoid: C1 to C3 Thyrohyoid: C1 and C2

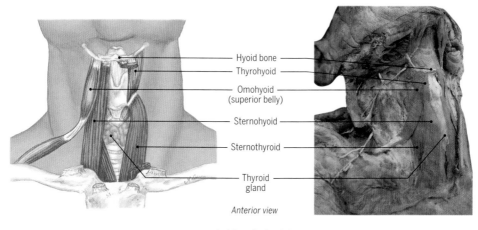

Hyoid bone
Thyrohyoid
Omohyoid (superior belly)
Sternohyoid
Sternothyroid
Thyroid gland

Anterior view

4.48 Infrahyoids

Extrinsic Muscles of the Tongue

Four extrinsic muscles originate on adjacent bones and act on the tongue:

- **genioglossus**—protrudes tongue
- **hyoglossus**—retracts and depresses tongue
- **styloglossus**—elevates sides of tongue for swallowing
- **palatoglossus**—elevates back of tongue for swallowing

Intrinsic Muscles of the Tongue

Originating and inserting within the tongue, four intrinsic muscles are oriented lengthwise along the tongue:

- **superior longitudinal**—elevates tip of tongue
- **inferior longitudinal**—depresses tip of tongue
- **vertical**—flattens and widens tongue
- **transverse**—narrows and protrudes tongue

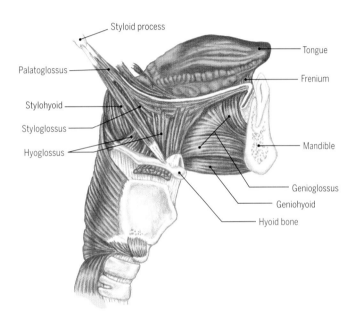

4.49 Extrinsic muscles of the tongue

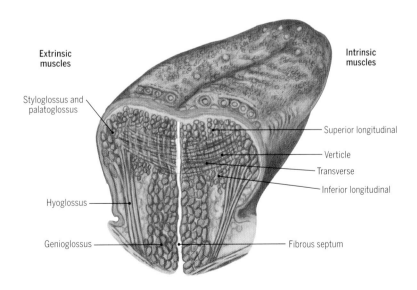

4.50 Muscles that form the tongue

Muscles of Eye Movement

The **extraocular** muscles are seven muscles that act to move the eye and one muscle that elevates the eyelid, called the **levator palpebrae**. These muscles, their attachments, and their actions on the eyeball are illustrated in Figure **4.51**.

The eyeballs move upward, downward, laterally, and medially, directing the pupil to scan the visual field. Did you know that your eyeball can also rotate to a certain degree? Think about lying down while watching TV. The image stays upright even though your head is tilted or horizontal.

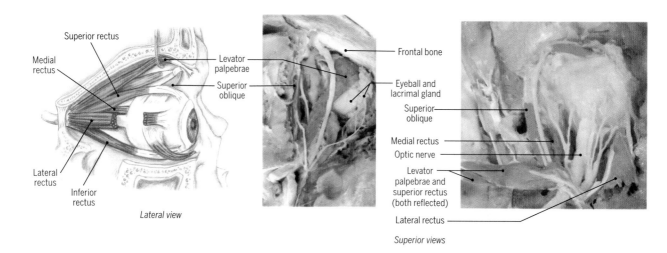

Lateral view

Superior views

4.51 Extraocular muscles of the eye

▶TRY IT

Much as preparatory exercises may be used to strengthen the hand for improved object manipulation, specific muscle groups of the face and mouth can be targeted in preparation for eating, swallowing, and communication, both verbal and nonverbal.

For example, if a client's goal is to drink out of a straw, you might have them prepare by puckering their lips and squeezing their cheeks together. What specific muscles would be targeted with this exercise? Would blowing through a straw be a beneficial activity? Why or why not?

Targeted elevation, depression, and lateral deviation of the jaw may facilitate chewing and swallowing food. Blinking the eyes, making patterned movements of the tongue in the mouth, and practicing various facial expressions may help in preparing for verbal and nonverbal communication.

Practicing in front of a mirror can provide visual feedback. Try this on your own: sit in front of a mirror and practice different facial expressions, patterns of speech, and chewing. What specific muscles are activated? What other activities could be used to support occupational performance? How might a mirror be used for interventions involving other regions of the body or specific functions?

Purposeful Movement of the Temporomandibular Joint

Recall that the TMJ is one of the only synovial joints in the head and is essential for eating, swallowing, and communication. Figures **4.52–4.55** outline its primary purposeful movements and related muscles, with prime movers listed first. Asterisks indicate muscles not shown.

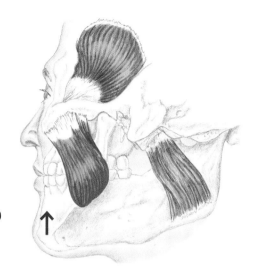

Posterior/lateral view

4.52 Elevation

Elevation
(*antagonists on depression*)
Masseter
Temporalis
Medial pterygoid

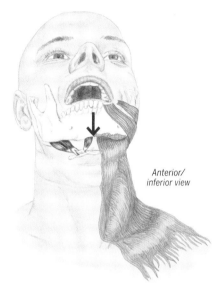

*Anterior/
inferior view*

4.53 Depression

Depression
(*antagonists on elevation*)
Geniohyoid*
Mylohyoid*
Stylohyoid
Digastric (with hyoid bone fixed)
Platysma (assists)

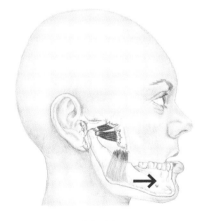

Lateral view

4.54 Protraction

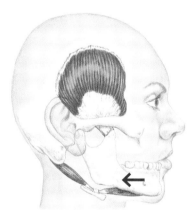

Lateral view

4.55 Retraction

Protraction
(*antagonists on retraction*)
Lateral pterygoid (bilaterally)
Medial pterygoid (bilaterally)
Masseter (assists)*

Retraction
(*antagonists on protraction*)
Temporalis
Digastric

▶TRY IT

The TMJ may be described as a hinge-type joint, but it is quite different from other synovial joints of the extremities. It connects the mandible to both sides of the skull, its center of rotation is not easy to visualize, and its motion is not typically measured with a goniometer.

Functional movement of this joint may be assessed by measuring the distance between the front teeth when opening, closing, protruding, retracting, or deviating the jaw. With a tape measure, measure the distance between your teeth with your mouth completely open. How much distance do you need to eat a meal?

Injuries to the TMJ may limit the movement of the jaw and impact speaking or eating. How might you adapt eating with limited mobility of the TMJ?

Occupational and Clinical Perspectives

As you can see, the head and face play a significant role in many motor and processing skills related to occupational performance. Let's explore some additional functional and clinical perspectives relating to this foundational functional anatomy.

Communication

Facial expression is a powerful nonverbal form of communication, often revealing the deeper emotional meaning behind the spoken word. Conveying and interpreting facial expression is an important part of occupational therapy practice. For example, a patient may not verbally express pain, but a grimace or muscle guarding (tension) could indicate that you should decrease the intensity or modify your approach.

Developing therapeutic rapport with patients also requires you to have self-awareness and intentionality with nonverbal communication. A warm smile, even on a bad day when you have to force it, is a much more inviting way to encourage patient engagement than a look of anxiety or concern (4.56). Both verbal and nonverbal communication are components of **therapeutic use of self**, integrating the therapist's unique personality and empathetic communication to enhance the therapeutic relationship.

Verbal communication begins with air in the lungs forced between the **vocal folds (cords)**, which are located within the larynx on the superior aspect of the trachea (4.57). Contraction and relaxation of the folds opens and closes the **rima glottidis** (often referred to just as the "glottis"). The air moving between the paired folds causes vibrations of the folds, resulting in the production of sound. The quality and pitch of the sound are adjusted by muscles that control the degree of closure and delicate movement of the folds.

Laryngitis, or inflammation of the larynx, can result from a common cold and cause someone to temporarily lose their voice. Although we have all experienced this temporary annoyance, for individuals such as performers, teachers, and public speakers, overtaxing the voice may result in chronic impairment and impact their role as a professional.

Certain cognitive or physical impairments affect the expression and understanding of communication. **Aphasia** refers to loss of ability to understand or express speech, generally referred to as **receptive** or **expressive aphasia**, respectively. For example, **Wernicke's aphasia** is loss of ability to understand spoken words, and **Broca's aphasia** is loss of ability to produce language (spoken or

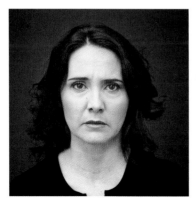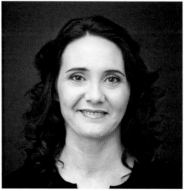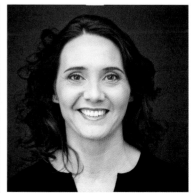

4.56 Nonverbal communication. How do facial expressions contribute to therapeutic use of self? What might each of these facial expressions communicate to a patient?

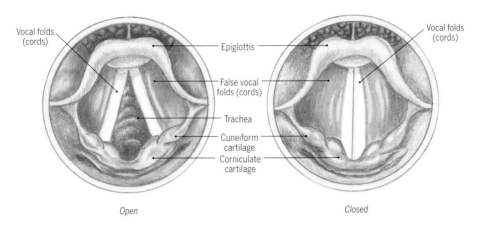

Vocal folds (cords)
Epiglottis
Vocal folds (cords)
False vocal folds (cords)
Trachea
Cuneiform cartilage
Corniculate cartilage

Open   *Closed*

4.57 Open and closed position of vocal folds. How do the vocal folds shape the pitch and volume of voice? What occupations might contribute to overuse of the vocal folds?

written). **Dysarthria** refers to any speech disorder caused by muscle weakness and can result from a neurological injury or general weakness of the face, tongue, or throat.

Occupational therapists and speech-language pathologists (SLPs) address these communication disorders by strengthening the muscles involved or working on adaptive ways to communicate, such as writing or using a communication board with various illustrations and letters (**4.58**).

Feeding, Eating, and Swallowing

The *Occupational Therapy Practice Framework*, fourth edition (OTPF-4) outlines feeding, eating, and swallowing within the scope of professional practice. Often referred to as self-feeding, this universal ADL involves moving food or drink to the mouth. It requires postural control as well as visual-motor integration, or the coordination of functional motor movements based on visual input. Eating involves keeping and manipulating food or fluid in the mouth. These are skills that occupational therapists are uniquely qualified to address, developing the necessary motor control or suggesting adaptive solutions.

Deglutition is the scientific term referring to moving food from the mouth to the stomach, or swallowing. When you are communicating informally with a patient, the terms *swallowing* and *feeding* will be more familiar. Deglutition is a patterned response involving both voluntary oral motor control and reflexive muscle actions coordinated between the mouth and throat.

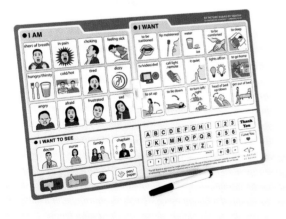

4.58 Communication board. How could this communication device offer an adaptive way of communicating for an individual who is nonverbal (cannot speak)?

CHARITY ROSE | After Charity's ER visit, she was referred to a neurologist who diagnosed her with **Bell's palsy**, or paralysis of the facial nerve. Charity is relieved to find her symptoms are not related to a stroke or other brain injury but is still concerned about how this diagnosis will affect her life. Do some research on this diagnosis and think about the following questions:

- What causes Bell's palsy?
- What is the prognosis for an individual diagnosed with Bell's palsy?
- How might this diagnosis impact Charity's occupational performance? Consider her motor, processing, and social interaction performance skills.

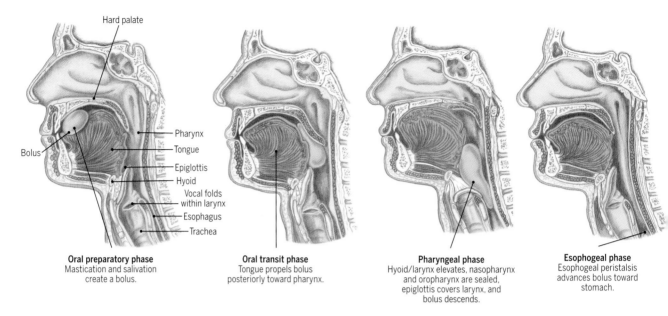

Oral preparatory phase
Mastication and salivation create a bolus.

Oral transit phase
Tongue propels bolus posteriorly toward pharynx.

Pharyngeal phase
Hyoid/larynx elevates, nasopharynx and oropharynx are sealed, epiglottis covers larynx, and bolus descends.

Esophogeal phase
Esophogeal peristalsis advances bolus toward stomach.

4.59 The phases of swallowing. How might occupational therapy practitioners and speech-language pathologists address issues with self-feeding and swallowing?

Self-feeding is initiated by bringing food or drink to the mouth. Once the food or drink enters the mouth, swallowing (deglutition) occurs in four distinct phases (**4.59**).[2]

1. The **oral preparatory phase** begins as food is mixed with saliva, if needed, and undergoes mastication (chewing and grinding) by the teeth to form a manageable bolus. This complex process involves precise timing, sensory recognition, and voluntary muscle control of the head and neck. Activation of the masseter provides the forceful elevation and deviation of the mandible for chewing food to form the bolus. The buccinator contracts to narrow the cheeks. The tongue moves from side to side, called **tongue lateralization**, to prevent food particles from being trapped below the gumline and direct the bolus toward the back of the oral cavity.

2. In the **oral transit phase**, the tongue propels the bolus posteriorly toward the pharynx—the final voluntary action of swallowing.

3. The **pharyngeal phase** begins with the formed bolus passing into the oropharynx. There, sensory receptors trigger a pattern of reflexes to ensure the bolus bypasses the nasopharynx and larynx to enter the esophagus. The soft palate elevates and tightens, sealing the nasopharynx, while the tongue thrusts posteriorly along the roof of the mouth to seal the oropharynx. The suprahyoid muscles reflexively contract to elevate the larynx, forcing it to open against the epiglottis, which tilts downward to prevent food and liquid from entering the airway. The vocal folds close to seal the airway as an additional protective measure, momentarily preventing breathing. As these passageways close, the pharyngeal muscles work in tandem to advance the bolus. The inner longitudinal muscles contract to shorten and widen the pharynx, while the outer constrictor muscles contract to propel the bolus downward, facilitated by gravity, toward the esophagus.

4. In the **esophageal phase**, esophageal peristalsis advances the bolus into the stomach to continue the digestive process.

Self-feeding is facilitated by visual-motor integration of the upper extremity and hand as well as an upright posture. Have you ever tried to swallow a drink while lying in bed? While it is possible, it is not easy, as optimal swallowing requires elevation of the upper body with a neutral head and neck. This position better aligns the pharynx and esophagus and enhances the effect of gravity to direct food to the stomach.

Dysphagia describes any impairment in swallowing and may involve either voluntary or involuntary mechanisms. Optimal self-feeding and swallowing require postural support with a neutral head and neck. Implementing adaptive seating systems for infants or individuals with low core muscle tone may improve trunk stability and swallowing.

Neuromuscular impairment may also limit visual-motor integration or functional grip, impairing a patient's ability to use their hand to bring food to their mouth. For conditions where the motor impairment is long-term, an adaptive or compensatory approach can help with function. For example, built-up grips on eating utensils or a universal cuff may compensate for the loss of grasp (**4.60**).

Beyond these voluntary contributions to swallowing, the reflexive pattern may also be impaired by general weakness or specific pathologies. When the precise biomechanics of reflexive swallowing are interrupted, **aspiration** can occur, with food or liquid descending beneath the vocal folds and potentially entering the trachea (windpipe).

Complete occlusion (blocking) of the trachea by a larger food particle or object is an emergency situation and may require the **Heimlich maneuver** to clear the life-threatening object from the windpipe and restore respiration.

Aspiration can also be insidious or silent, with small amounts of liquid entering the trachea and collecting in the lungs, increasing the risk of pneumonia and infection. Accurately diagnosing this type of aspiration may involve a **modified barium swallow study**, or radiologic imaging to examine the physiology of the swallow and identify aspiration (**4.61**).

Modified diets can increase thickness of foods and liquids, decreasing viscosity and the likelihood of aspiration. Other interventions target dysphagia to improve the pattern of swallowing.

Generalist occupational therapists are qualified to address postural and neuromuscular components of feeding, eating, and swallowing and, depending on the specific state practice act, may complete swallow studies. SLPs are qualified to address swallowing issues, and an interdisciplinary approach is recommended for best patient outcomes.

Toileting is also a necessary ADL involving functional mobility and underlying strength, coordination, and balance. Often the first step to safe toileting is navigating a potentially slippery bathroom floor under the duress of bowel or bladder distension. The Centers for Disease Control and Prevention (CDC) estimates more than 230,000 nonfatal bathroom injuries annually, with more than 14 percent occurring as a result of standing up, sitting down, or while sitting on the toilet.[3] Many of these injuries occur as a result of falls among the older adult population, who often have additional risk factors such as visual impairment, generalized weakness, or peripheral neuropathies.

Occupational therapy intervention might involve evaluating and modifying the bathroom environment. Additional lighting, grab bars, or an elevated toilet seat can help facilitate safe mobility and transfers (**4.62**).

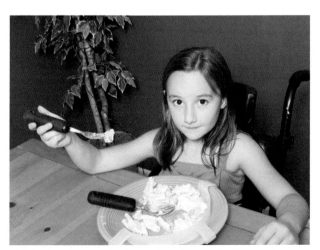

4.60 Adaptive utensils. How might these adaptive devices support independent self-feeding?

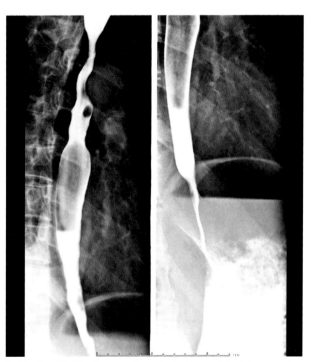

4.61 Modified barium swallow study. How might this type of study help to identify swallowing dysfunction?

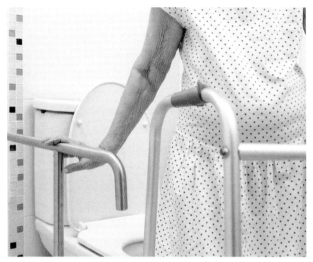

4.62 Toileting and transfer safety. How might grab bars improve safety with toileting and transfers? Would you recommend any other adaptations?

If possible, placing the toilet paper on the same side as the patient's dominant hand prevents the need to reach across and rotate the trunk when wiping, further enhancing safety.

Other pathologies impairing digestive function of the intestines, bowel, or bladder may require a colostomy bag or catheterization for safe elimination of waste. For example, an individual with a complete spinal cord injury relies on reflexive emptying of the bowels and bladder and might require long-term catheterization or a bowel program involving rectal stimulation. Additionally, prostate cancer and treatment may require use of a colostomy bag to empty the bowels and require training for use and sanitation.

The long-term impacts of meeting these needs can profoundly affect an individual's self-image, self-esteem, and general quality of life. Collaborative trust between the patient and therapist is essential to find solutions to promote occupational performance, self-efficacy, and dignity.

Vision

Visual input is a primary component of many ADLs and IADLs. Consider driving as an occupation with significant visual demands, such as scanning the horizon, interpreting the colors of a traffic light, or checking mirrors before changing lanes. While the loss of tactile sensation may restrict functional use of the hands, incomplete or inaccurate visual information can be life-threatening behind the wheel of a vehicle.

The fast-twitch extraocular muscles provide linear and rotary motion of the eyeball, allowing for scanning of the visual field and static fixation on stimuli. The **optokinetic reflex** stabilizes the visual field as the head moves through the surrounding environment. Symmetrical cooperation of the eye muscles is necessary for coordinated, simultaneous movements, producing complementary images from the right and left visual fields.

Unilateral weakness or paralysis can lead to **diplopia** (double vision), limiting the ability of the eyes to scan the visual field. Additionally, lesions affecting the optic nerve or cortical (occipital cortex) areas of visual processing will present with a somewhat predictable visual field loss.

Ptosis refers to drooping of the eyelid and may result from weakness of the levator palpebrae, a common symptom of oculomotor nerve impairment. The eyelids and surrounding fascia and muscles of the eye also begin to sag with age, occluding vision from the superior aspect of the eye.

There are also several predictable patterns of visual loss associated with lesions of the optic nerve. A complete lesion of the optic nerve anterior to the **optic chiasm** leads to complete ipsilateral (same-side) field loss. Lesions at the optic chiasm cause **bitemporal** deficits, or loss of peripheral vision on both sides (**4.63**).

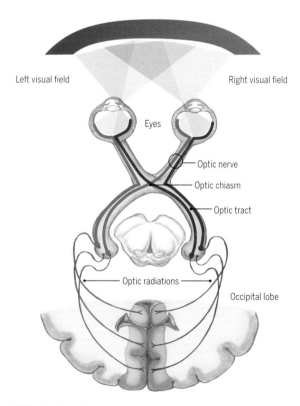

4.63 Visual pathway. How would a lesion at a specific portion of the visual pathway affect the visual field? How would these various visual deficits impact occupational performance?

Any lesions posterior to the optic chiasm or in the occipital lobe of the brain contribute to partial or full **homonymous hemianopsia**, loss of vision on the same side of each visual field, as some nerve fibers cross over to the opposite eye.

Pathologies that affect visual input have a profound impact on performance of ADLs and IADLs, as occupational performance relies heavily on visual-motor integration. This topic is broad and extends well beyond our discussion in this chapter. Here we are focused on a foundation for the underlying functional anatomy.

Individuals with visual field loss may benefit from cueing to scan the environment or from specialized prism glasses to "fill in" the missing visual field. Total visual loss may require use of other senses to compensate, such as the use of tactile sensation for reading (Braille).

As you can see, the underlying anatomy of the head and neck is complex, and its contribution to occupational performance is broad. For a generalist practitioner, understanding the foundational anatomy and its function is important. There are also several areas of advanced practice, such as low vision, feeding and swallowing, and vestibular rehabilitation, requiring significant additional specialty training and experience. Regardless of practice setting or population, an understanding of the unique structures and functions of the head and neck is necessary for a holistic approach to assessment and promotion of occupational performance.

APPLY AND REVIEW

Charity Rose

It has been several months since Charity's symptoms began, and she has noticed some improvement. The left side of her face is still weak, affecting her facial expressions, eating, and speech. The symptoms are distracting, and she feels self-conscious with social interaction.

Her physician told her to be patient as it might be quite a while before her symptoms resolve, if they resolve at all. The physician also offered to write a referral to occupational therapy.

Consider the following questions in relation to Charity and her diagnosis:

- How might occupational therapy address specific motor, processing, and social interaction performance skills?
- Do some research on interventions for Bell's palsy. What interventions does the evidence support as beneficial?

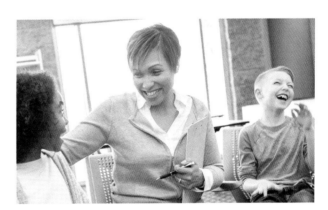

- What specific muscle groups should be targeted, or what activities should be implemented, to improve her speech, eating, and communication?
- Think about other client factors, such as emotional and psychosocial well-being or experience of self. How might an OT address these areas when working with Charity?

Review Questions

1. What term refers to the introduction of a solid or liquid into the trachea (windpipe)?
   a. aspiration
   b. aphasia
   c. reflux
   d. apraxia

2. Which of the following muscles is *not* a muscle of mastication?
   a. temporalis
   b. pterygoids
   c. orbicularis oculi
   d. masseter

3. What structure covers the trachea during swallowing to prevent food from entering?
   a. vocal folds
   b. uvula
   c. pharynx
   d. epiglottis

4. What condition, depending on its severity, can prevent sealing of the oral and nasal cavities during swallowing?
   a. aspiration
   b. cleft palate
   c. agnosia
   d. aphasia

5. What is the only synovial joint in the face and is essential for eating and speech?
   a. nasopharyngeal joint
   b. temporomandibular joint
   c. atlantooccipital joint
   d. zygapophyseal joint

6. Which of the following muscles does *not* directly attach to or move the eyeball?
   a. lateral rectus
   b. superior oblique
   c. medial rectus
   d. orbicularis oculi

7. A unilateral (on one side) lesion of the occipital lobe, posterior to the optic chiasm, contributes to which of the following visual field deficits?
   a. bitemporal visual loss
   b. homonymous hemianopsia
   c. loss of the entire right or left visual field
   d. loss of the entire visual field

8. Which muscle facilitates eating by narrowing the oral cavity and preventing food particles from descending below the gumline?
   a. masseter
   b. temporalis
   c. orbicularis oris
   d. buccinator

9. Which of the following marks the beginning of the involuntary phase of swallowing?
   a. oral preparatory phase
   b. oral transit phase
   c. pharyngeal phase
   d. esophageal phase

10. Which of the following may be the *best* adaptive way of communication for an individual with Broca's aphasia?
    a. speaking slowly and asking "yes" or "no" questions
    b. writing out words
    c. speaking louder
    d. pointing

See Answer Key in back of book.

Notes

1. Centers for Disease Control and Prevention, "Facts about Cleft Lip and Cleft Palate," Birth Defects, last reviewed December 5, 2019, https://www.cdc.gov/ncbddd/birthdefects/cleftlip.html.

2. American Speech-Language-Hearing Association, "Pediatric Dysphagia," The Practice Portal, accessed February 8, 2020, https://www.asha.org/Practice-Portal/Clinical-Topics/Pediatric-Dysphagia/.

3. Centers for Disease Control and Prevention, "Nonfatal Bathroom Injuries Among Persons Aged ≥15 Years—United States, 2008," *Morbidity and Mortality Weekly Report* 60, no. 22 (June 10, 2011): 729–33, https://www.jstor.org/stable/i23320723.

Bibliography

American Occupational Therapy Association. *Occupational Therapy Practice Framework: Domain and Process*. 4th ed. Bethesda, MD: AOTA Press, 2020.

American Speech-Language-Hearing Association. "Pediatric Dysphagia." The Practice Portal. Accessed February 8, 2020. https://www.asha.org/Practice-Portal/Clinical-Topics/Pediatric-Dysphagia/.

Biel, Andrew. *Trail Guide to Movement: Building the Body in Motion*. 2nd ed. Boulder, CO: Books of Discovery, 2019.

Biel, Andrew. *Trail Guide to the Body: A Hands-On Guide to Locating Muscles, Bones, and More*. 6th ed. Boulder, CO: Books of Discovery, 2019.

Centers for Disease Control and Prevention. "Facts about Cleft Lip and Cleft Palate." Birth Defects. Last reviewed December 5, 2019. https://www.cdc.gov/ncbddd/birthdefects/cleftlip.html.

Centers for Disease Control and Prevention. "Nonfatal Bathroom Injuries Among Persons Aged ≥15 Years—United States, 2008." *Morbidity and Mortality Weekly Report* 60, no. 22 (June 10, 2011): 729–33. https://www.jstor.org/stable/23320725.

Keough, Jeremy L., Susan J. Sain, and Carolyn L. Roller. *Kinesiology for the Occupational Therapy Assistant: Essential Components of Function and Movement*. 2nd ed. Thorofare, NJ: SLACK, 2017.

Lundy-Ekman, Laurie. *Neuroscience: Fundamentals for Rehabilitation*. 5th ed. St. Louis, MO: Elsevier, 2018.

Marcus, Sherna, and Suzanne Breton. *Infant and Child Feeding and Swallowing: Occupational Therapy Assessment and Intervention*. Bethesda, MD: American Occupational Therapy Association, 2013.

Oatis, Carol A. *Kinesiology: The Mechanics and Pathomechanics of Human Movement*. 3rd ed. Philadelphia: Wolters Kluwer, 2017.

Pendleton, Heidi McHugh, and Winifred Schultz-Krohn. *Pedretti's Occupational Therapy: Practice Skills for Physical Dysfunction*. 8th ed. St. Louis, MO: Elsevier, 2017.

Standring, Susan. *Gray's Anatomy: The Anatomical Basis of Clinical Practice, International Edition*. 41st ed. Cambridge, UK: Elsevier, 2016.

PART III

Upper Extremity

CHAPTER 5

Shoulder

Learning Objectives

- Describe the bones, joints, and muscles contributing to purposeful movement of the shoulder complex.

- Identify the primary purposeful movements of the shoulder within the context of occupational performance.

- Develop competency in goniometry and manual muscle testing (MMT) as clinical assessment techniques for the shoulder.

- Use clinical reasoning to identify limitations of the shoulder that may affect occupational performance.

Key Concepts

adhesive capsulitis

bicipital tendinitis

dynamic stability

fall on outstretched hands (FOOSH)

glenohumeral subluxation

hemiparesis

rotator cuff

scaption

scapular dyskinesis

scapular plane

scapular winging

scapulohumeral rhythm

shoulder separation

static stability

subacromial impingement

thoracic outlet syndrome (TOS)

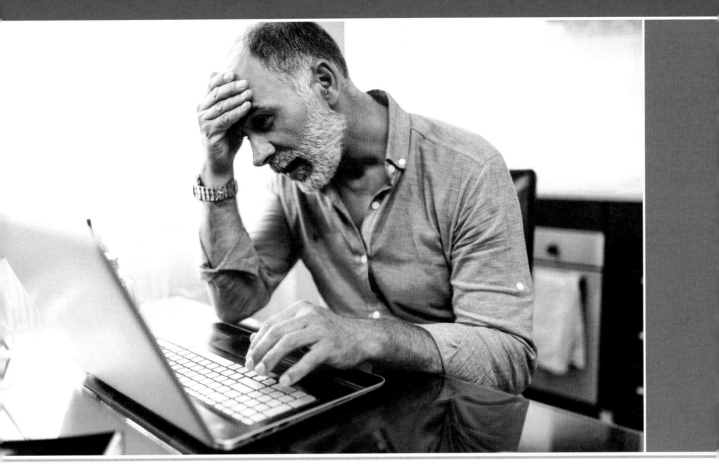

 Occupational Profile: Taylor Schultz

TAYLOR SCHULTZ is a fifty-six-year-old account executive with a commercial insurance company. He spends the majority of his day, sometimes eight to ten hours, at his computer workstation. Recently, he began experiencing pain in his dominant (right) shoulder, particularly with overhead motion. He does not recall a specific injury, just gradually increasing pain.

The symptoms are now affecting his golf game—his primary leisure occupation—and, more importantly, the way he spends time with his teenage son. Additionally, he is having trouble with upper body dressing and showering. He has also noticed an impact on his job performance. The pain is keeping him from sleeping at night, and he feels less productive and has lower energy levels. He has an annual report due next month, and his supervisor has been putting pressure on him to complete it.

Fortunately, Taylor's primary care physician (PCP) has referred him to occupational therapy in an outpatient setting—your office. Before he comes into the clinic, let's take a look at the underlying anatomy of the shoulder.

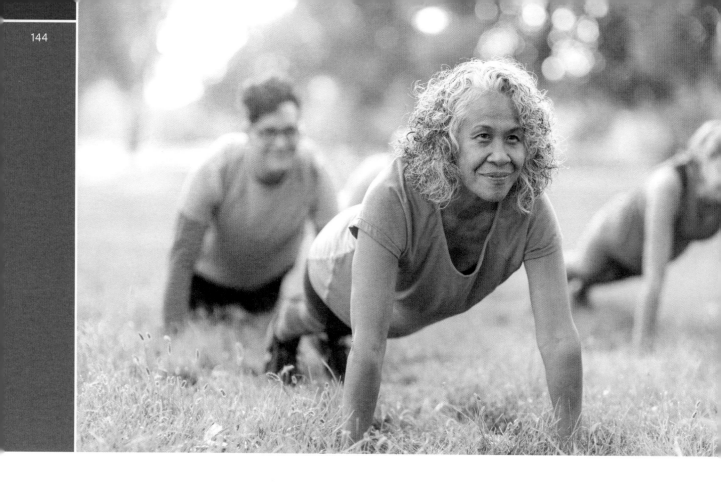

The Shoulder: A Functional Link

When you want to relax and unwind after a stressful week, what is your favorite leisure occupation? Do you enjoy yoga, biking, or kayaking? Or maybe you prefer an artistic pursuit like playing an instrument or painting?

Consider the position and movement of your upper limb for these activities. For your hand to manipulate objects as a component of occupational performance, you must move and stabilize it in the appropriate position. What provides this gross positioning and stability? The answer is your shoulder.

TAYLOR SCHULTZ | As we follow Taylor throughout this chapter, think about what factors may be affecting his occupational performance. (You might find it helpful to refer to the *Occupational Therapy Practice Framework*, fourth edition [OTPF-4] as you go.[1]) Consider using the **Person-Environment-Occupation (PEO) Model** to identify the relationships between Taylor, his environment, and specific occupations.

Keeping Taylor's occupational profile in mind, let's explore the osteology (bones) of the shoulder.

Similar to how an artist's hand stabilizes a paintbrush from above to depict minute detail in the painting below, the shoulder aligns and positions the hand in space for precise object manipulation. It is a primary component of reaching, such as when showering, lifting, or completing personal hygiene. The shoulder is the functional connection between the trunk and upper extremity (limb), providing gross motion and stability to position the arm for occupational performance.

For practitioners, understanding the broader role of the shoulder complex in occupational performance starts with learning its underlying anatomy. This chapter describes the functional anatomy of the entire shoulder complex, which includes several bones and joints. Using the digital palpation resources will help you better understand these skeletal structures. After examining muscles and joint motions, we will practice goniometry and manual muscle testing (MMT) using the *OT Guide to Goniometry & MMT* eTextbook. Think about how the application of the functional anatomy of this region relates to the case study of Taylor Schultz.

Osteology: Bones of the Shoulder Complex

The scapula, humerus, and clavicle supply the skeletal structure for movement of the shoulder complex related to occupational performance (**5.1**). Motion in this region is complex. Identifying and palpating bony landmarks will lay the foundation for understanding the muscle attachments and movements presented later in the chapter.

Scapula

The **scapula** is a flat triangular bone located on the back, overlying the second through seventh ribs. It is part of the shoulder joint complex, also known as the shoulder girdle (**5.2**).

Featuring three borders and three angles, the scapula provides attachment points for numerous muscles, including muscles that stabilize the scapula against the rib cage and those that supply dynamic stability for humeral motion at the glenohumeral joint (see **5.1**).

Bony Landmarks of the Scapula

The scapula features many bony landmarks that are clinically useful and are often easy to palpate just beneath the skin. The **medial (vertebral) border** of the scapula is parallel to the vertebral column (**5.3**). This is the longest border of the scapula and serves as an anchor for muscles that rotate, adduct, and abduct the scapula.

The thick inferolateral border of the scapula is the **lateral (axillary) border**. The **superior border** refers to the superior edge of the scapula. This border provides an attachment site for muscles that elevate and upwardly rotate the scapula.

At the lateral end of the superior border is a deep semicircular notch called the **suprascapular (superior) notch**. The **superior angle** is at the junction of the vertebral and superior borders. The **inferior angle** is at the junction of the vertebral and axillary borders.

The junction of the superior and lateral borders forms the **lateral angle**. This angle includes the **glenoid fossa (cavity)**, a shallow socket that, with the head of

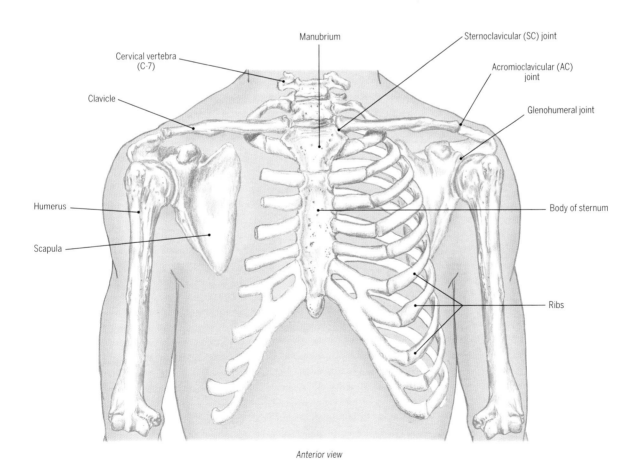

Anterior view

5.1 Bones of the shoulder and arm with ribs removed on the right side

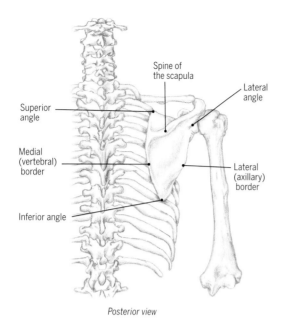

Posterior view

5.2 Posterior aspect of the scapula positioned on the rib cage

the humerus, forms the bony components of the glenohumeral joint.

The **infraglenoid tubercle** and **supraglenoid tubercle** are on the bottom and top of the glenoid fossa. They serve as attachment sites for the major flexor and extensor muscles of the elbow (long heads of biceps and triceps).

Immediately medial to the glenoid fossa, along the top of the bone, arises the **coracoid process (5.4)**.

CLINICAL APPLICATION
Manual Scapular Mobilization

The borders and many of the bony landmarks of the scapula are easily palpated just beneath the skin and superficial trapezius muscles. Palpation and manual mobilization of the scapula are often used in assessment and intervention because scapular mobility is vital to overall upper extremity motion and occupational performance.

For instance, an individual who has had a CVA (stroke) may experience generalized weakness of the scapular muscles. As a clinician, you might need to facilitate overhead motion by using passive assistance.

Or, after a period of immobilization due to an injury, the muscles surrounding the scapula may demonstrate adaptive shortening and tightness due to lack of elongation. Manual (passive) mobilization of the scapula can help to restore scapular mobility as a component of functional scapulohumeral rhythm (presented in detail later in this chapter). In what direction would you passively (manually) mobilize the scapula to facilitate overhead motion of the shoulder?

This process serves as an anterior attachment site for muscles and ligaments that are critical to maintaining the bony connection between the clavicle and the acromion (AC joint).

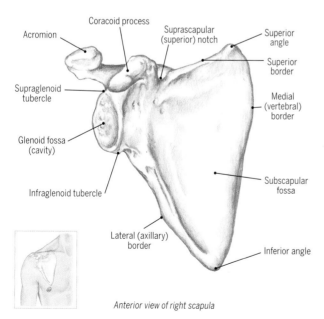

Anterior view of right scapula

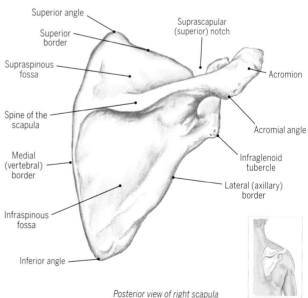

Posterior view of right scapula

5.3 Bony landmarks of the scapula

The scapula has two major projections: the spine and the crest. The spine projects from the posterior aspect of the bone along a line extending from the vertebral border almost to the glenoid fossa. The crest of the spine extends laterally beyond the body of the spine as the large **acromion**, which overlies the glenoid fossa (**5.5**). Muscles that attach to the scapula are often named relative to its bony landmarks. For example, the supraspinatus lies *above the spine* of the scapula while the infraspinatus lies *below the spine*.

The scapula serves to position the glenoid fossa for humeral motion. In the anatomical position, it is rotated forward, approximately 30°–40° anterior to the frontal plane, referred to as the **scapular plane**. Movement in this plane, midway between the sagittal and frontal planes, is called **scaption**. Scaption is a more natural movement than purely flexion or abduction. It also positions the arms and hands in front of the body, where function typically occurs.

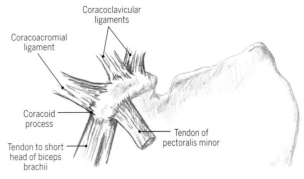

Anterior view of right scapula

5.4 Coracoid process

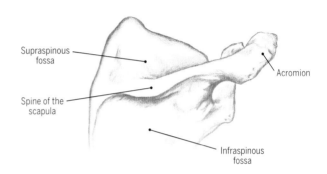

5.5 Spine and acromion of scapula

CLINICAL APPLICATION
Scapular Plane (Scaption)

Rarely do we go about our day moving our arms in single planes of flexion (sagittal) or abduction (frontal). When we interact with our surrounding environment or lift and carry objects in front of our bodies, the humerus generally elevates, aligned with the scapula, at some point between these two planes.

The scapular plane is often more comfortable for patients when they are performing overhead activities or receiving passive range of motion (PROM) as an intervention to support occupational performance. For example, postoperative shoulder conditions such as rotator cuff repair (discussed later in this chapter) often involve PROM to maintain joint mobility with the patient lying supine (on their back). Placing a pillow or towel roll beneath the scapula supports the shoulder in the scapular plane, preventing undue strain to the anterior shoulder resting against the mat (**5.6**). The patient should be more comfortable in this position and may tolerate passive motion with less pain.

This principle also applies to individuals after neurological injuries like a stroke with hemiparesis (weakness) of the upper extremity. A lap pillow or tray table placed under the forearm may support the shoulder complex in its natural resting position (scaption) when sitting up. Pillows or towel rolls may be appropriate when sleeping in supine or side lying.

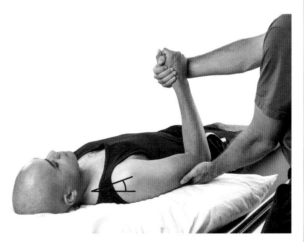

5.6 Scapula supported in the scapular plane for passive range of motion of the shoulder

▶TRY IT

To illustrate functional movement in the scapular plane, raise your arm overhead as if giving someone a high five. Now, note the position of the humerus. Is it in flexion (sagittal plane) or abduction (frontal plane)? Likely it is midway between in the scapular plane.

Put yourself in a future patient's shoes: You just had a painful shoulder surgery a few days ago and are coming to your first OT appointment. Lie in supine on the floor, a mat, or your bed with your posterior shoulder flat against the surface. Do you feel the strain in the muscles of the anterior shoulder? Now place a small cushion or towel roll behind your shoulder while lying in supine. Do you notice the difference with your shoulder supported in the more natural scapular plane? Your patients will too!

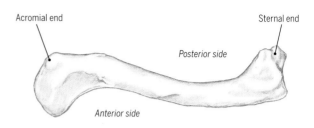

Superior view of right clavicle

Clavicle

The **clavicle** (collarbone) is S-shaped (**5.7**). Palpate your own clavicle and you can verify that the medial third is convex anteriorly, whereas the lateral third is concave anteriorly. Functionally, the clavicle acts as a longitudinal strut, linking the chest and upper arm and, along with the scapula, positioning the humerus laterally away from the upper body.

Bony Landmarks of the Clavicle

The medial (sternal) end of the clavicle has a flat surface (**5.7**). This surface articulates with a fibrocartilaginous disc between the clavicle and the **manubrium**, the upper part of the sternum (**5.8**). The medial end of the clavicle is much larger than the articular surface on the manubrium, so it extends considerably higher than the upper edge of the manubrium, deepening the jugular notch.

The lateral portion of the clavicle is flattened from top to bottom. It presents an ovoid, or egg-shaped, surface for articulation with the medial border of the acromion.

Humerus

The **humerus**, the connection between the trunk and forearm, has a long, slender shaft that expands at each end (**5.9**). The proximal end of the humerus consists of a nearly hemispherical head that articulates with the glenoid fossa of the scapula.

Bony Landmarks of the Humerus

Opposite to the humeral head, the lateral aspect of the proximal humerus has a prominence, the **greater**

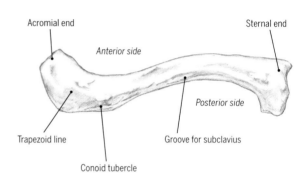

Inferior view of right clavicle

5.7 Clavicle

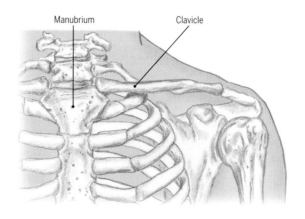

5.8 Manubrium and clavicle

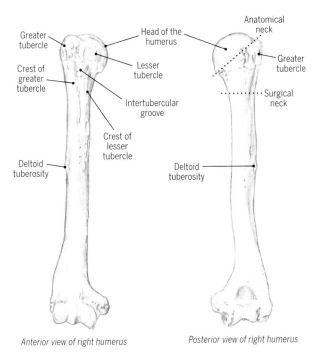

Greater tubercle · Head of the humerus · Anatomical neck · Lesser tubercle · Greater tubercle · Crest of greater tubercle · Intertubercular groove · Surgical neck · Crest of lesser tubercle · Deltoid tuberosity · Deltoid tuberosity

Anterior view of right humerus   *Posterior view of right humerus*

5.9 Humerus

tubercle. Here also is the anteriorly located **lesser tubercle** (**5.9**). The groove between the head and the tubercles is a part of the **anatomical neck**.

Between the lesser and greater tubercles is a narrow **intertubercular groove** (**5.11**). A transverse humeral ligament, running from one tubercle to the other, converts this groove into a tunnel. Traversing through this tunnel is the long head of the biceps brachii tendon, which arises from the superior aspect of the glenoid fossa and its fibrous outer rim, the **glenoid labrum**. (We will revisit this labrum when we discuss joints.)

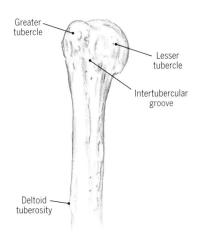

Greater tubercle · Lesser tubercle · Intertubercular groove · Deltoid tuberosity

5.11 Intertubercular groove and deltoid tuberosity

 CLINICAL APPLICATION
What Is the Surgical Neck?

The anatomical neck is distinguished from the **surgical neck**, the region of the shaft immediately below the head and tubercles where the humerus begins to narrow. The surgical neck is named as such because it is much more susceptible to fracture.

In young adults, surgical neck fractures may occur as a result of a high-impact athletic injury. For older adults, the cause is often a fall. Nondisplaced fractures may heal with immobilization, whereas more complex or displaced fractures may require surgical fixation (**5.10**).

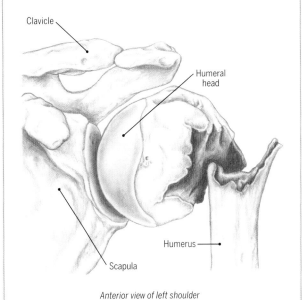

Clavicle · Humeral head · Humerus · Scapula

Anterior view of left shoulder

5.10 Fracture of the proximal humerus. Why would the surgical neck of the humerus be more susceptible to fracture?

At about midshaft laterally, there is a rough area of bone called the **deltoid tuberosity**, which marks the site of insertion of the deltoid muscle. Posterior to the deltoid tuberosity is a shallow depression in the humeral shaft, the radial groove, which creates a pathway for the radial nerve as it wraps around the humerus (see Figure **6.24** in Chapter 6). Because the radial nerve lies against the bone at this site, a midhumeral fracture may damage this nerve. This can result in a condition known as wrist-drop, with paralysis of the radially innervated wrist, thumb, and digital extensor muscles (see Chapter 7).

CLINICAL APPLICATION
Humeral Fractures

Certain types of injuries are more likely to fracture specific parts of the humerus. Geographical location also plays a part: in certain parts of the country you may see humeral fractures from skiing or bull-riding injuries. (As a clinician in New Mexico, the author worked with someone who had a completely displaced midshaft humerus fracture from a bull-riding injury that went untreated for five years.)

A **fall-on-outstretched-hands (FOOSH)** injury may result in a proximal humerus fracture as force is transferred upward through the extended elbow. High-impact force applied directly to the humerus, such as in a motor vehicle accident (MVA), is more likely to cause a midshaft or distal humerus fracture.

The radial nerve is susceptible to injury with a midshaft fracture, as the nerve wraps around the midshaft of the humerus (see Figure **6.24** in Chapter 6). What specific motor or sensory deficits might indicate an injury to the radial nerve? (You might want to refer to Chapter 2.)

TAYLOR SCHULTZ | Before we discuss the joints of the shoulder complex, let's consider Taylor. Look at the photo of Taylor at work.

- Describe the posture of his upper body as he sits at his desk.
- Note that the shoulder functions best with the trunk upright (straight) and scapulae stabilized against the rib cage in a neutral position (not tilting forward). How are Taylor's scapulae positioned? What impact might this have on the orientation of the glenoid fossa?

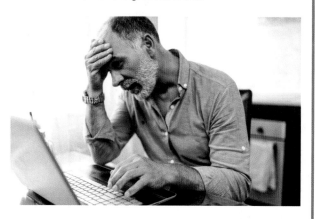

Joints

The shoulder complex is formed by the scapulothoracic (ST), sternoclavicular (SC), acromioclavicular (AC), and glenohumeral joints (**5.12**). Together they provide integrated, interdependent movement of the scapula, clavicle, and humerus. Before we examine the muscles that generate the forces of motion within the shoulder complex, let's discuss the structure and function of each joint.

Scapulothoracic Joint

Structural/functional classification: atypical
Movements:
- *Gliding:* elevation, depression, abduction, adduction
- *Rotation:* internal, external, upward, downward
- *Tilt:* anterior, posterior

The **scapulothoracic (ST) joint** is not a typical synovial joint because there is no direct connection between the bones of the rib cage and scapula (**5.12**). Rather, the rib cage and anterior surface of the scapula are separated by muscle tissue—specifically the subscapularis and serratus anterior muscles. Many other muscles attach to its dorsal surface and borders, allowing the scapula to translate (glide), rotate, and tilt relative to the rib cage (**5.13**).

These motions of the scapula position the glenoid fossa to facilitate motion of the glenohumeral joint. For example, overhead flexion of the humerus at the glenohumeral joint, as when casting a fishing line, requires upward rotation of the scapula.

Often, combinations of scapular motions serve as the foundation of the kinetic chain of upper extremity motion. Many functional activities involve a combination of scapular movements. For example, scapular retraction, as when pulling a door open, is a combination of scapular adduction and posterior tilt.

The pattern of movement between the scapula and humerus, called *scapulohumeral rhythm*, is described later in this chapter.

Get in the habit of analyzing scapular movement while completing your ADLs and IADLs and observing the functional activities of others. Your ability to visualize and understand the contribution of the scapula to purposeful activity of the upper extremity will better serve your future patients.

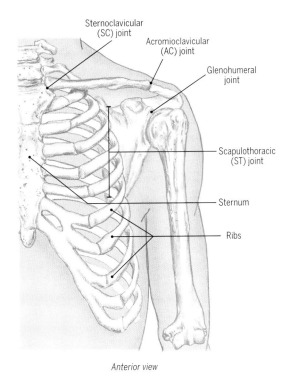

Anterior view

5.12 Joints of the shoulder and humerus

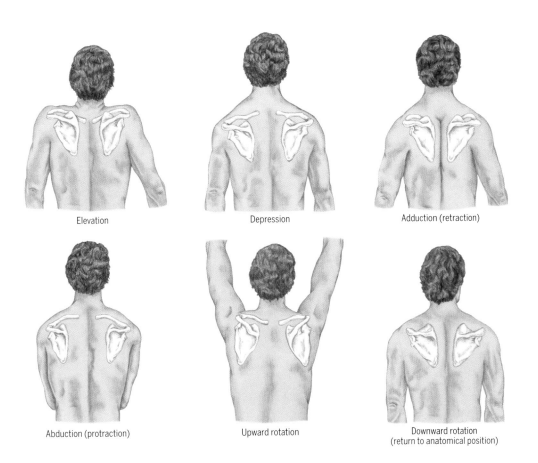

5.13 Scapulothoracic joint movements

▶TRY IT

To develop an appreciation of scapular motion as a component of upper extremity function, palpate the scapula on a partner while they simulate different functional movements.

You might palpate the superior aspect of the acromion or the spine of the scapula as a starting point. Have your partner simulate putting on a shirt overhead, rowing a boat, or throwing a baseball. What do you notice about the position and movement of the scapula?

Now have your partner reach into their back pocket or scratch their low back. How do the scapular movement and position change? Think about how these scapular movements position and facilitate purposeful movement of the humerus.

Sternoclavicular Joint

Structural classification: saddle or ball-and-socket
Functional (mechanical) classification: triaxial
Movements: elevation, depression, protraction, retraction, posterior rotation, anterior rotation

The **sternoclavicular (SC) joint** represents the only direct bony attachment of the shoulder complex to the axial skeleton. The bony parts of this joint are formed by the medial end of the clavicle and the superolateral corner of the manubrium (**5.14**).

The SC joint cooperates with the scapula as it translates and rotates to facilitate motion of the humerus. To conceptualize this pattern, think about cleaning a tall window with large upward and downward motions of the arm. As the humerus flexes, the scapula elevates and upwardly rotates, while the clavicle elevates and rotates posteriorly. When the humerus extends, moving the hand downward on the window, the scapula depresses and downwardly rotates, while the clavicle depresses and rotates anteriorly.

Mimic this window-washing motion and palpate near the middle of your clavicle. Can you feel the elevation and rotation that occur? Limitations in SC mobility will have an effect on ST mobility and overall shoulder function.

The SC joint contains a fibrocartilaginous articular disc that divides it into two separate synovial cavities. The disc acts as a ligament that prevents the clavicle from being driven medially and upward off the articular surface of the manubrium when large forces are exerted on the upper limb, as when falling on the lateral shoulder. This type of injury is common when falling sideways without your arms to cushion the fall, as when falling off a bicycle or during a contact sport.

In addition to the fibrous articular capsule, the SC joint has an **interclavicular ligament** between the clavicles (**5.14**). This ligament becomes tense when the lateral end of the clavicle is depressed, as when you are carrying a heavy object.

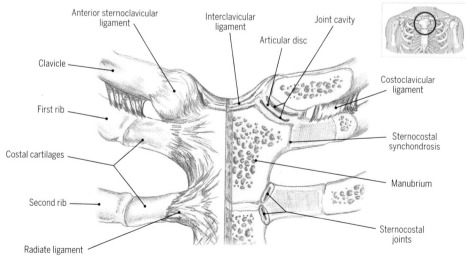

Anterior view of superior portion of sternum

5.14 Sternoclavicular joint

Acromioclavicular Joint

Structural classification: gliding

Functional (mechanical) classification: biaxial

Movements: anterior/posterior and superior/inferior
gliding

The **acromioclavicular (AC) joint** permits a small amount of motion, primarily anterior/posterior and superior/inferior translation between the acromion and clavicle (**5.15**).

These small gliding motions occur synchronously and in proportion to ST and SC movements, facilitating motion of the entire shoulder complex (**5.16**). For example, when putting dishes away in an overhead cabinet, the ST and SC joints upwardly rotate while the acromion glides superior relative to the clavicle.

There are two ligaments that are intrinsic to the scapula (connecting points within the scapula itself). The larger of these is the **coracoacromial ligament**, extending between the acromion and the coracoid process. Notice in Figure **5.15** that this ligament forms a roof over the proximal humerus, called the **coracoacromial arch**. A smaller **suprascapular ligament** bridges across the suprascapular notch, converting it into a foramen for the passage of the suprascapular nerve.

Also notice the incline between the lateral end of the clavicle and the acromion (**5.15**, **5.16**). This incline

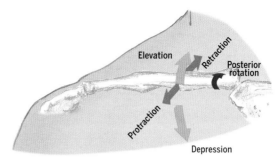

Anterior view of right clavicle

5.16 Motion of the acromioclavicular and sternoclavicular joints

makes the AC joint susceptible to dislocation with direct medial force. This type of AC dislocation is popularly called a **shoulder separation** and may occur as a result of a fall directly on the lateral shoulder. The clavicle typically migrates superiorly in relation to the acromion due to ligament laxity.

Clinically, if a dislocated clavicle is manually reduced (pressed) back to the acromion, it may elevate when released, similar to a piano key. Because the capsule of the AC joint is weak, it depends on the **coracoclavicular ligament** to prevent shoulder separation. These ligaments run from the crest of the coracoid process to the clavicle.

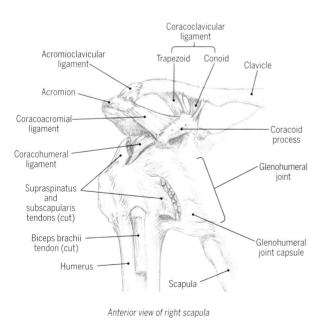

Anterior view of right scapula

5.15 Acromioclavicular joint

TAYLOR SCHULTZ | Look again at how Taylor is sitting at his desk.

- How are his ST, SC, and AC joints positioned?
- He mentioned difficulty with overhead dressing and showering. What purposeful movements are required at these joints to complete these essential ADLs?

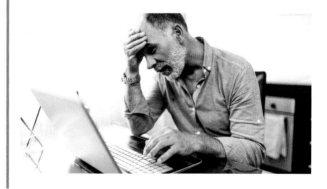

Glenohumeral (Shoulder) Joint

Structural classification: ball-and-socket
Functional (mechanical) classification: triaxial
Movements: flexion, extension, abduction (including horizontal abduction), adduction (including horizontal adduction), internal (medial) rotation, external (lateral) rotation

The **glenohumeral joint (GHJ)** is often the individual joint referred to as the shoulder, though the shoulder complex includes several joints. The GHJ is located between the glenoid fossa of the scapula and the head of the humerus (**5.17**).

The convex humeral head is much larger than the concave glenoid fossa, much like a golf ball on a tee (**5.18**). The shallowness of the glenoid fossa, coupled with the large hemisphere of the humeral head, affords great joint mobility: it can move in six directions around three axes.

However, this arrangement allows for minimal contact between the surfaces of the bones, which sacrifices bony congruity and joint stability. Without inherent joint stability from bony congruence, the surrounding muscles of the shoulder have to provide the stability needed for functional motion.

The glenoid fossa is slightly deepened by an attached fibrous rim, the **glenoid labrum**, which increases joint surface contact and stability (**5.19**).

The posterior part of this labrum is continuous with the tendon of the long head of the biceps brachii

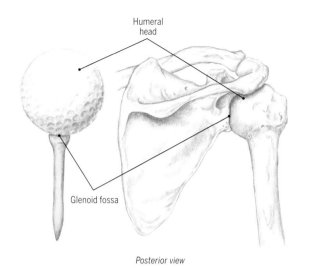

Posterior view

5.18 Humeral head and glenoid fossa

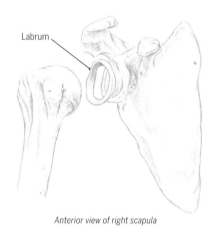

Anterior view of right scapula

5.19 Glenoid labrum at the glenohumeral joint (shown separated)

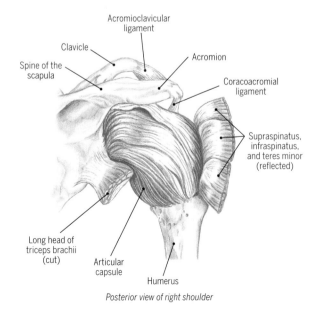

Posterior view of right shoulder

5.17 Glenohumeral joint capsule

(biceps anchor). The anterior part is continuous with the thickened regions of the joint capsule called the **glenohumeral ligaments** (**5.20**). If the humerus is dislocated, the labrum is often damaged as a result, with significant impairment to joint stability.

When the arm is in neutral position at the side of the body, the inferior portion of the GHJ capsule is lax (loose). This allows the capsule to expand with humeral elevation. **Adhesive capsulitis**, or frozen shoulder, is a pathology that involves thickening and tightness of the GHJ capsule, significantly limiting mobility and function.

Combined abduction and external rotation increase the tension on the supporting capsule and ligaments, contributing to a close-pack position. Functionally, this position is involved with washing your hair or winding up to throw a ball. The open-pack position is 40°–50°

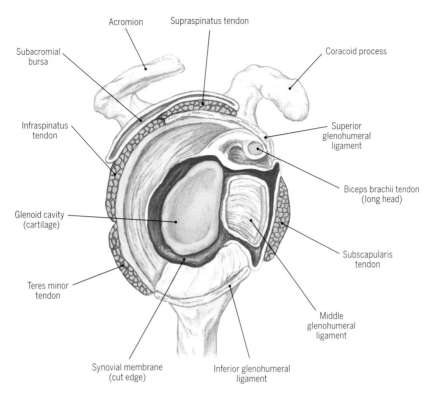

Lateral view of right shoulder, joint opened and humerus removed

5.20 Glenoid fossa and surrounding soft tissues

abduction with 30° horizontal adduction, as when reaching for a seat belt.

Because of the structural instability of the shoulder joint, it can dislocate. Thus, it depends on surrounding muscles for stability with motion. These layers of supportive muscle provide **dynamic stability**, contracting to maintain the position of the humeral head as the shoulder moves through its wide range of motion. Later in this chapter we will look at causes and implications of shoulder dislocations.

Without the surrounding contractile rotator cuff and deltoid muscles to hold the humeral head in place, the joint capsule is subject to excessive strain. For example, a person who has paralysis of the surrounding muscles due to a CVA may experience painful stretching of the joint capsule due to the effect of gravity on the shoulder without muscular support.

The long head of the biceps brachii traverses the GHJ capsule and is surrounded by a synovial membrane sleeve. Repeated stress on this tendon can result in inflammation and pain upon movement (bicipital tendinitis).

The narrow space between the humeral head and the underside of the acromion is the **subacromial space**.

The long head of the biceps, tendons of infraspinatus and supraspinatus, and the **subacromial (subdeltoid) bursae** lie within and are susceptible to compressive forces with repetitive overhead motion (**5.21**). Inflammation of these tissues and associated pain is called *subacromial impingement* and may be related to postural

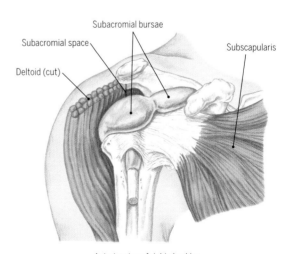

Anterior view of right shoulder

5.21 Subacromial bursae of the glenohumeral joint

compromise or rotator cuff weakness (described later in this chapter).

Glenohumeral arthrokinematics have been studied extensively, but identifying the exact pattern of this complex joint has proven challenging. Although the GHJ is technically a convex-on-concave joint (as you learned in Chapter 1), it does not adhere to the same rules regarding rotation and translation as other joints with this arrangement. Most studies confirm that there is some degree of axial rotation and translation of the humerus during elevation, but the magnitude and direction are disputed. It is generally clinically accepted that translation (gliding) must be addressed to restore full motion of the GHJ. But with rotator cuff weakness and joint instability, excessive superior gliding may be present, potentially leading to subacromial impingement.[2]

Musculature and Movement

Distinct muscle groups contribute to the complex and integrated movements of the scapula, clavicle, and humerus (5.22, 5.23). As you study the arrangement and attachments of each muscle, think about that muscle in a functional context.

- How does the muscle support purposeful movement of the shoulder for occupational performance?
- How do movement and positioning of the shoulder contribute to function of the entire upper extremity?

After you have familiarized yourself with the muscles and movements of the shoulder, we will take it a step further and practice goniometry and MMT for specific motions of the scapula and GHJ.

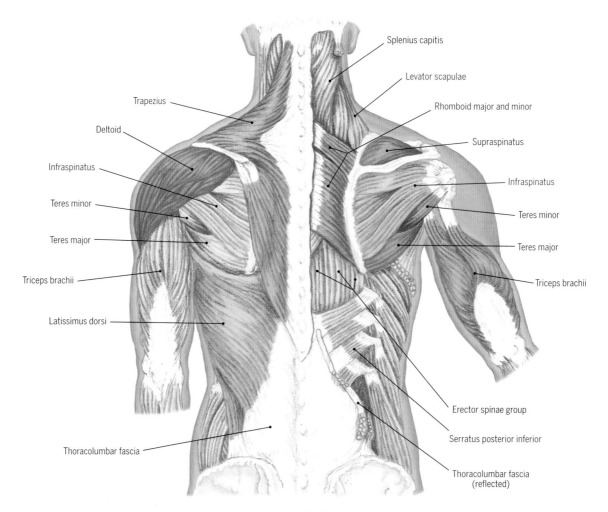

Splenius capitis

Levator scapulae

Rhomboid major and minor

Supraspinatus

Infraspinatus

Teres minor

Teres major

Triceps brachii

Erector spinae group

Serratus posterior inferior

Thoracolumbar fascia
(reflected)

Trapezius

Deltoid

Infraspinatus

Teres minor

Teres major

Triceps brachii

Latissimus dorsi

Thoracolumbar fascia

Posterior view

5.22 Posterior view of shoulder and back. The latissimus dorsi, trapezius, and deltoid are removed on the right side.

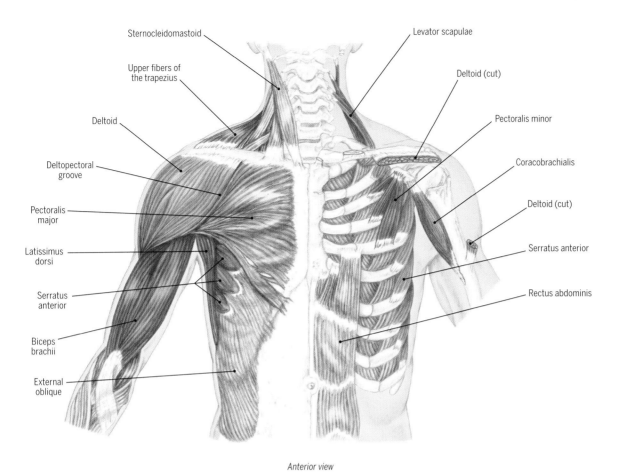

Anterior view

5.23 Anterior view of shoulder and chest. The pectoralis major, deltoid, and biceps brachii are removed on the left side.

TAYLOR SCHULTZ | Now that you know more about the anatomy of the shoulder complex, let's return to Taylor. He says his shoulder pain is worse after a long day at work. Sometimes it even hurts to bring his hands to the steering wheel to drive home. He also complains of pain in his upper back and neck. Once he arrives home, he usually takes an over-the-counter (OTC) pain reliever and wants to relax and watch television. He notices that he has been a little less patient and more irritable.

Take a look again at his posture when sitting at his desk. Note the specific position of his trunk.

- How does this trunk posture affect the position of his scapulae?
- How might his posture and the position of his scapula affect motion of the humerus?
- How might his habits, roles, or routines, outlined in his occupational profile, contribute to or be affected by his symptoms?

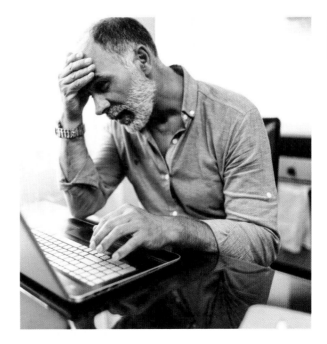

Axioscapular Muscles

Trapezius

Levator scapulae and rhomboids

Serratus anterior

Pectoralis minor

As noted earlier, there is no direct skeletal link (synovial joint) attaching the scapula to the skeleton. Instead, the *axioscapular muscles* anchor the scapula to the posterior vertebral column and rib cage (axial skeleton). Two of these muscles—the serratus anterior and pectoralis minor—also attach the scapula to the anterior rib cage. The dorsal axioscapular muscles are arranged in layers, from superficial to deep.

Trapezius

The most superficial dorsal axioscapular muscle is the broad **trapezius**, with its upper, middle, and lower fibers serving to stabilize and mobilize the scapula in relation to the spine. To help form the trapezoid shape, muscle fibers that originate from the vertebrae project in two directions: from superior downward, attaching

to the clavicle, and from inferior upward, attaching to the scapula (**5.24**).

The trapezius is a good example of a muscle that anatomically appears to be a single muscle but functionally is at least three muscles:

- The upper fibers provide elevation and upward rotation of the scapula, facilitating humeral elevation for overhead activity.
- The middle fibers, horizontally oriented, adduct the scapula toward the spine, a component of functional retraction.
- The inferior (lower) fibers also assist with upward rotation or depression of the scapula as a force couple with other muscles.

The trapezius helps stabilize and mobilize the scapula for effective positioning of the proximal upper extremity.

Posterior view

5.24 The trapezius is the most superficial muscle of the posterior upper back and shoulder.

Labels on figure: Superior nuchal line of the occiput; Upper fibers; Middle fibers; Lower fibers

TRAPEZIUS

Purposeful Activity

P Reaching for an object overhead (upper/lower trapezius), rowing a kayak or canoe (middle trapezius)

A UPPER FIBERS
Bilaterally:
Extend the head and neck
Unilaterally:
Laterally flex the head and neck to the same side
Rotate the head and neck to the opposite side
Elevate the scapula (ST joint)
Upwardly rotate the scapula (ST joint)

MIDDLE FIBERS
Adduct the scapula (ST joint)
Stabilize the scapula (ST joint)

LOWER FIBERS
Depress the scapula (ST joint)
Upwardly rotate the scapula (ST joint)

O External occipital protuberance, medial portion of superior nuchal line of the occiput, ligamentum nuchae, and spinous processes of C-7 through T-12

I Lateral one-third of clavicle, acromion, and spine of the scapula

N Spinal portion of cranial nerve XI (accessory) and ventral ramus C2 to C4

Levator Scapulae and Rhomboids

Deep to the trapezius, from superior to inferior, lie the **levator scapulae**, **rhomboid minor**, and **rhomboid major** (**5.25**).

Collectively, these muscles act to elevate and downwardly rotate the scapula, providing a counterbalance to the muscles that upwardly rotate (upper/lower trapezius and serratus anterior). The rhomboids, along with the middle deltoid, also play an important role in adducting the scapula and preventing excessive abduction or protraction.

TAYLOR SCHULTZ | Based on what you know so far, do you think targeted strengthening of the rhomboids and middle trapezius would have any value as an exercise to promote occupational performance for Taylor? Why or why not?

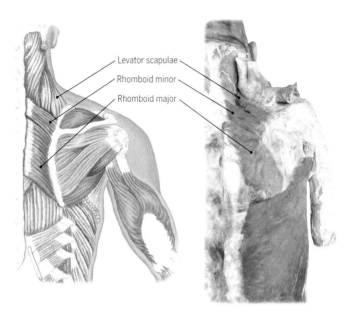

Posterior view

5.25 The levator scapulae and rhomboids lie deep to the trapezius.

LEVATOR SCAPULAE
Purposeful Activity

P Shrugging shoulders (nonverbal communication) or carrying a briefcase

A *Unilaterally:*
Elevate the scapula (ST joint)
Downwardly rotate the scapula (ST joint)
Laterally flex the head and neck
Rotate the head and neck to the same side
Bilaterally:
Extend the head and neck

O Transverse processes of first through fourth cervical vertebrae

I Medial border of scapula between superior angle and superior portion of spine of scapula

N Cervical C3 and C4, and dorsal scapular C4 and C5

RHOMBOID MAJOR AND MINOR
Purposeful Activity

P Reaching into a back pocket

A **Adduct** the scapula (ST joint)
Elevate the scapula (ST joint)
Downwardly rotate the scapula (ST joint)

O Major: Spinous processes of T-2 to T-5
Minor: Spinous processes of C-7 and T-1

I Major: Medial border of the scapula between the spine of the scapula and inferior angle
Minor: Upper portion of medial border of the scapula, across from spine of the scapula

N Dorsal scapular C4 and C5

Serratus Anterior

The muscle that anchors the medial border of the scapula to the rib cage is known as the **serratus anterior** (5.26). The serratus anterior is extremely important for maintaining the position of the scapula against the rib cage.

Damage to the long thoracic nerve, which innervates this muscle, may lead to *scapular winging* (discussed later in this chapter). In this condition, the medial border of the scapula becomes unstable and migrates away from the rib cage dorsally (winging).

SERRATUS ANTERIOR
Purposeful Activity

P **Pushing open a heavy door**

A *With the origin fixed:*
Abduct the scapula (ST joint)
Upwardly rotate the scapula (ST joint)
Depress the scapula (ST joint)
Hold the medial border of the scapula against the rib cage

With the scapula fixed:
May act to **elevate** the thorax during forced inhalation

O External surfaces of upper eight or nine ribs

I Anterior surface of medial border of the scapula

N Long thoracic C5 to C8

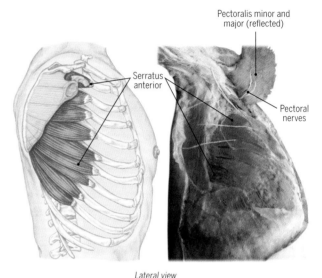

Lateral view

5.26 Serratus anterior

Pectoralis Minor

The coracoid process of the scapula serves as an anchor for an additional muscle that stabilizes the scapula anteriorly against the rib cage, the **pectoralis minor** (5.27).

PECTORALIS MINOR
Purposeful Activity

P **Taking a deep breath, walking with crutches**

A **Depress** the scapula (ST joint)
Abduct the scapula (ST joint)
Downwardly rotate the scapula (ST joint)

With the scapula fixed:
Assist to **elevate** the thorax during forced inhalation

O Third, fourth, and fifth ribs

I Medial surface of coracoid process of the scapula

N Medial pectoral, with fibers from a communicating branch of the lateral pectoral C6 to C8, T1

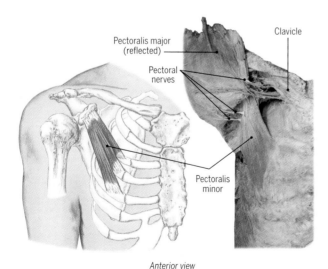

Anterior view

5.27 Pectoralis minor

CLINICAL APPLICATION
What Happens When the Clavicle Breaks?

As mentioned earlier, the clavicle acts partially as a strut, or a structure that resists longitudinal compression along its length. If you break your clavicle, the shoulder joint complex becomes unstable, and all arm movements become very painful. The left side of Figure **5.28** shows the clavicle acting as a strut, keeping the shoulder joint away from the body. After clavicular fracture (shown on the right side of the figure), however, the following occurs:

1. Gravity (indicated by the blue arrows) pulls downward on the lateral fragment.
2. Muscles that attach to the clavicle—including the trapezius, depending on where the fracture occurs—pull the medial clavicle upward.
3. The fibers of the pectoralis major adduct the humerus.

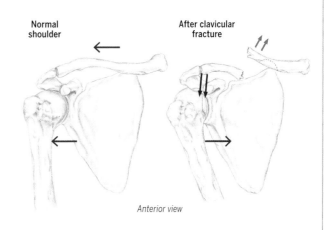

Anterior view

5.28 Impact of a clavicular fracture on the shoulder complex. How does the clavicle serve to position the humerus for functional motion?

Purposeful Movement of the Scapula

The four primary motions of the scapula in the frontal plane are generally considered to be elevation, depression, abduction, and adduction. However, functional movement of the scapula is not confined to the frontal plane; often it also involves rotation or tilting of the scapula relative to the rib cage. For example, reaching in front of the body with the arm involves scapular protraction, a combination of abduction and anterior tilt. As a student and future clinician, you should be familiar with the anatomical movements in the frontal plane as well the combined functional movements:

- protraction—abduction with anterior tilt
- retraction—adduction with posterior tilt
- upward rotation—elevation with abduction
- downward rotation—depression with adduction

In a sense, the scapula positions the glenoid fossa to facilitate movement of the humerus, similar to a gear rotating the hand of a clock (**5.29**). Full flexion and abduction (elevation) of the humerus require

Scapulohumeral rhythm can be conceptualized as the relative movement between the gear (scapula) and hand (humerus) of a clock.

For the first 30° of humeral elevation (flexion or abduction), or 6 to 7 on the clock, the scapula (gear) remains stationary.

As the humerus elevates from 30° to 180°, or 7 to 12 on the clock, the scapula upwardly rotates 1° for every 2° of humeral elevation.

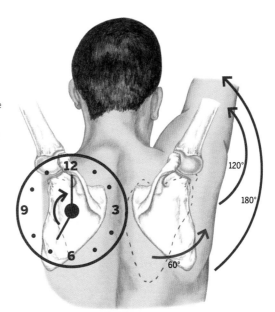

5.29 Scapulohumeral rhythm as a gear rotating the hand of a clock

upward rotation of the scapula. The scapula positions the glenoid fossa in the direction of humeral motion and allows clearance of the humeral head beneath the acromion.

Many of the muscles of the scapula work together in synergy, acting in opposing directions but contributing to the same motion. For example, the serratus anterior, upper trapezius, and lower trapezius all contribute to upward rotation of the scapula, but their attachments and direction of pull are very different. Other muscles form force couples that act as antagonists to counterbalance and stabilize the scapula. For example, the rhomboids and levator scapulae downwardly rotate the scapula to counterbalance the muscles that contribute to upward rotation.

As you read about the specific motions, what other force couples can you identify for scapular elevation, depression, or downward rotation? Now take it to the functional level: What scapular motion(s) and specific muscles are involved when you reach into your back pocket, push open a heavy door, or throw a football?

Figures **5.30–5.34** feature the muscles that act on the scapula in a functional context, with prime movers listed first. Asterisks indicate muscles not shown.

Elevation

(*antagonists on depression*)
Trapezius (upper fibers, unilaterally)
Rhomboid major
Rhomboid minor
Levator scapulae (unilaterally)

5.30 Scapular elevation

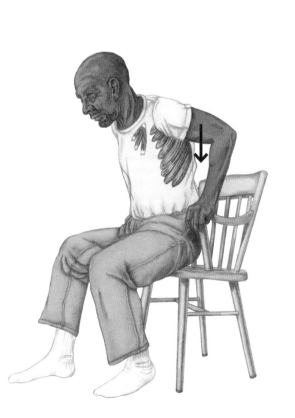

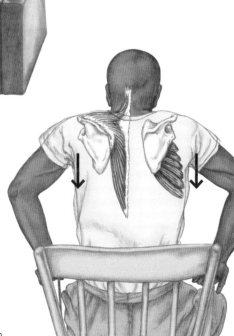

Depression

(*antagonists on elevation*)
Trapezius (lower fibers)
Serratus anterior
  (with the origin fixed)
Pectoralis minor

5.31 Scapular depression

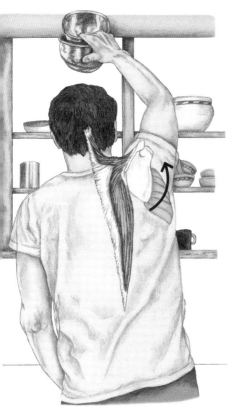

Upward Rotation of the Scapula
(*antagonists on downward rotation*)
Trapezius (upper and lower fibers)
Serratus anterior (with the origin fixed)

Downward Rotation of the Scapula
(*antagonists on upward rotation*)
Rhomboid major
Rhomboid minor
Levator scapulae
Pectoralis minor

5.32 Scapular upward rotation

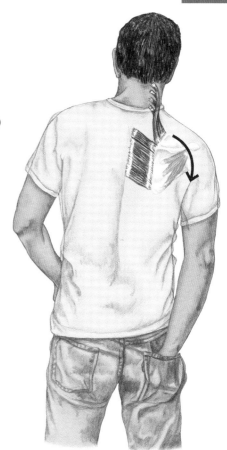

5.33 Scapular downward rotation

Protraction (abduction with anterior tilt)
(*antagonists on adduction*)
Serratus anterior (with the origin fixed)*
Pectoralis minor*

Retraction (adduction with posterior tilt)
(*antagonists on abduction*)
Trapezius (middle fibers)
Rhomboid major
Rhomboid minor

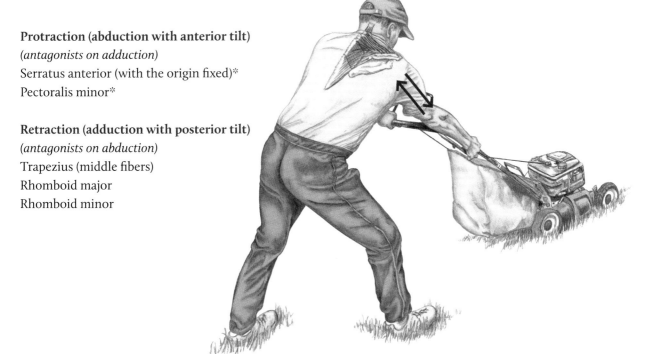

5.34 Scapular protraction and retraction

▶TRY IT

As complex patterns of movement for an atypical joint, scapular protraction and retraction are difficult to measure. Some sources suggest measuring the distance between the scapular border and the spine. A recently developed technique uses the superior angle and acromion as anatomical landmarks to measure scapular protraction and retraction relative to the frontal plane (**5.35A**). The axis of the goniometer is aligned with the superior angle, the static arm remains fixed in the frontal plane, and the moving arm follows the acromion as the scapula protracts or retracts.

Take a look at Figure **5.35**. Use the technique described above to measure the scapula at rest (**B**), in protraction (**C**), and in retraction (**D**). The technique is still being researched but has demonstrated a high degree of interrater reliability, meaning two different clinicians using the technique can obtain similar measurements.[3] What do you think?

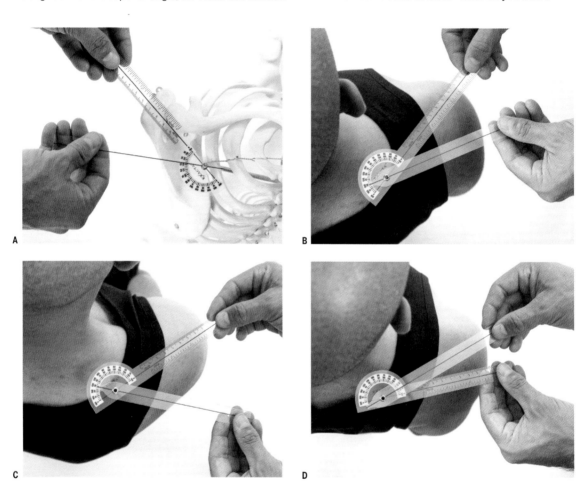

5.35 Goniometric measurement of scapular protraction and retraction

Scapulohumeral Muscles

Rotator cuff

Deltoid

Teres major

The scapula serves as the link between the trunk and humerus, providing a balance of stability and mobility to facilitate humeral motion. The next functional muscle group includes muscles that connect the scapula and proximal humerus, or the *scapulohumeral muscles*.

These muscles stabilize the humeral head against the glenoid fossa and supply force for elevation and rotation. They are active when the shoulder is moving in space, such as when reaching, placing, or throwing.

Rotator Cuff

Infraspinatus
Teres minor
Subscapularis
Supraspinatus

The **rotator cuff** group—infraspinatus, teres minor, subscapularis, and supraspinatus—creates an anatomical cuff around the shoulder joint, enveloping the humeral head almost in its entirety (the cuff is deficient inferiorly). The muscles not only produce motion of the arm but also maintain the functional integrity of the GHJ by keeping the head of the humerus stabilized in the glenoid fossa.

The long head of the biceps brachii also helps to stabilize the joint. It is sometimes referred to as the fifth rotator cuff muscle. The long head of the triceps brachii offers minimal support to the inferior aspect of the joint.

The posterior aspect of the cuff is composed of the **infraspinatus** and **teres minor**, which insert into the greater tubercle (**5.36**). These muscles contribute primarily to external rotation of the humerus, as when reaching behind the head or upper back for bathing.

The posterior cuff is balanced by its anterior antagonist, the **subscapularis** (**5.37**). This muscle serves to internally rotate the humerus, as when putting on a

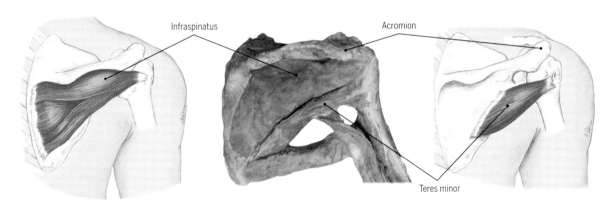

Posterior view

5.36 Infraspinatus and teres minor

INFRASPINATUS	TERES MINOR
Purposeful Activity	**Purposeful Activity**
P Playing racket sports or table tennis	**P** Washing the back of the head and neck
A Externally (laterally) rotate the shoulder (GHJ) Adduct the shoulder (GHJ) Stabilize the head of humerus in glenoid cavity	**A** Externally (laterally) rotate the shoulder (GHJ) Adduct the shoulder (GHJ) Stabilize the head of humerus in glenoid cavity
O Infraspinous fossa of the scapula	**O** Upper two-thirds of lateral border of the scapula
I Greater tubercle of the humerus	**I** Greater tubercle of the humerus
N Suprascapular C4 to C6	**N** Axillary C5 and C6

bra or toileting (remember that these movements are defined relative to the anatomical position).

The **supraspinatus**—perhaps the most well-known (and commonly injured) rotator cuff muscle—lies supe-rior on the scapula, passing beneath the acromion to insert into the greater tubercle (**5.38**). In synergy with the deltoid, the supraspinatus abducts the humerus.

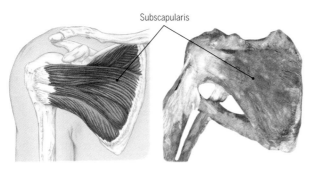

Subscapularis

Anterior view

5.37 Subscapularis

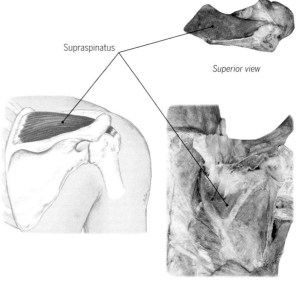

Supraspinatus

Superior view

Posterior view

5.38 Supraspinatus

SUBSCAPULARIS	
Purposeful Activity	
P	Toileting, donning a bra, or throwing a baseball
A	**Internally (medially) rotate** the shoulder (GHJ) **Stabilize** the head of humerus in glenoid cavity
O	Subscapular fossa of the scapula
I	Lesser tubercle of the humerus
N	Upper and lower subscapular C5 to C7

TAYLOR SCHULTZ | How might the supraspinatus be involved in Taylor's situation? Consider its pathway beneath the acromion and the pain he feels when using his arms overhead.

SUPRASPINATUS	
Purposeful Activity	
P	Painting overhead or washing your hair
A	**Abduct** the shoulder (GHJ) **Stabilize** the head of humerus in glenoid cavity
O	Supraspinous fossa of the scapula
I	Greater tubercle of the humerus
N	Suprascapular C4 to C6

Deltoid

The **deltoid** is a superficial muscle that caps the proximal humerus from above (superiorly). Its superior orientation and distinct anterior, middle, and posterior fibers
supply force for flexion, abduction, and extension (**5.39**).

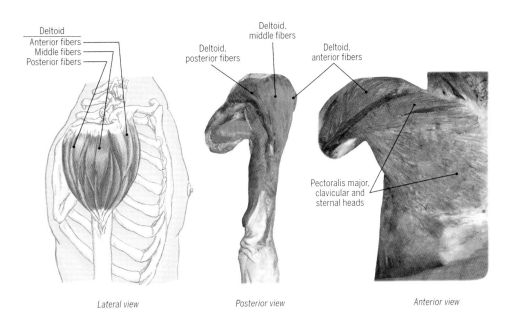

Lateral view   *Posterior view*   *Anterior view*

5.39 Deltoid

DELTOID

Purposeful Activity

P   Doing yoga poses with arms overhead (all fibers),
    reaching for (anterior fibers) and putting on (posterior
    fibers) a seat belt

A   *All fibers:*
    Abduct the shoulder (GHJ)

    Anterior fibers:
    Flex the shoulder (GHJ)
    Internally (medially) rotate the shoulder (GHJ)
    Horizontally adduct the shoulder (GHJ)

    Posterior fibers:
    Extend the shoulder (GHJ)
    Externally (laterally) rotate the shoulder (GHJ)
    Horizontally abduct the shoulder (GHJ)

O   Lateral one-third of clavicle, acromion, and spine of scapula

I   Deltoid tuberosity

N   Axillary C5 and C6

Teres Major

The **teres major** is also known as the "lat's (latissimus dorsi's) little helper" because it has similar actions of adduction and internal rotation (**5.40**).

TERES MAJOR	
Purposeful Activity	
P	Toileting and perineal care
A	**Extend** the shoulder (GHJ) **Adduct** the shoulder (GHJ) **Internally (medially) rotate** the shoulder (GHJ)
O	Inferior angle and lower one-third of lateral border of the scapula
I	Crest of the lesser tubercle of the humerus
N	Lower subscapular C5 to C7

As we begin to discuss purposeful movement of the GHJ, let's think about force couples at this joint. One of the classic musculoskeletal force couples involves the supraspinatus and the deltoid. First, identify their attachment sites and the direction of force applied to the humerus. Next, answer the following questions:

- If both of these muscles act simultaneously, what specific motion will occur?
- What occupations would involve this force couple?
- How might occupational performance be impacted with weakness of these muscles?

The general term "shoulder" often refers to the GHJ, but remember the shoulder involves four distinct joints.

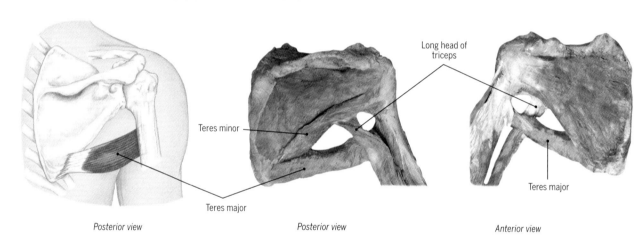

Teres minor

Teres major

Long head of triceps

Teres major

Posterior view   *Posterior view*   *Anterior view*

5.40 Teres major

Purposeful Movement of the Glenohumeral Joint

Movement of the humerus at the GHJ depends on the stability and mobility of the scapula and clavicle. For example, painting a ceiling involves shoulder flexion, which requires upward rotation of the scapula.

Figures **5.41–5.47** feature muscles that act on the glenohumeral joint in a functional context, with prime movers listed first. Asterisks indicate muscles not shown.

Abduction
(antagonists on adduction)
Deltoid (all fibers)
Supraspinatus*

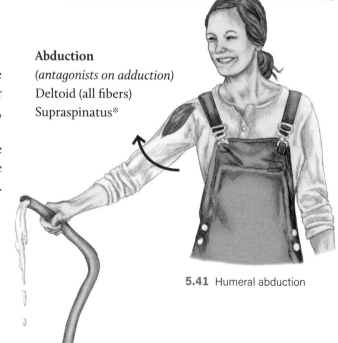

5.41 Humeral abduction

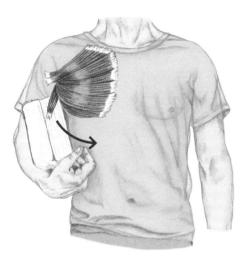

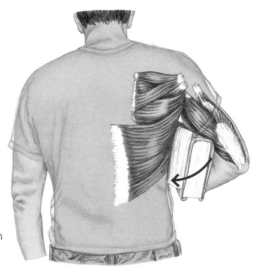

5.42 Humeral adduction

Adduction

(antagonists on abduction)

Latissimus dorsi

Teres major

Infraspinatus

Teres minor

Pectoralis major (all fibers)

Triceps brachii (long head)

Coracobrachialis

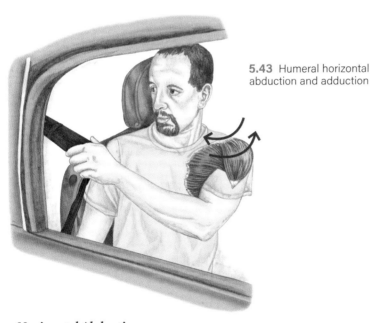

5.43 Humeral horizontal abduction and adduction

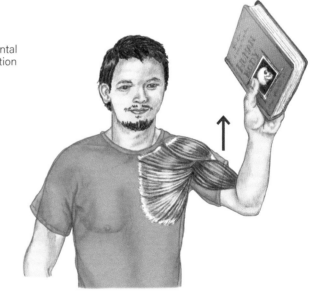

5.44 Humeral flexion

Horizontal Abduction

(antagonist on horizontal adduction)

Deltoid (posterior fibers)

Horizontal Adduction

(antagonists on horizontal abduction)

Deltoid (anterior fibers)

Pectoralis major (upper fibers)

Flexion

(antagonists on extension)

Deltoid (anterior fibers)

Pectoralis major (clavicular fibers)

Biceps brachii

Coracobrachialis*

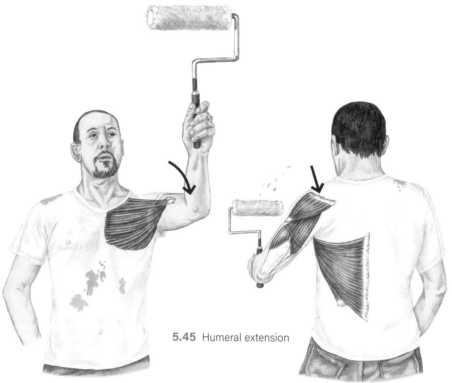

Extension
(*antagonists on flexion*)
Deltoid (posterior fibers)
Latissimus dorsi
Teres major*
Pectoralis major (sternal fibers)
Triceps brachii (long head)

5.45 Humeral extension

External Rotation (lateral rotation)
(*antagonists on internal rotation*)
Deltoid (posterior fibers)
Infraspinatus
Teres minor

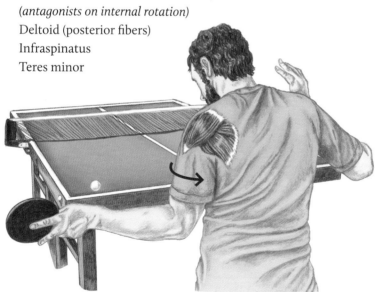

5.46 Humeral external (lateral) rotation

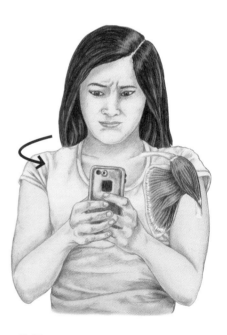

5.47 Humeral internal (medial) rotation

Internal Rotation (medial rotation)
(*antagonists on external rotation*)
Deltoid (anterior fibers)
Latissimus dorsi*
Teres major*
Subscapularis
Pectoralis major (all fibers)*

OT Guide to Goniometry & MMT: Shoulder

Now that you have examined the muscles acting on the shoulder complex and have thought about specific movements from a functional perspective, let's practice goniometry and MMT techniques using the *OT Guide to Goniometry & MMT* eTextbook.

Review the techniques described for the ST and glenohumeral joints. Describe the various muscles and force couples involved with specific movements. As you practice, describe the motions of the scapula, clavicle, and humerus at the ST, SC, AC, and glenohumeral joints. How do these motions serve to position and stabilize the upper extremity for functional activity?

Also, narrate the actions of various muscles and force couples involved with specific motions. This will take practice due to the intricacy of the shoulder complex. You might start with the scapula: "Upward rotation of the scapula facilitates the abduction and flexion of the humerus and recruits the upper and lower trapezius as well as the serratus anterior..." Then build on this foundational scapular motion as you describe the muscles flexing the humerus.

Take some goniometry measurements for specific occupations. How much horizontal adduction of the humerus is needed to put on a seat belt? How much internal rotation is required for toileting? Think of others and describe the purposeful movements necessary for occupational performance.

Occupational and Clinical Perspectives

Now that you have an understanding of the bones, joints, and muscles that generate force for purposeful movement of the shoulder complex, let's apply this knowledge through the lens of occupation and clinical reasoning. The following sections further integrate the functional anatomy of this region into occupational performance and explain several common pathologies you may encounter as a future practitioner.

Scapula: The Foundation of Upper Extremity Motion

The scapula serves as the beginning of a chain of interconnected links of the upper extremity. It offers a base of support for the GHJ to position the arm in space for functional activity.

Many ADLs require shoulder elevation (flexion or abduction), including personal hygiene/grooming, upper body dressing, and bathing (**5.48**). Work and leisure occupations often include forceful or resisted shoulder elevation. Consider a warehouse employee stocking overhead shelves or a volleyball player spiking the ball over the net. These purposeful movements require complex cooperation of multiple scapular and humeral muscle groups.

To be an effective therapist, you must be able to discern patterns of dysfunctional motion that impede occupational performance. This requires a thorough understand-

TAYLOR SCHULTZ | Let's get back to Taylor. You'll remember that he spends much of his day at a computer workstation, a specific environmental context. Consider again the position of his trunk and scapula when using a computer. You might even Google some images of workstation posture.

- What musculoskeletal imbalance can occur due to workstation posture?
- What muscles might be in a shortened position and susceptible to tightness?
- What muscles might be elongated, eventually becoming weaker? How might this pattern contribute to shoulder pain?
- How might this specific environmental context support or inhibit occupational performance?

Keep these thoughts in mind as we explore some occupational and clinical perspectives that can help you work effectively with Taylor.

ing of the underlying functional anatomy and the typical movement patterns that occur in the shoulder complex.

There is no bony articulation between the scapula and rib cage. The scapula translates (glides) and rotates within soft tissues. This arrangement affords a balance of scapular stability and mobility necessary for upper extremity function. However, weakness of specific muscles or an imbalance of forces may contribute to **scapular dyskinesis**, an alteration in the resting or active position of the scapula.

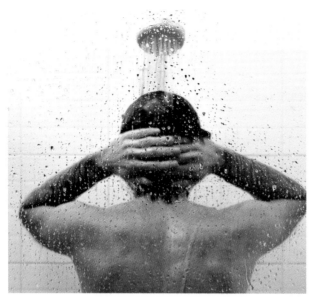

5.48 Washing your hair. What specific movements of the joints of the shoulder complex are required for this ADL?

Weakness of the serratus anterior, which stabilizes the scapula against the rib cage, may lead to **scapular winging (5.49)**. With this condition, the medial border of the scapula tilts posteriorly away from the rib cage due to the unrestrained dorsal pull of the trapezius. As a result, scapular mobility is impaired, which interrupts the functional movement of the shoulder. A client with mild winging due to weakness of the scapular stabilizers may benefit from strengthening of the serratus anterior and other scapular stabilizers.

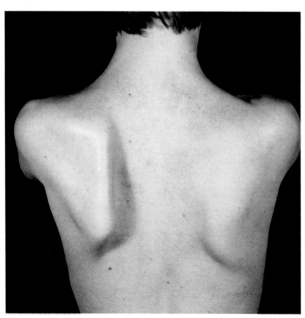

5.49 Winged scapula. What specific muscle(s) are weak?

More severe winging may be related to paralysis due to a neurological impairment such as a stroke or injury to the long thoracic nerve. In these cases, rehabilitative measures may involve manual mobilization of the scapula with upper extremity motion, and the practitioner should support the hemiparetic (weak) arm to avoid strain of weakened soft tissues.

The scapula facilitates motion of the humerus at the GHJ, and the two bones must work together for functional elevation of the upper extremity. Also recall that the SC and AC joints must proportionally elevate, depress, and rotate (SC joint only) the clavicle to facilitate scapular movement. This cooperative mechanical pattern is called **scapulohumeral rhythm**. Proportional scapular and humeral motion maintains optimal anatomical alignment of the bones of the shoulder complex with dynamic activity.

This means, for instance, that scapular protraction and retraction magnify forward and backward reaching with the arm, while upward rotation supports overhead elevation. The scapula remains relatively stable for the initial 30° of humeral elevation (flexion or abduction). Then it begins to upwardly rotate at a 1:2 ratio (scapular rotation relative to glenohumeral rotation), contributing approximately 60° to the total 180° excursion at end-range overhead motion (**5.50**).

Co-contraction of the surrounding muscles stabilizes the scapula and proximal upper extremity for closed-chain functional activities like gymnastics or rock climbing (**5.51**). Functional activity that requires reaching forward

▶TRY IT

To better understand the link between scapular and humeral mobility, roll (slouch) your shoulders forward as far as possible and then try to raise your arms overhead. Does it seem difficult? It should. The absence of scapular rotation in this position limits your overall humeral mobility. Why do you think it is difficult to raise your arm in this position?

Now simulate limited scapular mobility and its impact on function with a partner. Have your partner stand upright and place your hand firmly on the superior aspect of their scapula. As they slowly try to raise their arm, prevent the scapula from moving. Be careful as this may be uncomfortable for your partner. How high were they able to raise their arm?[4] How might limited scapular mobility affect ADLs, IADLs, work, and leisure?

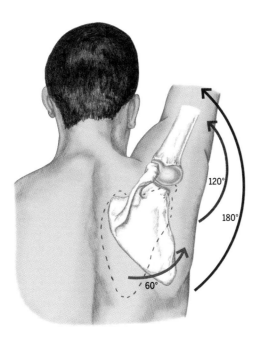

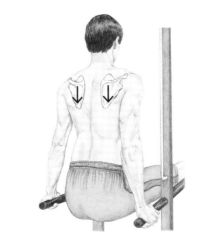

5.50 Scapulohumeral rhythm. Beyond 30° flexion, the scapula and humerus move at a 1:2 ratio. Full flexion or abduction of the shoulder involves approximately 60° scapular rotation and 120° humeral flexion.

or backward *below* shoulder level involves scapular protraction and retraction with respective flexion and extension of the humerus. For an example of alternating protraction and retraction, consider the action of rowing a boat (**5.52**). As a rower begins the cycle, her trunk flexes forward while the scapula *protracts* with simultaneous *flexion* of the humerus to reach forward into the water with the handle of the oar. Pulling the handle backward in the water, the rower's trunk extends while her scapula *retracts* with simultaneous *extension* of the humerus.

When the arm is functioning at or below the level of the shoulder, the scapula is well positioned to transfer powerful force from core muscles through the arm to generate "push" or "pull." Think of playing tug-of-war. With your arms at your sides, you can generate forceful pull through the rope, pulling your team to victory.

In contrast, with the arm functioning overhead, as when lifting a child for a ride on your shoulders, the humerus relies on much smaller muscles—primarily the supraspinatus and deltoid, which lie superiorly—to support the arm in this elevated position. This is why the supraspinatus is the most commonly injured rotator cuff muscle: it is relatively small but under significant strain in the overhead position without the support of the scapular stabilizers.

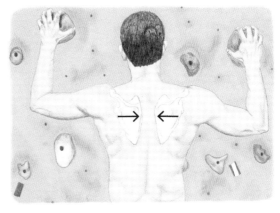

5.51 Describe the scapular position or movement that facilitates upper extremity function for these activities.

TAYLOR SCHULTZ | How can you apply the concept of scapulohumeral rhythm to Taylor's case? How might his scapular mobility, as a component of overhead activity, be limited?

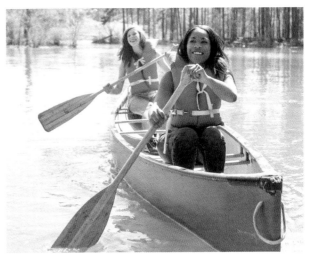

5.52 Canoeing. What scapular motions are involved with paddling?

A boxer throwing a jab illustrates the force production available at the scapula (**5.53**). With the humerus elevated, the serratus anterior forcefully protracts the scapula as the boxer's trunk rotates forward, generating forward momentum to thrust his hand into the punching bag. In this example, the arm essentially acts as a conduit to transfer force from the lower extremities, trunk, and scapula. Similar mechanics are at work when a shopper pushes a grocery cart.

Other functional activities involve a static scapula, such as replacing a light bulb overhead. The scapula remains in a fixed, upwardly rotated position to support the distal joints of the upper extremity, providing more precise movement to complete the task.

Overhead use of the shoulder against gravity exerts more strain on the rotator cuff—specifically the supraspinatus—and should be limited in frequency and resistance to avoid injury.

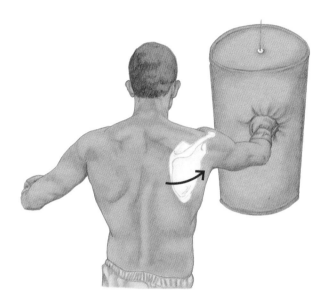

5.53 Hitting a punching bag. What specific movement of the scapula is involved in a punching motion of the upper extremity? What muscle(s) are involved?

Postural Compromise and Shoulder Dysfunction

Maintaining balanced, upright posture of the trunk and scapula is essential for maintaining musculoskeletal balance and promoting purposeful movement of the shoulder. After sitting too long at a workstation or in class, the core muscles (abdominals and back) may begin to fatigue, leading to flexion of the trunk as well as protraction and anterior scapular tilt (slouching). In fact, you may be in this position as you read this text.

Consistently slouched posture may lead to tightening of the pectoralis major and minor as well as stretching and weakness of the scapular stabilizers, exacerbating postural imbalance (**5.54**).

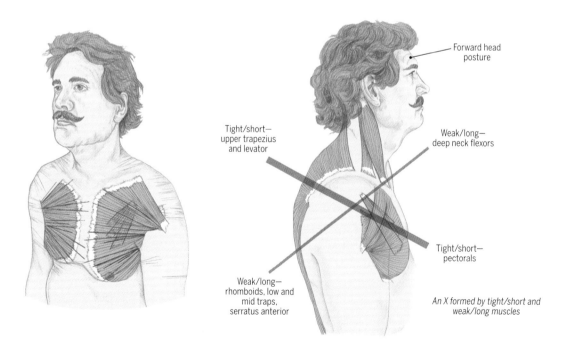

Forward head posture

Tight/short— upper trapezius and levator

Weak/long— deep neck flexors

Weak/long— rhomboids, low and mid traps, serratus anterior

Tight/short— pectorals

An X formed by tight/short and weak/long muscles

5.54 Upper crossed syndrome. How would you address this pattern of muscle imbalance? Does this pattern relate to Taylor's case? Why or why not?

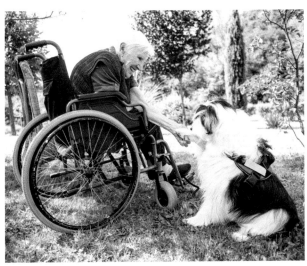

5.55 Wheelchair mobility. How might prolonged sitting in a wheelchair impact the posture and function of the shoulder? How would this position affect other body systems (cardiovascular, respiratory) and specific occupations—ADLs, IADLs, or social participation?

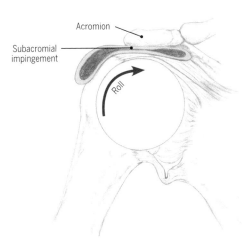

Anterior view of right shoulder

5.56 Subacromial impingement. Can you describe this condition as if explaining it to a future patient?

Optimal shoulder posture depends on musculoskeletal balance throughout the entire body. Asymmetry of the lower extremities or pelvis, curvature of the spine, or core instability will impact functional positioning of the shoulders (see Chapter 10 for a full discussion).

Older adults who use wheelchairs for functional mobility are particularly susceptible to this pattern of postural compromise. The imbalance may impair their respiratory function as well as their interaction with the environment because of the downward orientation of the head and neck (**5.55**).

Prolonged postural compromise can lead to several upper extremity pathologies of the shoulder. One of these is **subacromial impingement**, or compression of the soft tissues between the acromion and humeral head (**5.56**).

As the scapula abducts and tilts anteriorly, the glenoid fossa and acromion are oriented downward, which narrows the subacromial space, increasing pressure and limiting humeral mobility as the humeral head rotates, or rolls, to produce shoulder motion. Repetitive movements involving abduction and internal rotation, a position known to narrow the subacromial space and common in swimmers, may also contribute to impingement.

Remember from Chapter 2 that the nerves of the brachial plexus pass beneath the clavicle and pectoralis minor insertion. Slouched posture may also lead to anatomical compression of these structures, known as **thoracic outlet syndrome (TOS)** (**5.57**).

Some occupational therapy interventions for these pathologies include postural education, workstation or task modification, and exercises or activities to counteract the postural compromise and contribute to occupational performance.

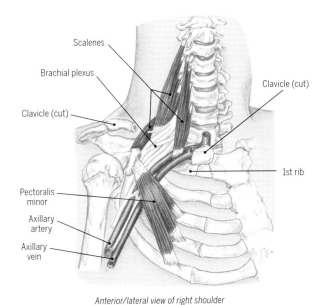

Anterior/lateral view of right shoulder and cervical spine

5.57 Sites of thoracic outlet syndrome (TOS). What symptoms would you expect in the upper extremity with compression of the brachial plexus, or TOS?

Glenohumeral Joint Function

The ball-and-socket design of the GHJ supplies vast mobility, allowing for motion and positioning of the upper extremity through all planes of motion for functional tasks.

Anatomically, the humeral head has minimal surface contact with the glenoid fossa, like a golf ball on a tee, allowing freedom of movement but limiting inherent stability. Without bony congruence, the GHJ relies primarily on noncontractile soft tissues for **static stability**, or stability at rest. The outermost rim of the glenoid fossa, the labrum, increases the depth of the fossa to accommodate the humeral head.

The joint capsule creates a layer of ligamentous tissue to maintain the position of the humeral head relative to the glenoid fossa. Whereas the contractile tissues (muscles) of the shoulder give it dynamic stability, it is the thick encompassing joint capsule that enhances static stability when the GHJ is at rest. The capsule and its anterior thickenings compose the glenohumeral ligaments, providing multidirectional support to the humeral head.

Hemiparesis, or weakness of one side of the body, due to neurological injury such as CVA or traumatic brain injury (TBI) may contribute to strain of the joint capsule as the weight of gravity pulls downward on the arm without opposition from muscle force. Eventually, this pulling may elongate the ligamentous fibers of the capsule and allow the humeral head to partially dislocate inferiorly, also known as **glenohumeral subluxation** (**5.58**). As the innervated capsule is overstretched, pain receptors are activated, leading to considerable shoulder pain.

Orthotics may offer external support to prevent this painful strain on the capsule (**5.59**). A wheelchair user may benefit from a tray that supports underneath the arm and helps the humeral head maintain a more neutral position.

The rotator cuff muscles supply much needed stability to the humeral head as the most important layer of dynamic support (**5.60**). As the humerus elevates, these muscles contract to provide dynamic stability for complex functional motions such as washing your upper back or casting a fishing line.

The rotator cuff muscle group is active during many ADLs that involve reaching behind the head or back, such as upper body dressing and toileting. Leisure activities that involve throwing a ball or swinging a racket

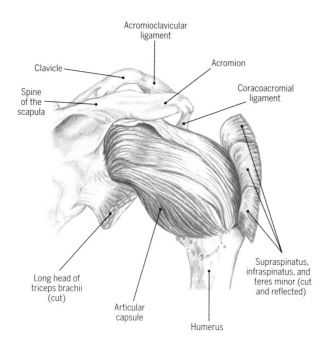

Posterior view of right shoulder

5.58 Subluxation of the glenohumeral joint. What holds the humeral head in place when the surrounding muscles are weak or paralyzed (passive stability)?

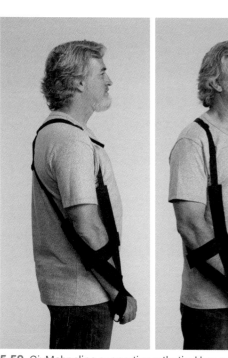

5.59 GivMohr sling supportive orthotic. How would this orthosis address subluxation of the glenohumeral joint related to hemiparesis after a stroke?

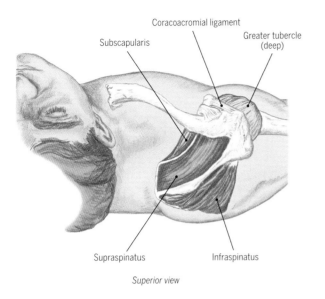

Coracoacromial ligament
Subscapularis
Greater tubercle (deep)
Supraspinatus
Infraspinatus

Superior view

5.60 Superior view of the rotator cuff muscles. How do these muscles support stability and mobility of the humerus?

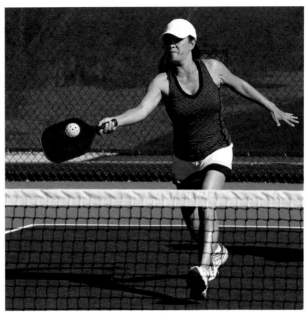

5.61 Describe the movements of the joints of the shoulder when playing pickleball.

rely on the rotator cuff, in cooperation with the core and lower extremities, to generate high-velocity motion (**5.61**). Pitching a baseball highlights end-range external rotation during the windup, followed by forceful internal rotation to accelerate the ball.

The rotator cuff generates essential motion but also plays an important role in stabilizing the humeral head in the glenoid fossa. Weakness of the rotator cuff can contribute to impingement, as the humeral head may migrate superiorly in the fossa, compressing tissues against the inferior acromion and AC ligament.

The deltoid and supraspinatus form an important force couple for overhead shoulder motion, particularly abduction. If the deltoid muscle is weak, the supraspinatus must exert more force to elevate the humerus, increasing the risk of a rotator cuff injury.

With rotator cuff weakness, the long head of the biceps may become inflamed as it supplies compensatory force for shoulder elevation. Repetitive shoulder flexion, such as when painting an overhead wall, may contribute to this condition, known as **bicipital tendinitis**.

The broad latissimus dorsi and pectoralis major generate strength for motion at the scapula and humerus. The latissimus dorsi's primary motion is shoulder extension from an elevated position, such as swinging a sledgehammer (**5.62**).

The pectoralis major, with its sternal and clavicular portions, generates strong adduction of the humerus (sternal

fibers) as well as flexion (clavicular fibers). You can get an idea of the function of pectoralis major when you reach for a seat belt with your humerus in midrange flexion.

These powerful muscles work in synergy to exert inferior (downward) force at the humeral head, counteracting external upward (superior) forces. For example, think of someone walking with crutches. Functional mobility with crutches substitutes weight-bearing through the lower extremities with upper extremity

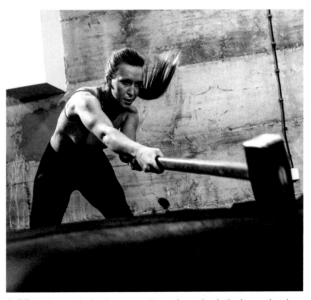

5.62 Using a sledgehammer. How does the latissimus dorsi contribute to swinging the hammer downward?

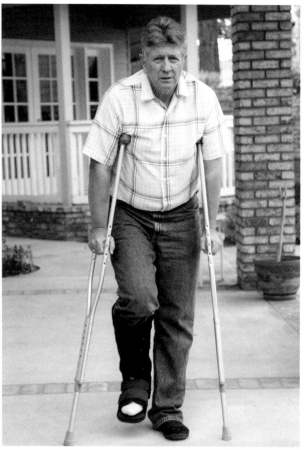

5.63 Using crutches to aid functional mobility. How do the muscles of the shoulder counteract the upward force generated through the shoulder girdle by the crutches?

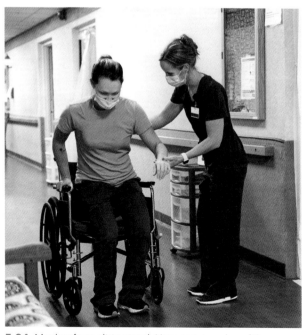

5.64 Moving from sit to stand. How can muscles of the shoulder help someone move from a seated position to standing?

force applied downward through the crutches (**5.63**). The combined force of these two axiohumeral muscles exerts counteractive downward humeral force, in conjunction with the scapular depressors (pectoralis minor, lower trapezius), to elevate the body on the crutches and allow for modified mobility.

With a fixed humerus, as when braced on the arms of a chair, the latissimus dorsi can work in the opposite direction through its broad origin on the lower trunk, exerting superior force on the trunk and pelvis to help raise the body from a seated position (**5.64**).

For older adults, maintaining strength of the latissimus dorsi along with the quadriceps femoris (for knee extension) contributes to more independent and safe transfers, particularly on lower surfaces such as a traditional commode.

Rotator Cuff Tear

As with many musculoskeletal pathologies, the risk of a rotator cuff tear increases with age as flexibility and muscle mass decrease. Rotator cuff tears may be attritional, or developing slowly due to friction over time, as with subacromial impingement. Or they may result from a single traumatic incident. Injuries often involve forceful loading of the shoulder in the elevated position, with the supraspinatus most commonly injured (**5.65**), as when lifting an object into an overhead cabinet.

Glenohumeral Joint Dislocation

The GHJ, with its limited surface contact between the humeral head and glenoid fossa, is the most commonly dislocated joint in the human body. Repetitive activities involving end-range glenohumeral motion, such as swimming, can lead to elongation of the joint capsule with general instability and eventual dislocation.

Injuries involving force through the proximal humerus with the arm in a closed-chain weight-bearing position can result in traumatic dislocation. Many dislocations occur anteriorly, often due to traumatic external rotation in the abducted position, or the 90/90 position, with the shoulder and elbow at right angles. These types of injuries are common in sports with forced end-range joint positions, such as martial arts or wrestling.

Dislocation of the shoulder may also involve damage to the labrum, the protective rim around the glenoid, leading to further instability. Labral tears are classified according to the portion of the labrum involved—for example, a superior labrum anterior to posterior (SLAP)

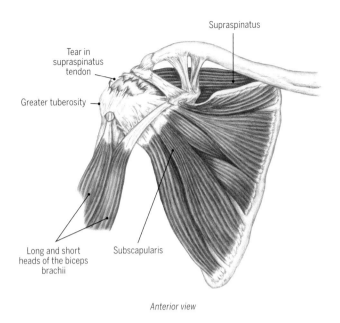

Tear in
supraspinatus
tendon

Supraspinatus

Greater tuberosity

Long and short
heads of the biceps
brachii

Subscapularis

Anterior view

5.65 Tear of the supraspinatus tendon. How might this injury impact purposeful movement of the shoulder? What specific occupations would be affected?

tear (**5.66**). This injury also involves the long head of the biceps. Depending on their severity, these injuries may require surgical intervention, with functional stability as the primary goal for postoperative rehabilitation.

With any dislocation, the surrounding capsule and muscles are often elongated, increasing instability and chance of reinjury. Conservative interventions may include strengthening of the rotator cuff to enhance dynamic stability of the shoulder and contribute to occupational performance.

Osteoarthritis

As with any synovial joint, the shoulder is susceptible to osteoarthritis (OA) with repetitive use over time (**5.67**). Coupled with weakness of the rotator cuff, glenohumeral elevation can be significantly limited and may require activity modification or adaptive equipment such as a reacher to compensate for painful motion. Shoulder arthroplasty (replacement) may be an option for individuals with advanced joint degeneration to address debilitating pain and restore basic functional motion.

Long head of
biceps tendon   Normal labrum

SLAP tear

Anterior view, right glenohumeral joint

5.66 Superior labrum anterior to posterior (SLAP) injury. How would this injury affect the stability of the glenohumeral joint?

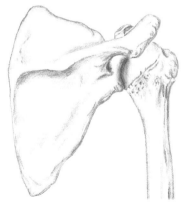

Posterior view

5.67 Osteoarthritis of the glenohumeral joint. How might this condition of the shoulder impact occupational performance?

As an OT practitioner, you will develop keen awareness of shoulder girdle symmetry and muscle imbalance. You also will learn how to use palpation and clinical assessments to identify musculoskeletal limitations to occupation. Because the upper extremity is a kinetic chain, motion between joints is interdependent for functional tasks.

General principles you can follow when assessing the upper extremity are to work (1) proximal to distal and (2) broad to more specific. For example, if a patient has full passive motion at the GHJ but is limited to 90° active flexion against gravity, this would indicate muscular weakness as opposed to joint limitation or impingement.

Full passive motion rules out bony restriction (impingement), while limited active motion, powered by the muscles of the patient, suggests muscular weakness. Gross MMT may identify weakness of the posterior rotator cuff, with more advanced orthopedic special tests used to isolate individual muscles. For example, the empty can test is used to isolate the supraspinatus and indicate rotator cuff pathology. These orthopedic tests of the shoulder inform clinical reasoning, guiding assessment and intervention. Developing more advanced clinical assessment skills depends on mastering the foundational techniques described in the *OT Guide to Goniometry & MMT* eTextbook.

APPLY AND REVIEW

Taylor Schultz

Taylor comes to see you, the OT practitioner, for his first OT visit, or initial evaluation. You listen carefully as he describes his symptoms and their impact on his daily life. Refer back to Taylor's occupational profile, an important component of the subjective portion of the evaluation. Think back to the performance skills, performance patterns, client factors, and contexts you identified.

The objective part of your evaluation includes goniometry and MMT (refer to the *OT Guide to Goniometry & MMT* eTextbook). Taylor demonstrates active motion of approximately 120° flexion and 100° abduction at the glenohumeral joint, with significant pain beyond that point. He has full external and internal rotation with the arm at the side. MMT reveals a 5/5 muscle grade in all planes of shoulder motion, with isolated testing of the rotator cuff muscles demonstrating a grade 5/5 as well. You note a rounded posture of the shoulders with the scapula abducted and tilted anteriorly.

- What do you suspect is causing his pain, specifically with overhead motion?
- Clinicians also use orthopedic special tests to further identify the source of musculoskeletal symptoms. Research Hawkins-Kennedy and Neer's tests. How might these exams help to identify the specific issue Taylor is having in his shoulder?

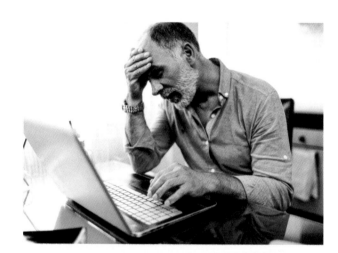

- What anatomical structures are likely involved?
- What strategies could be implemented to restore Taylor's occupational performance and prevent further symptoms and limitations?
- Taylor is very concerned that he cannot sleep at night and worries about the impact it is having on his job performance. What recommendations do you have to prevent his symptoms and restore his sleep and rest?
- How might you educate or modify the work environment to prevent similar symptoms for an entire group of employees working at workstations?

Review Questions

1. Which of the following muscle(s) contribute(s) to upward rotation of the scapula?
   a. upper trapezius
   b. lower trapezius
   c. serratus anterior
   d. all of the above

2. Which of the following occupations would be *most* difficult to complete with a rotator cuff tear involving the supraspinatus and infraspinatus tendons?
   a. lower body dressing
   b. upper body dressing
   c. sewing
   d. simple meal preparation

3. Which shoulder muscles should be strengthened to promote independence and safety when transitioning from sitting to standing?
   a. biceps
   b. supraspinatus
   c. latissimus dorsi
   d. subscapularis

4. You are working with a patient who sustained a stroke (CVA) with right hemiparesis of the upper extremity about a month ago. She is complaining of severe right shoulder pain. You notice a gap between the acromion and humeral head of about two finger widths. Which of the following *best* describes this clinical presentation?
   a. rotator cuff weakness
   b. bicipital tendinitis
   c. subacromial impingement
   d. glenohumeral subluxation

5. Which rotator cuff muscle is *most* important for internal rotation of the humerus to complete toileting?
   a. subscapularis
   b. supraspinatus
   c. teres minor
   d. infraspinatus

6. A patient is receiving occupational therapy services after surgical repair of the right rotator cuff. The physician's order specifies active range of motion (AROM) below 90° elevation. Which of the following would be an appropriate occupation-based intervention for this individual?
   a. pulleys
   b. nonresisted arm bike
   c. washing windows below shoulder level
   d. upper body dressing

7. An older adult presents with limited internal rotation of his dominant right glenohumeral joint, limiting completion of his ADLs. Which of the following specific ADLs do you anticipate would be *most* limited?
   a. hygiene
   b. upper body dressing
   c. self-feeding
   d. toileting

8. Which of the following muscle(s) contribute(s) to extension of the glenohumeral joint to facilitate dressing?
   a. triceps
   b. posterior deltoid
   c. latissimus dorsi
   d. all of the above

9. What scapular movement is necessary to facilitate overhead flexion of the glenohumeral joint for ADLs such as dressing or bathing?
   a. downward rotation
   b. adduction
   c. retraction
   d. upward rotation

10. Paralysis of this muscle may contribute to scapular winging, which impairs scapulohumeral rhythm and functional use of the upper extremity:
    a. supraspinatus
    b. subscapularis
    c. serratus anterior
    d. latissimus dorsi

See Answer Key in back of book.

Notes

1. American Occupational Therapy Association, *Occupational Therapy Practice Framework: Domain and Process*, 4th ed. (Bethesda, MD: AOTA Press, 2020).

2. Carol A. Oatis, *Kinesiology: The Mechanics and Pathomechanics of Human Movement*, 3rd ed. (Philadelphia: Wolters Kluwer, 2017).

3. Nathan Short et al., "Proposed Method for Goniometric Measurement of Scapular Protraction and Retraction," preprint, submitted August 31, 2019, https://doi.org/10.1016/j.jht.2019.02.002; Nathan Short et al., "Inter-rater Reliability of Goniometric Technique to Measure Scapular Protraction and Retraction," *American Journal of Occupational Therapy* 75 (forthcoming).

4. Adapted from David Paul Greene and Susan L. Roberts, *Kinesiology: Movement in the Context of Activity*, 3rd ed. (St. Louis, MO: Elsevier, 2017).

Bibliography

American Occupational Therapy Association. *Occupational Therapy Practice Framework: Domain and Process.* 4th ed. Bethesda, MD: AOTA Press, 2020.

Avers, Dale, and Marybeth Brown. *Daniels and Worthingham's Muscle Testing: Techniques of Manual Examination and Performance Testing.* 10th ed. St. Louis, MO: Saunders, 2019.

Biel, Andrew. *Trail Guide to Movement: Building the Body in Motion.* 2nd ed. Boulder, CO: Books of Discovery, 2019.

Biel, Andrew. *Trail Guide to the Body: A Hands-On Guide to Locating Muscles, Bones, and More.* 6th ed. Boulder, CO: Books of Discovery, 2019.

Clarkson, Hazel M. *Joint Motion, Muscle Length, and Function Assessment: A Research-Based Practical Guide.* 2nd ed. Philadelphia: Wolters Kluwer, 2020.

Greene, David Paul, and Susan L. Roberts. *Kinesiology: Movement in the Context of Activity.* 3rd ed. St. Louis, MO: Elsevier, 2017.

Keough, Jeremy L., Susan J. Sain, and Carolyn L. Roller. *Kinesiology for the Occupational Therapy Assistant: Essential Components of Function and Movement.* 2nd ed. Thorofare, NJ: SLACK, 2017.

Lundy-Ekman, Laurie. *Neuroscience: Fundamentals for Rehabilitation.* 5th ed. St. Louis, MO: Elsevier, 2018.

Oatis, Carol A. *Kinesiology: The Mechanics and Pathomechanics of Human Movement.* 3rd ed. Philadelphia: Wolters Kluwer, 2017.

Short, Nathan, Michelle Mays, Ruth Ford, and Ethan Fahrney. "Proposed Method for Goniometric Measurement of Scapular Protraction and Retraction." Preprint, submitted August 31, 2019. https://doi.org/10.1016/j.jht.2019.02.002.

Short, Nathan, Abigail Baist, Tony Clifton, Adam Horty, Micaela Kosty, Courtney Olson, and Riddhi Patel. "Inter-rater Reliability of Goniometric Technique to Measure Scapular Protraction and Retraction." *American Journal of Occupational Therapy* 75 (forthcoming).

Standring, Susan. *Gray's Anatomy: The Anatomical Basis of Clinical Practice, International Edition.* 41st ed. Cambridge, UK: Elsevier, 2016.

CHAPTER 6

Elbow and Forearm

Learning Objectives

- Describe the bones, joints, and muscles contributing to purposeful movement of the elbow and forearm.

- Identify the primary purposeful movements of the elbow and forearm within the context of occupational performance.

- Develop competency in goniometry and manual muscle testing (MMT) as clinical assessment techniques for the elbow and forearm.

- Use clinical reasoning to identify limitations of the elbow and forearm that may affect occupational performance.

Key Concepts

acquired amputation	cumulative trauma disorder (CTD)
bony congruity	flexion contracture
carrying angle	lateral epicondylosis
cubital tunnel syndrome	medial epicondylosis
cubitus valgus	pronator teres syndrome
cubitus varus	upper limb amputation

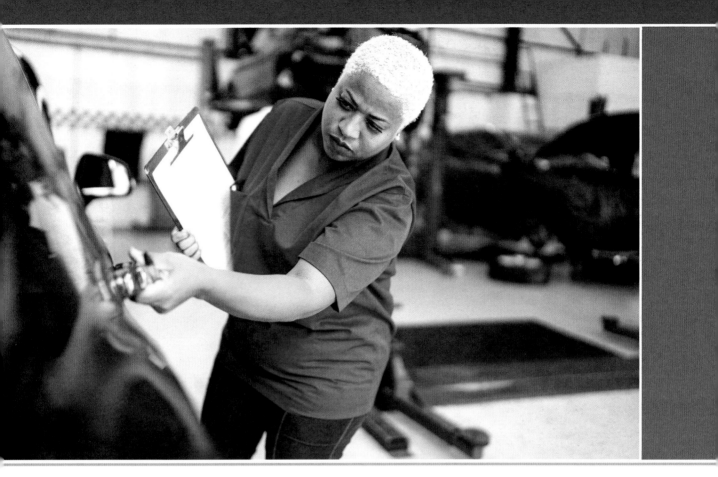

 Occupational Profile: Jamie Robbins

JAMIE ROBBINS is a forty-five-year-old female who works full-time on an assembly line installing doors on midsize trucks using a variety of power tools. Recently, she has been experiencing pain in her dominant left elbow, particularly when using tools at work.

She is still able to complete all ADLs, but the symptoms are beginning to affect her primary leisure occupations of pickleball and gardening. She also has some difficulty taking care of her Labrador retriever, Socks—specifically, holding the leash for their evening walks, which often requires both hands.

She has taken sick leave for the next few weeks and has received a referral for occupational therapy. She is concerned about returning to work, as she lives alone with no other source of income and must be able to complete all essential job tasks during her eight-hour shifts.

We'll talk more about Jamie as we explore the anatomy of the elbow and forearm.

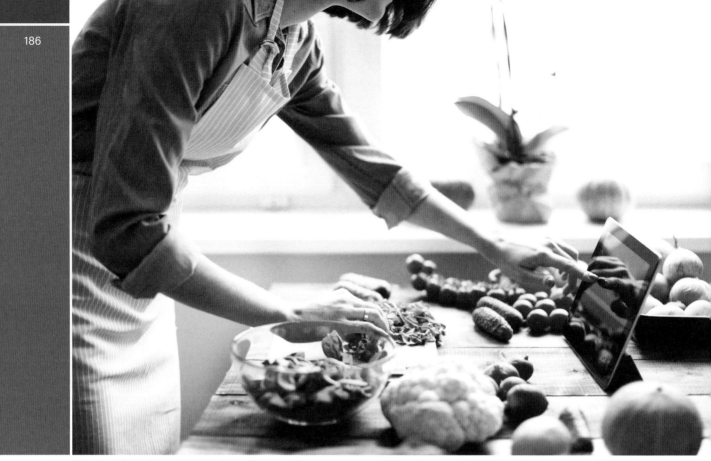

6.1 Coordinated movements of the elbow and forearm are essential for ADLs and IADLs.

Elbow and Forearm: A Rotating Hinge

Flipping pancakes with a spatula, using a screwdriver to assemble a woodworking project, turning on the hot water for a morning shower—these activities all require purposeful movement of the elbow and forearm.

As the functional link between the upper arm and hand, the elbow and forearm serve as a rotating hinge, bringing the hand to or away from the body with the palm up or down to facilitate occupational performance. These functional motions may occur simultaneously or separately, quickly or slowly, depending on the occupation.

Elbow flexion is needed for many self-care tasks, including hygiene, self-feeding, and bathing. Elbow extension is often involved with weight-bearing through the upper extremity, such as when pushing down on the armrests of a chair to stand up. Turning functional objects like keys, knobs, and dials relies on rotation of the forearm.

The elbow and forearm supply proximal attachment sites for the muscles that act on the wrist and hand, creating intricate functional links between these segments of the upper extremity. Think of the hand as a puppet controlled by strings (tendons) extending from the elbow

and forearm. Each tendon has a specific action on the hand that requires a balance of forces for functional motion and interaction with objects in the surrounding environment.

For instance, say you are swiping on a tablet to follow a recipe while preparing a meal (**6.1**). Your forearm is pronated with your fingertip touching the screen as your wrist moves laterally (ulnar deviation) or medially (radial deviation) to swipe. This simple motion involves coordination of multiple wrist and finger muscles, which are anchored by their proximal origins on the elbow and forearm.

This chapter describes the anatomy underlying purposeful movement of the elbow and forearm. As our examination of functional anatomy moves closer to the hand, you will notice the movements become more precise. As you study and apply this knowledge, continue to think about the contribution of the elbow and forearm to hand function in the broader context of occupational performance. In particular, use the case study of Jamie Robbins, the assembly line worker, to develop your clinical reasoning.

Osteology: Bones of the Elbow and Forearm

The bones of the elbow and forearm, with their distinct bony landmarks, form the skeletal structure supporting the muscles that act on the forearm, wrist, and hand (**6.2**).

Spend some time using the digital palpation resources accompanying this text to identify key features of these bones, which will also be referenced when you use the *OT Guide to Goniometry & MMT* eTextbook to practice your clinical assessment skills.

Humerus

You know from Chapter 5 that the **humerus** connects the trunk and the forearm and has a long, slender shaft that expands at each end (**6.3**). In that chapter, we focused on the proximal end and its role in shoulder function. Now let's explore the other end: the distal expansion, featuring the articular surfaces for the forearm bones (the ulna medially and the radius laterally, in the anatomical position).

JAMIE ROBBINS | Jamie is clearly facing some challenges to her occupational roles. Revisit her occupational profile and gather some additional information:

- How is her occupational performance specifically being affected? Refer to the *Occupational Therapy Practice Framework*, fourth edition (OTPF-4) and identify specific occupations, performance skills, roles, habits, and routines.[1]
- Do some research on different OT models of practice such as the Person-Environment-Occupation (PEO) Model or the Model of Human Occupation (MOHO). Think about how you could use these models in Jamie's case. Which one helps you to best conceptualize the various factors contributing to or inhibiting Jamie's occupational performance?

Keep these questions and your findings in mind as you read the chapter. Let's start with the bones.

Bony Landmarks of the Humerus

The medial surface of the distal humerus is called the **trochlea**, a bony wheel that supplies the articular surface

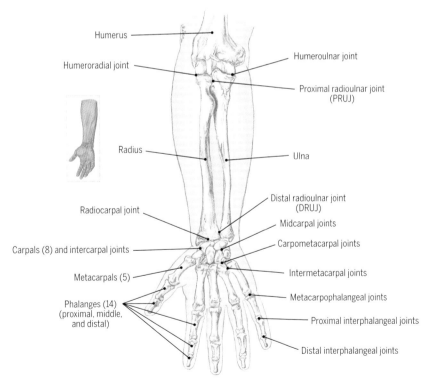

Anterior (volar) view of right forearm and hand

6.2 Bones of the elbow, forearm, and hand

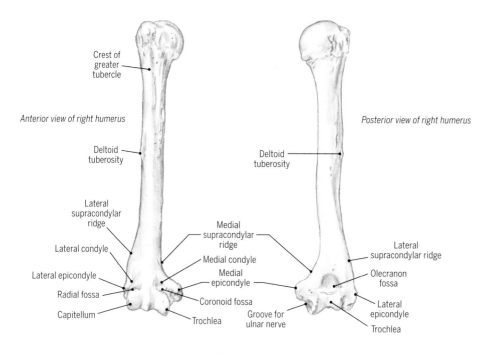

Crest of greater tubercle

Anterior view of right humerus

Posterior view of right humerus

Deltoid tuberosity

Deltoid tuberosity

Lateral supracondylar ridge

Medial supracondylar ridge

Lateral supracondylar ridge

Lateral condyle

Medial condyle

Olecranon fossa

Lateral epicondyle

Medial epicondyle

Radial fossa

Coronoid fossa

Lateral epicondyle

Capitellum

Trochlea

Groove for ulnar nerve

Trochlea

6.3 Humerus

for the ulna. A shallow groove separates the lateral lip of the trochlea from the rounded **capitellum (capitulum)**, the articular surface between the humerus and radius (**6.3**).

Because the trochlea extends farther distally than the capitellum, the bones of the forearm (radius and ulna) are positioned anatomically in 5°–15° of **valgus**, angled laterally away from midline relative to the humerus (**6.4**).

This angle is referred to as the **carrying angle** and is typically greater in females, allowing the arms to clear the hips during ambulation (walking or running). The angle may also be greater in repetitive throwing athletes, like baseball pitchers, with elongation of the ulnar collateral ligament (UCL). We will talk more about this ligament later in the chapter.

Additionally, the carrying angle encourages the hands to move away from the body with elbow extension, as when carrying a bucket, and toward the body with elbow flexion, as when brushing your teeth or eating.

Bony projections, or epicondyles, are found medially and laterally at the distal humerus. The **medial** and **lateral epicondyles** are the origins for many of the flexor and extensor muscles of the forearm, wrist, and fingers. Extending superiorly from these epicondyles are the **medial** and **lateral supracondylar ridges** (**6.5**).

Two depressions mark the anterior aspect of the humerus immediately proximal to its distal articular

surface: the **coronoid fossa** is superior to the trochlea, and the **radial fossa** is superior to the capitellum. A third, larger depression called the **olecranon fossa** is

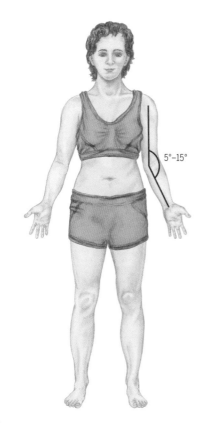

5°–15°

6.4 Valgus angulation at the elbow forms its carrying angle.

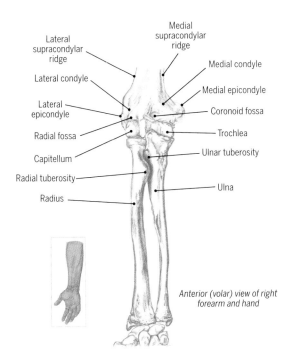
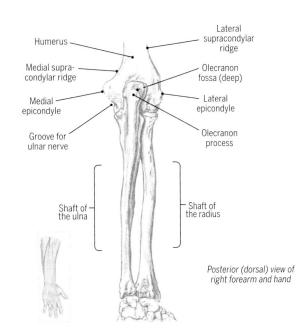

6.5 Features of the distal humerus and proximal radius and ulna

found in the posterior surface immediately proximal to the trochlea.

These three concave features of the distal humerus provide articular surfaces for the bony projections of the proximal radius and ulna. Like pieces of a puzzle, they fit together to enhance stability and function of the elbow. In musculoskeletal terms, this is referred to as **bony congruity**, a concept presented in Chapter 1. What impact does bony congruity have on joint mobility?

Ulna

The **ulna** is the largest bone of the forearm and serves as a stable base for elbow flexion and forearm rotation (**6.6**). The proximal end of the ulna is specialized for articulation with both the humeral trochlea and the head of the radius.

Bony Landmarks of the Ulna

The bony landmarks of the ulna contribute to the congruity and stability of the elbow and serve as attachment sites for the muscles in this region (**6.6**).

The ulnar socket that articulates with the trochlea is called the **trochlear notch**. The pronounced posterior projection of the ulna at the upper portion of the notch is the **olecranon process**. The lower portion of the trochlear notch features a wedge of bone that projects anteriorly, the **coronoid process**.

The olecranon and coronoid resemble a claw, "grasping" the rounded trochlea, and enhance the stability of the humeroulnar joint. A fracture of the olecranon or coronoid may compromise elbow stability.

The lateral surface of the coronoid process contains a shallow cup-shaped articular surface for the head of the radius, the **radial notch of the ulna**. The distal end of the ulna, or **head of the ulna**, articulates with both the radius and the intra-articular disc (triangular fibrocartilage complex, or TFCC) of the wrist joint. The TFCC is between the ulna and the carpus, or wrist (we'll talk more about the TFCC in Chapter 7).

JAMIE ROBBINS | Let's return to Jamie for a moment. Her pain seems to be focused near the epicondyles of her elbow. She takes over-the-counter (OTC) pain medication, which allows her to work a full shift.

Her pain intensifies later in the evening and is now interrupting her sleep. Lately she has been feeling some fatigue and stiffness at the beginning of her work shift.

- Based on what you know of her daily roles and performance patterns, why do you think her pain is located in this area?
- How might her pain affect her process or social interaction skills?

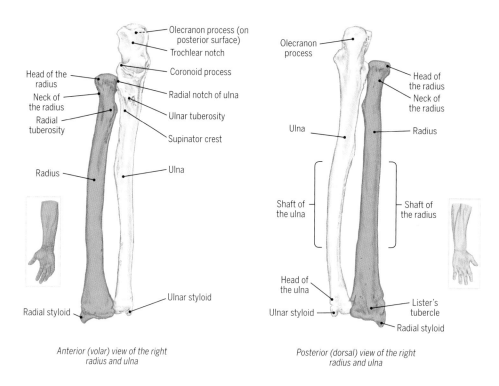

Anterior (volar) view of the right
radius and ulna

Posterior (dorsal) view of the right
radius and ulna

6.6 Ulna and radius

The posterior (subcutaneous) border of the shaft of the ulna continues distally beyond the head as the **ulnar styloid**.

Along its anterolateral surface, the ulna has a sharp ridge called the **interosseous border**. This border serves as the attachment for the **interosseous membrane** (**6.7**), which spans the length of the ulna and radius.

In addition to binding the forearm bones, the interosseous membrane protects the humeroradial joint from excessive compression by transmitting any force tending to drive the radius proximally, such as from a fall on an outstretched hand, across to the ulna.

Radius

The **radius** is the smaller of the two bones of the forearm. It rotates around the more stable ulna with forearm pronation and supination (**6.6**, **6.8**). The proximal end (head) of the radius is disclike and articulates (rotates) with both the radial notch and the capitellum of the humerus.

Bony Landmarks of the Radius

The **head of the radius** is a bony cylinder contributing to rotation of the radius around the ulna. The part of the radial shaft immediately distal to the head is called

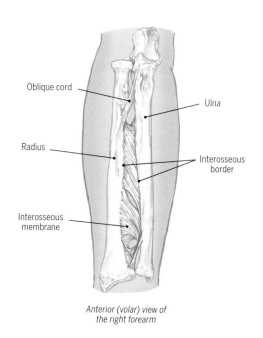

Anterior (volar) view of
the right forearm

6.7 Interosseous membrane

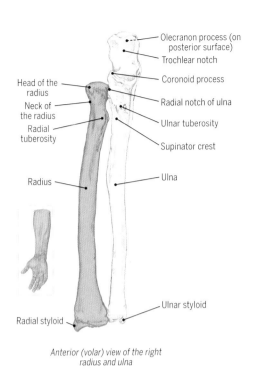

Olecranon process (on posterior surface)
Trochlear notch
Head of the radius
Coronoid process
Neck of the radius
Radial notch of ulna
Radial tuberosity
Ulnar tuberosity
Supinator crest
Radius
Ulna
Ulnar styloid
Radial styloid

Anterior (volar) view of the right radius and ulna

6.8 Bony landmarks of the radius and ulna

the neck (**6.8**). The neck is two to three centimeters long, ending at a site where the medial surface of the shaft bulges to form the **radial** (bicipital) **tuberosity**, the insertion site of the biceps tendon.

The medial border of the radius is characterized by a sharp interosseous border similar to the anterolateral border of the ulna. The distal end of the radius expands, and the extreme lateral part bulges outward and downward to form the **radial styloid**. The medial surface of the distal radius contains a shallow depression, called the **ulnar notch of radius**, for articulation with the head of the ulna.

Joints

As noted earlier, the elbow and forearm work together like a rotating hinge. Functionally, the joints cooperate to move the hand either closer to or farther away from the body while also turning the palm up or down—essential movements for ADL and IADL performance.

The joints in this region include the humeroulnar joint, humeroradial joint, and proximal radioulnar joint (**6.10**).

CLINICAL APPLICATION
Upper Limb Amputations

An **upper limb** (extremity) **amputation** may occur due to trauma or a disease process. Surgical removal is known as **acquired amputation**.

Amputations near the elbow and proximal forearm are classified in one of three ways: A **transhumeral** (long) amputation is through the distal humerus. An **elbow disarticulation** is at the elbow joint itself. A **transradial** (short) amputation is through the radius and ulna at the forearm.

As a practitioner, you may work with an individual after amputation on **preprosthetic training** by preparing the **residual limb** for a prosthetic device, helping the patient adjust to the loss of the limb, and working on ADL retraining with adaptive and compensatory strategies. If the patient's dominant limb has been amputated, training emphasizes a change in hand dominance, as the prosthetic device will have limited fine motor control.

The **prosthetic training** phase of recovery involves the functional integration of the prosthetic into daily occupations and roles. There are many different types of prosthetics designed for the elbow and forearm (**6.9**). Some are powered by movements of remaining proximal joints (body powered), and others are controlled by motor signals of remaining muscles via electrodes placed on the skin (myoelectric).

Do some additional research on the role of occupational therapy for individuals with upper limb amputation. What are the unique contributions of occupational therapy in each phase of rehabilitation?

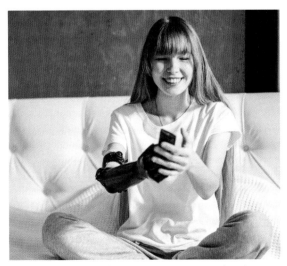

6.9 A prosthetic device may support occupational performance after upper limb amputation.

Elbow Joint (Humeroulnar and Humeroradial Joints)

Humeroulnar

Structural classification: hinge
Functional (mechanical) classification: uniaxial
Movements: flexion, extension

Humeroradial

Structural classification: modified hinge
Functional (mechanical) classification: biaxial
Movements: flexion, extension, rotation

The elbow refers to the combined humeroulnar and humeroradial joints (**6.10**). Together, the joints contribute to the functional hinge of the elbow with flexion and extension. The humeroulnar joint is the "true hinge" (limited to flexion and extension), while the humeroradial joint also pivots relative to the capitellum with forearm rotation. These cooperative motions contribute to a wide variety of ADLs and IADLs, such as painting, cooking, playing an instrument, and typing, to name a few.

The elbow joints are located within the same synovial cavity that contains the proximal radioulnar joint (PRUJ). The PRUJ, however, is distinct from the elbow joint (we'll explore it separately in a later section).

The **humeroulnar joint** acts as the primary hinge of the elbow (**6.11**). This joint demonstrates relatively more bony congruity than a ball-and-socket design, with the bony surfaces interlocked and constraining movement to flexion and extension with virtually no translation.[2]

The close-pack position of the elbow is in full extension, where it is most stable for weight-bearing, and the open-pack position is in approximately 70° of flexion. After an elbow injury, the most comfortable position for the patient is often to keep the elbow flexed. This avoids tension on the surrounding ligaments and joint capsule, which may lead to stiffness.

The **ulnar** (medial) **collateral ligament (UCL)** attaches to the medial epicondyle and fans out to a distal attachment on the olecranon and coronoid processes (**6.12**). This ligament prevents excessive valgus (lateral angulation) at the elbow.

The weaker **radial** (lateral) **collateral ligament (RCL)** runs from the lateral epicondyle to the annular ligament of the radius. The RCL and the lateral aspect of the joint capsule prevent **varus** (medial angulation) at the elbow.

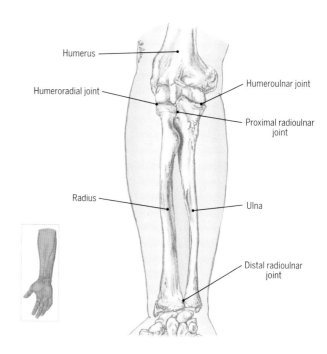

6.10 Joints of the elbow and forearm

We noted earlier that the elbow is anatomically positioned in 5°–15° of valgus. However, this angle may be different due to a congenital difference or injury.

- **Cubitus varus** indicates an angulation of the elbow positioning the forearm closer to the body (medial) than normal.
- **Cubitus valgus** describes an angulation of the elbow positioning the forearm farther away (lateral) from the body than normal (**6.13**).

While the humeroulnar joint is the primary articulation for flexion and extension of the elbow, the

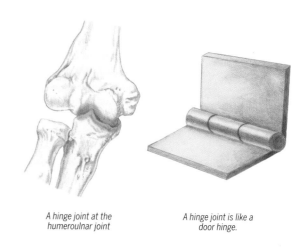

A hinge joint at the humeroulnar joint

A hinge joint is like a door hinge.

6.11 The humeroulnar joint is a hinge joint.

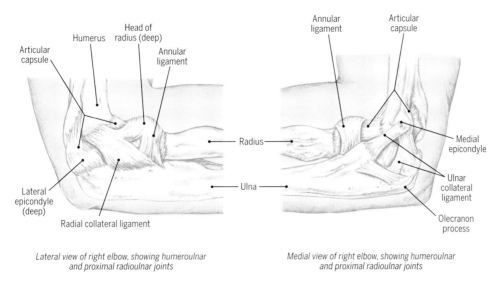

Lateral view of right elbow, showing humeroulnar and proximal radioulnar joints

Medial view of right elbow, showing humeroulnar and proximal radioulnar joints

6.12 Ligaments of the elbow

humeroradial joint also flexes and extends around the capitellum as a component of the overall elbow hinge. However, there is less bony surface contact and congruity compared to the humeroulnar joint and the radial head pivots relative to the capitellum with forearm rotation (**6.14**). This axis of motion is relatively fixed, passing through the heads of the radius and ulna.[3]

The humeroradial joint's most stable (close-pack) position is in full supination with the elbow extended, and its most mobile (open-pack) position is in slight supination beyond neutral with the elbow flexed. These joint dynamics contribute to the balance of stability and mobility necessary for motor performance, such as when lifting, carrying, and manipulating objects.

The annular ligament, which is part of the elbow joint capsule, is primarily responsible for maintaining the position of the head of the radius within the elbow joint (preventing inferior displacement). We will learn more about this ligament in the next section.

6.13 Cubitus varus (right elbow) and cubitus valgus (left elbow)

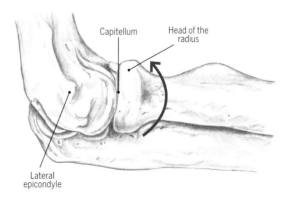

6.14 Humeroradial joint. The radial head rotates with forearm supination and pronation.

Proximal Radioulnar Joint

Structural classification: pivot

Functional (mechanical) classification: uniaxial

Movements: pronation, supination

The **proximal radioulnar joint (PRUJ)** is a pivot joint, permitting only axial rotation. This motion results in pronation and supination of the forearm and hand, which is carried along with rotation of the radius around the ulna.

The radial head, a component of the PRUJ, is held in the radial notch of the ulna by the **annular ligament** of the radius (**6.15**). This ligament wraps around the circumference of the radial head.

The annular ligament has an inferior rim that is important for preventing a distal dislocation of the

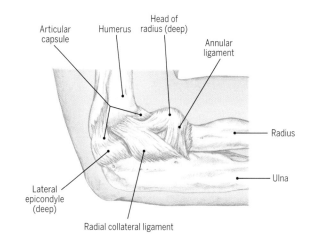

Lateral view of right elbow, showing humeroulnar and proximal radioulnar joints

6.15 Ligaments of the elbow

CLINICAL APPLICATION
Elbow Dislocation

Many patient injuries to the upper extremity that you may encounter as a future clinician occur as a result of a fall. Elbow dislocations are frequently related to a fall-on-outstretched-hands (FOOSH) injury or other trauma that forces the ulna posterior relative to the distal humerus (**6.16**).

Elbow joint dislocation is almost always posterior. This injury is a clinical emergency because of the many neurovascular structures that cross the joint. Nerves and blood vessels move relatively freely in the soft tissues of the upper arm. However, the upper arm narrows as it moves toward the elbow, creating an anatomical choke point for these neurovascular structures as they pass through to the forearm. Dislocation disrupts these tightly engineered spaces and can place damaging tension or compression on the ulnar, radial, or median nerves, with potentially long-term functional consequences. Closed reduction or surgical repair attempts to restore the anatomical position and stability of the elbow while preserving neurovascular function.

Rehabilitation often involves a period of immobilization to encourage stability of the joint, followed by interventions to safely restore motion, strength, and function. What functional limitations would an individual experience with stiffness of the elbow and forearm after immobilization? What compensatory or adaptive techniques might be beneficial?

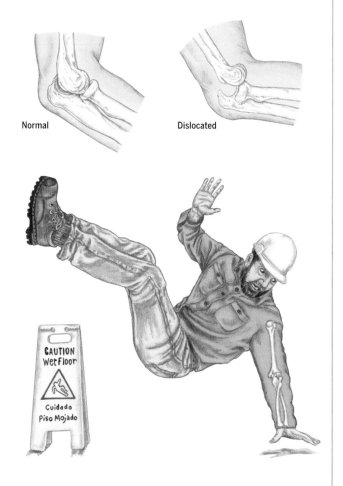

6.16 Fall on outstretched hands (FOOSH) resulting in a posterior elbow dislocation

PRUJ, or the radius being displaced distally. However, in young children, the head of the radius is still largely cartilaginous and, consequently, deformable. If a child's muscles are relaxed, a strong distal pull on the forearm can result in a partial descent of the radial head through the inferior opening in the annular ligament. This condition is traditionally called "nursemaid's elbow" because it often arose from an impatient caregiver yanking on a child's hand in an upward motion or swinging the child around by the arms, creating traction of the radius.

Limitations of individual or multiple joints involved in forearm rotation—the humeroradial joint, PRUJ, and distal radioulnar joint (DRUJ) (see Chapter 7)—may limit functional motion of the entire forearm. Functional rotation of the forearm and associated compensatory patterns are described later in this chapter.

Musculature and Movement

The muscles of the elbow and forearm (6.17–6.19) relate to occupational performance beyond simply lifting or carrying objects. Consider their broader capabilities: How might these muscle groups enable the motor performance skills involved in ADLs or IADLs as well as functional mobility? As you work through this section, think of additional functional examples.

▶TRY IT

Let's explore self-feeding as an ADL that requires simultaneous elbow and forearm motion. First, find an apple or other piece of fruit. What motions are involved with simply picking up the fruit and taking a bite? Mimic these actions as you conceptualize them.

Now consider a patient who has sustained an injury with significant limitations in forearm rotation. Try to pick up the fruit and take a bite while keeping your forearm in a neutral position without rotating it (thumbs up). What happens?

Did you notice your shoulder naturally begin to compensate? What shoulder motions might compensate for a loss of forearm pronation or supination?

In your future practice, if you are working with a patient to restore true forearm rotation, you may want to prevent this compensatory pattern of shoulder motion. For someone with more permanent loss of forearm mobility, how might this substitute movement serve as a beneficial compensatory strategy?

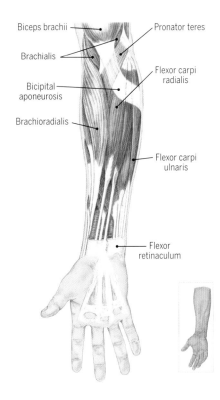

6.17 Anterior view of right forearm

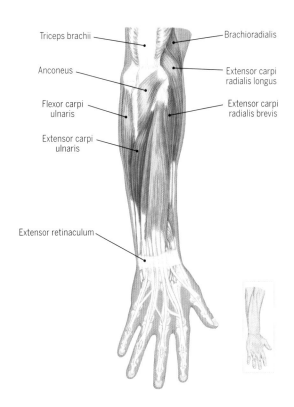

6.18 Posterior view of right forearm

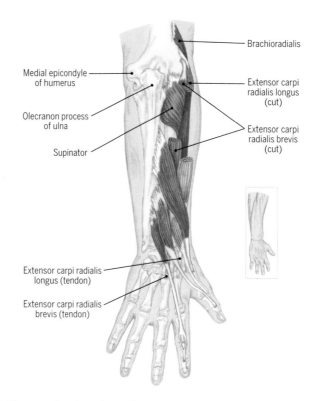

6.19 Posterior view of right forearm, showing deep layer of muscles

Flexors of the Elbow

Biceps brachii
Brachialis
Brachioradialis

The flexors of the elbow bring the hand closer to the body to facilitate personal hygiene, self-feeding, lifting objects, and similar functional activities (**6.20**).

Biceps Brachii

The **biceps brachii**, mentioned in Chapter 5, is featured again here because it is a two-joint muscle, exerting force at both the shoulder and elbow joints (**6.21**).

Look carefully at Figure **6.21** and you will see two distinct tendons—the long and short heads—that serve as dual origins on the scapula. The long head of the biceps crosses and contributes to flexion of the glenohumeral joint. Now follow the muscle fibers as they pass downward across the anterior humerus. Did you notice they converge into a single insertion?

In addition, some fibers of the biceps brachii tendon sweep away from the medial edge of the tendon and insert into the deep fascia along the anteromedial aspect

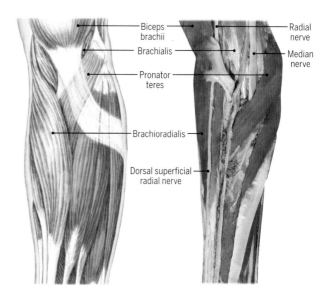

Anterior (volar) view

6.20 Flexors of the elbow

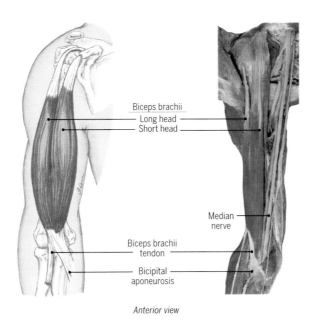

Biceps brachii
Long head
Short head

Median
nerve

Biceps brachii
tendon

Bicipital
aponeurosis

Anterior view

6.21 Biceps brachii

of the forearm. This tendinous expansion is called the **bicipital aponeurosis**.

Take a close look at the pathway of the median nerve as it crosses the elbow. It runs beneath the bicipital aponeurosis, along with the brachial artery, which helps to protect these delicate neurovascular structures from injury or during surgery. For this reason, the thick fascia is sometimes referred to as the grâce à Dieu (praise to God) fascia.

The primary function of the biceps brachii is elbow flexion. But with its insertion into the radial tuberosity, it also acts on the proximal radioulnar joint as a supinator. The biceps brachii can generate more force for supination with the elbow in a flexed position, as when turning a doorknob, as opposed to functional motion with the elbow extended, as when tightening a screw overhead with a manual screwdriver in the right hand.

If the biceps ruptures, supination is often more affected than flexion, as there are other strong elbow flexors, such as the brachialis and brachioradialis. Also, the biceps is a stronger supinator than the supinator itself due to its larger cross-sectional area.

The biceps is most effective as a flexor of the elbow with the forearm supinated, as when you bring a washcloth toward your face. It is inhibited when flexing the elbow with the forearm pronated, such as when putting on glasses, preventing undesired supination.

This is one reason that a chin-up is easier to perform than a pull-up. With a chin-up, the forearm is supinated, permitting the biceps to aid in flexion of the elbow joint. For a pull-up, the forearms remain pronated, and the biceps are of limited use relative to the lifting.

BICEPS BRACHII	
Purposeful Activity	
P	Combing your hair, eating an apple, washing your face (elbow flexion with the forearm supinated)
A	**Flex** the elbow (humeroulnar joint) **Supinate** the forearm (radioulnar joints) **Flex** the shoulder (glenohumeral joint)
O	Short head: Coracoid process of scapula Long head: Supraglenoid tubercle of scapula
I	Radial tuberosity and bicipital aponeurosis
N	Musculocutaneous C5 and C6

▶TRY IT

Let's palpate to compare biceps muscle recruitment with the elbow flexed and extended. With your elbow flexed, palpate your biceps muscle while forcefully supinating your forearm. What happens?

Did you notice the strong contraction? Try the same thing with the elbow extended with your arm overhead. Did you notice any difference?

Brachialis

The **brachialis** is a deep muscle arising from the anterior humeral shaft distal to the deltoid tuberosity (**6.22**). The fibers of the brachialis cross the elbow to insert into the coronoid process and the anterior aspect of the ulnar shaft that is immediately distal to it (ulnar tuberosity).

Because the brachialis crosses only the elbow joint and inserts into the stable (nonrotating) proximal ulna, it is a pure flexor of this joint. Referred to as the "workhorse of elbow flexion," the brachialis is active regardless of forearm position. Think about Jamie's case study and how the action of this muscle relates to completion of her daily work tasks.

Brachioradialis

Originating from the upper two-thirds of the lateral supracondylar ridge of the humerus, the **brachioradialis** crosses the anterolateral aspect of the elbow (**6.23**). Its fibers continue distally as a tendon along the radial aspect of the forearm and insert into the radial styloid.

The brachioradialis acts to flex the elbow joint. This muscle can also rotate the forearm to neutral (thumb up) from the supinated or pronated position but not beyond. It can best flex the elbow with the forearm neutral. The brachioradialis is active during self-feeding or drinking. You might think of it as the coffee-drinking muscle.

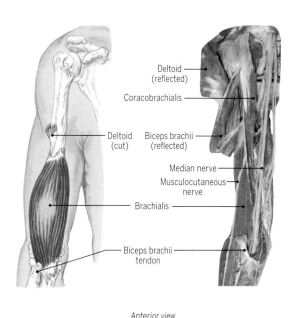

Anterior view

6.22 Brachialis

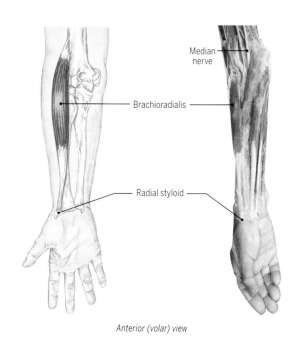

Anterior (volar) view

6.23 Brachioradialis

BRACHIALIS	
Purposeful Activity	
P	Eating soup, brushing your teeth (elbow flexion with the forearm pronated)
A	Flex the elbow (humeroulnar joint)
O	Distal half of anterior surface of humerus
I	Ulnar tuberosity and coronoid process of ulna
N	Musculocutaneous, small branch from radial C5 and C6

BRACHIORADIALIS	
Purposeful Activity	
P	Hammering a nail, playing a drum (elbow flexion with the forearm neutral)
A	Flex the elbow (humeroulnar joint) Assist to **pronate** and **supinate** the forearm when these movements are resisted (humeroradial joints)
O	Proximal two-thirds of the lateral supracondylar ridge of humerus
I	Radial styloid
N	Radial C5 and C6

Extensors of the Elbow

Triceps brachii
Anconeus

The extensors of the elbow move the hand away from the body for activities involving open-chain motion, such as casting a fishing line. This muscle group is also important for functional mobility when using the upper extremities in a closed-chain pattern to support movement or positioning of the body. Some examples include pushing down on the arms of a chair to stand up or using a cane to improve stability while walking.

Triceps Brachii

The **triceps brachii** is composed of three bellies—the long, lateral, and medial heads—with separate origins and a common tendinous insertion into the olecranon process of the ulna (**6.24**).

The long and lateral heads are superficial while the medial head is relatively deeper. The long head crosses both the shoulder and elbow joints and, as a result, can extend both of these joints. The medial and lateral heads supply the forces for moderate extension, as when placing a book on a high shelf. The long head is recruited for higher resistance, such as when doing a push-up.

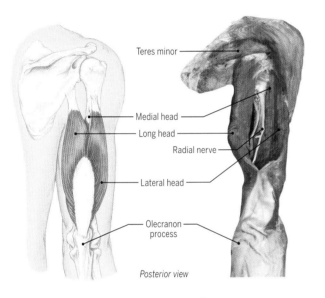

6.24 Triceps brachii

TRICEPS BRACHII	
Purposeful Activity	
P	Transfers (pushing up from the arms of a chair), wheelchair mobility
A	All heads: **Extend** the elbow (humeroulnar joint) Long head: **Extend** the shoulder (GHJ) **Adduct** the shoulder (GHJ)
O	Long head: Infraglenoid tubercle of the scapula Lateral head: Posterior surface of proximal half of the humerus Medial head: Posterior surface of distal half of the humerus
I	Olecranon process of the ulna
N	Radial C6 to C8, T1

Anconeus

The **anconeus** arises from a small area on the posterolateral aspect of the humerus (**6.25**). Its fibers run inferomedially, fanning out and inserting on the superolateral surface of the ulna, including the olecranon process.

Based on its size and attachments, the anconeus is described as a weak extensor of the elbow, contributing to functional movements similar to those of the triceps.

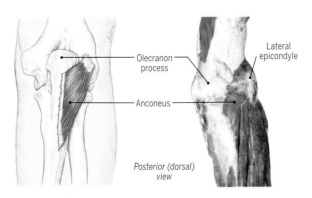

6.25 Anconeus

ANCONEUS	
Purposeful Activity	
P	Casting a fishing line, throwing a football
A	**Extend** the elbow (humeroulnar joint)
O	Lateral epicondyle of the humerus
I	Olecranon process and posterior, proximal surface of ulna
N	Radial C7 and C8

CLINICAL APPLICATION
Cubital Tunnel Syndrome

Refer to Figure **6.26** and take a close look at the ulnar nerve pathway. Do you notice how it disappears from view once it enters the elbow? The **cubital tunnel** is a bony passageway posterior to the medial epicondyle of the elbow. The roof of this tunnel is elastic and formed by a retinaculum called the **ligament of Osborne**. Chronic compression or tension on the ulnar nerve within the tunnel is known as **cubital tunnel syndrome**.

This syndrome is generally considered a cumulative trauma disorder (CTD). Daily habits or routines involving prolonged elbow flexion, such as texting while lying in bed, may increase internal pressure within the cubital tunnel and can place tension on the nerve, leading to distinct paresthesia (tingling) in the ring and small fingers. How might you modify an individual's habits or routines to prevent these symptoms?

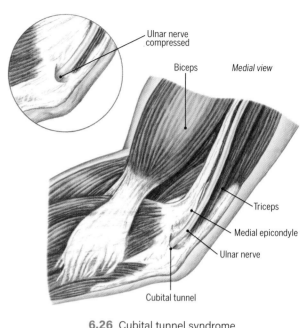

6.26 Cubital tunnel syndrome

Primary Rotators of the Forearm

Biceps brachii (see flexors of the elbow)
Supinator
Pronator teres
Pronator quadratus

The primary rotator muscles supply the forces to specifically rotate the forearm for object manipulation, such as when turning a smartphone faceup to read a text message or opening a letter.

Supinator

The **supinator** lies deep to the extensor muscles. Take a close look at the way its fibers are arranged on the dorsolateral forearm (**6.27**).

Do you notice how the supinator crosses the forearm diagonally from the lateral epicondyle of the humerus to the proximal radius? This arrangement is a clear example of structure determining function: the diagonal, or oblique, alignment of the supinator fibers allows

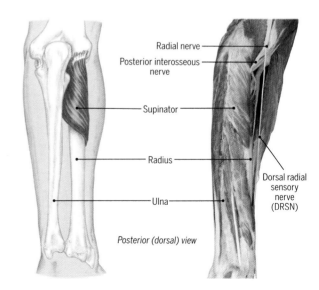

JAMIE ROBBINS | Review Jamie's case so far, along with the Clinical Application feature on cubital tunnel syndrome. Jamie is now complaining of occasional numbness and tingling, mainly in her ring and small fingers. How might these symptoms be related to her daily roles, habits, and routines?

6.27 Supinator

the muscle to rotate the forearm. These motions often occur simultaneously, such as when you use your smartphone to respond to the text message you just received.

The forearm can generate considerably more strength for supination than it can for pronation due to the force generated by the biceps brachii. This is the reason, along with the preponderance of right-handedness, that screws are designed to be tightened by supination as opposed to pronation.

Refer again to the cadaver figure (6.27, right). Do you see the nerve that passes beneath the proximal edge of the supinator? This is the deep branch of the radial nerve, which becomes the posterior interosseous nerve (PIN), or motor branch of the radial nerve. As it passes beneath the supinator, the PIN may become compressed, leading to pain and eventual weakness of the extensor muscles of the wrist and fingers. This condition is known as PIN syndrome and may be caused by repetitive forearm rotation with resistance. Can you think of specific work or leisure activities that might increase the risk of PIN syndrome? The superficial branch of the radial nerve, also referred to as the dorsal radial sensory nerve (DRSN), splits off of the main radial pathway. This nerve provides sensory innervation to the radial aspect of the dorsal wrist and thumb.

SUPINATOR
Purposeful Activity

P Using a screwdriver, turning a doorknob

A Supinate the forearm (radioulnar joints)

O Lateral epicondyle of humerus, radial collateral ligament, annular ligament, and supinator crest of the ulna

I Anterior, lateral surface of proximal one-third of radial shaft

N Radial C5 to C7

Pronator Teres

The **pronator teres** originates primarily from the medial supracondylar ridge of the humerus (6.28).

Notice that, similar to the supinator, the **pronator teres** has fibers that are oriented diagonally (oblique), attaching to the radius. However, this muscle is positioned on the anterior forearm and, unlike the supinator, originates on the medial epicondyle. As a result—and as you probably guessed from its name—this muscle pronates the forearm, as when throwing an object into a wastebasket.

Notice on the cadaver figure how the median nerve enters the forearm between the two heads of this muscle (6.28, right). Compression of the median nerve beneath these muscle fibers describes a condition known as **pronator teres syndrome**, which may cause a similar pattern of numbness and tingling in the hand as carpal tunnel syndrome.

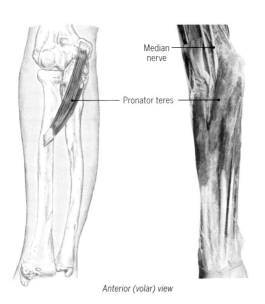

Median nerve
Pronator teres

Anterior (volar) view

6.28 Pronator teres

PRONATOR TERES
Purposeful Activity

P Knitting, pouring coffee

A Pronate the forearm (radioulnar joints)
   Assist to flex the elbow (humeroulnar joint)

O Common flexor tendon from medial epicondyle of humerus and coronoid process of the ulna

I Middle of lateral surface of the radius

N Median C6 and C7

Severe compression or severance of the median nerve at this level may result in a pattern of motor loss known as the hand of benediction, which involves lack of flexion of the thumb, index, and middle fingers when making a fist, similar to a priest offering the sign of blessing (see Chapter 7).

Pronator Quadratus

Pronator quadratus is a deeply placed muscle lying just proximal to the wrist (**6.29**). It is active for all forearm pronation and is particularly important for pronation with the elbow fully flexed, as this position shortens and inhibits the pronator quadratus. For example, you use this motion when shaving or putting on makeup.

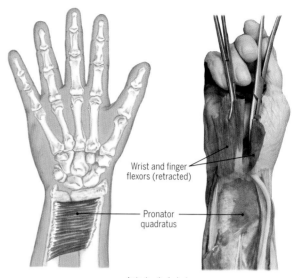

Anterior (volar) view

6.29 Pronator quadratus

JAMIE ROBBINS | Now that we know more about the muscles of the elbow and forearm, let's think more about Jamie. Do some activity analysis:

- What motor performance skills are required for Jamie's IADLs, work, and leisure occupations?
- How might performance of these occupations align with the symptoms she described in her occupational profile?
- What muscles of the elbow or forearm are involved?

PRONATOR QUADRATUS	
Purposeful Activity	
P	**Replacing an overhead light bulb, unlocking a combination lock**
A	**Pronate** the forearm (radioulnar joints)
O	Medial, anterior surface of distal ulna
I	Lateral, anterior surface of distal radius
N	Median C7 and C8, T1

▶ TRY IT

The elbow is an important site of origin for the muscles that act on the wrist and fingers. Many of the flexor muscles originate at the medial epicondyle, along with the pronator teres. The extensors originate predominantly at the lateral epicondyle with the supinator.

With your palm up, palpate the medial and lateral elbow just distal to the epicondyles (the sharp bony points on either side of the joint). Now flex and extend your wrist and fingers.

Did you notice the lateral muscles (extensors) contract with extension and medial muscles (flexors) contract with flexion? Now keep your wrist still and make a tight fist. What happens?

Did you notice both sides contract? Why would both the flexors and extensors contract when flexing the fingers only? Think about the wrist stability needed for grasping.

Imagine thousands of contractions of these muscle groups on a daily basis as we grip, type, use tools, text, and play video games, to name a few repetitive activities. This continuous use over time can cause cumulative trauma, or wear and tear, on soft tissues. Eventually, the soft tissues may fatigue, leading to painful CTDs like lateral or medial epicondylosis. Common CTDs in the elbow region are discussed later in this chapter.

Purposeful Movement of the Elbow and Forearm

Motions of the elbow and forearm are often simultaneous, rotating the hand while moving it closer to or farther from the body. Analyze the individual movements of the elbow and forearm and their integration into motion of the entire upper extremity for occupational performance. In Figures **6.30**–**6.33**, prime movers are listed first, with asterisks indicating muscles not shown.

Flexion

(*antagonists on extension*)
Biceps brachii
Brachialis
Brachioradialis
Flexor carpi radialis (assists)*
Flexor carpi ulnaris (assists)*
Palmaris longus (assists)*
Pronator teres (assists)*
Extensor carpi radialis
longus (assists)*
Extensor carpi radialis brevis
(assists)*

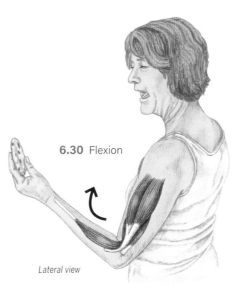

6.30 Flexion

Lateral view

Extension

(*antagonists on flexion*)
Triceps brachii (all heads)
Anconeus*

Posterior view

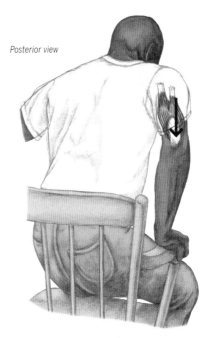

6.31 Extension

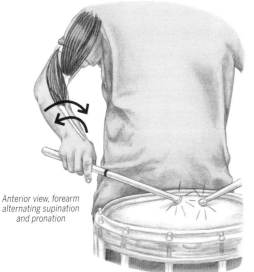

Anterior view, forearm alternating supination and pronation

6.32 Supination

Supination

(*antagonists on pronation*)
Biceps brachii
Supinator*
Brachioradialis (assists)

Pronation

(*antagonists on supination*)
Pronator teres
Pronator quadratus*
Brachioradialis (assists)

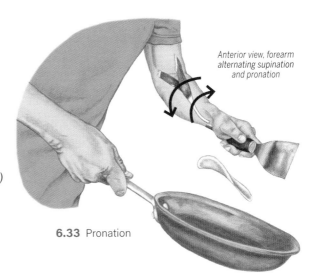

Anterior view, forearm alternating supination and pronation

6.33 Pronation

OT Guide to Goniometry & MMT: Elbow and Forearm

Now that you know the underlying anatomy and movements of the elbow and forearm, let's practice goniometry and MMT using the *OT Guide to Goniometry & MMT* eTextbook.

Practice narrating the underlying anatomy and related functional tasks associated with the particular motions. This will help to solidify your knowledge, make connections between anatomy and occupation, and prepare you to better educate your future patients. For example, while measuring forearm supination with the arm at the side, you might say, "This motion is often used for turning dials and knobs or flipping pancakes. The muscles that contribute to this motion are the biceps brachii and supinator." Think about the functional examples provided, but also think of other examples.

Once you are comfortable with each technique, take it a step further and compare the *typical* range of motion available at each joint to the *functional* range needed for specific ADLs or IADLs. How much elbow flexion is required to shave? How much pronation is needed to type on a keyboard? Also consider how you might use these values to set specific occupation-based goals for an individual with a deficit in motion or strength.

Occupational and Clinical Perspectives

The following sections explore several occupational and clinical applications of the underlying anatomy and purposeful movement of the elbow and forearm. These motions contribute to the motor performance skills needed for ADLs like self-feeding and hygiene, as well as for IADLs involving carrying or manipulating objects.

Elbow and Self-Care

The elbow joint positions the hand in space for prehensile (grasp or pinch) activities and object manipulation. As the only joint in the upper extremity that can bring the hand inward in the sagittal plane, toward the body, the elbow is especially significant for occupation, specifically for ADLs.

Without functional flexion and extension of the elbow, basic self-care tasks such as self-feeding and hygiene (shaving, brushing teeth) are severely limited. Imagine a joint contracture of the elbow limiting active flexion to 30°. Simply bringing the hand to the mouth for self-feeding or brushing teeth would become impossible (**6.34**).

Additionally, the PRUJ allows for rotation of the radius around a longitudinal axis, in cooperation with the DRUJ, such as when opening a medicine bottle or jar of peanut butter. Three distinct articulations—humeroulnar joint, humeroradial joint, and PRUJ—are configured for isolated or combined elbow flexion or extension with forearm rotation (along with the DRUJ).

Consider using a spoon to eat soup (**6.35**). The elbow is initially held in static flexion to hold the hand over

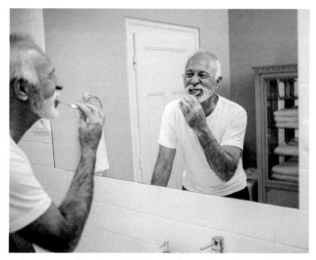

6.34 Personal hygiene. What muscles and motions of the elbow and forearm are involved when brushing your teeth?

the bowl, while the forearm pronates to dip the spoon into the soup. The forearm then supinates to neutral to balance the liquid on the spoon, while the elbow flexes and then brings the spoon to the mouth. The elbow flexes at the humeroulnar joint, with the olecranon and coronoid processes clutching the trochlea of the distal humerus like a claw. Forearm rotation occurs as the proximal radius revolves relative to the capitellum (superiorly) as well as the adjacent proximal ulna (PRUJ). The radius and ulna articulate just proximal to the wrist at the DRUJ, which pivots and glides proportional to the PRUJ for functional rotation of the forearm.

Think about and practice describing in your own words the movement and underlying anatomy required for other ADLs involving the elbow and forearm.

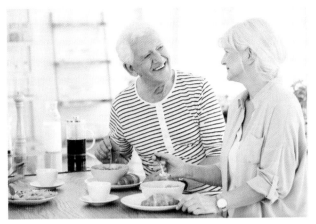

6.35 Self-feeding. What specific coordinated movements of the elbow and forearm are involved when eating soup?

Functional Forearm Rotation

True forearm rotation occurs with the elbow fixed in space, such as when turning a doorknob with the elbow against the side of the body. At the proximal forearm, the radius rotates around a fixed ulna, while distally, near the wrist, the radius rotates as the ulna moves (translates) laterally with pronation and medially with supination (**6.36**).

When the elbow and forearm are moving freely in space, as opposed to in a fixed position, shoulder movements may enhance, or compensate for a deficit of, forearm

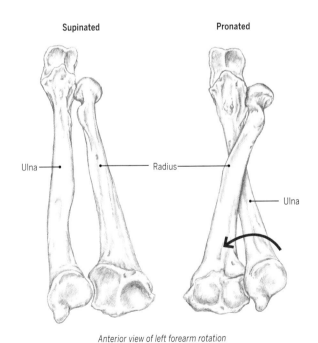

Supinated   Pronated

Ulna — | — Radius — | — Ulna

Anterior view of left forearm rotation

6.36 The radius and ulna contribute to forearm rotation. How does the relative position of these bones change with the forearm supinated, pronated, and neutral (thumbs up)?

▶**TRY IT**

Let's compare movement of the ulna during forearm rotation at the proximal and distal forearm.

First, stabilize your elbow against your side to prevent the compensatory shoulder motions mentioned earlier. Now, place your hand on the proximal ulna while rotating your forearm. Then place your hand on the distal ulna with the same motion.

Can you feel the difference in ulnar mobility? How would you describe it?

rotation. Shoulder abduction and internal rotation increase the ability of the palm to turn downward (pronation), whereas shoulder adduction and external rotation turn the hand upward (supination) (**6.37**).

As a practitioner assessing the range of motion of an individual's forearm rotation, you'll want to be sure to maintain the elbow in a flexed position against the side of the body. This allows you to measure true forearm rotation and prevent compensatory motion. Also remember that forearm rotation involves cooperation of the PRUJ and DRUJ. Restrictions in either or both of these joints may limit overall forearm rotation.

Forearm position affects individual muscle force (sufficiency) for various functional movements of the elbow and forearm. For example, with the forearm supinated (anatomical position), the biceps brachii has a strong moment to flex the elbow. A neutral or pronated forearm relies more on the brachioradialis or brachialis for elbow flexion, lessening the demand on the biceps.

These are important considerations, specifically when analyzing repetitive forceful movements of the elbow and forearm. For example, if a worker who lifts and carries

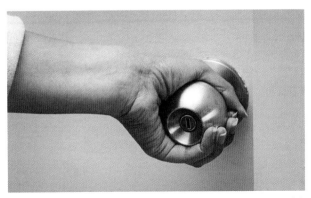

6.37 Turning a doorknob. What motions of the shoulder could compensate for a loss of forearm rotation for this functional task?

heavy objects frequently experiences bicipital tendinitis, or inflammation of the long head of the biceps (see Chapter 5), how might you recommend they modify their lifting technique to decrease these symptoms?

Encouraging an individual to lift with the forearm neutral (thumbs up) or pronated, if possible, may limit recruitment of the biceps and decrease the repetitive stress that is contributing to the symptoms.

When supinating the forearm with the shoulder flexed and elbow extended, as when changing a light bulb, the supinator is recruited first. The biceps becomes involved when increasing speed or strength is needed (6.38). Addressing the pace and strength required for functional activities may also lessen harmful repetitive forces to specific muscles or muscle groups. How might this relate to Jamie's situation in the case study?

Scapular Depression Transfer

The unique design of the elbow joint allows scapular movements to compensate for a loss of active elbow extension to perform transfers. Bony congruity contributes to elbow stability in the fully extended position with the elbow "locked" (the olecranon process stabilized in its fossa, its close-pack position). Articular stability decreases as the elbow flexes, decreasing bony

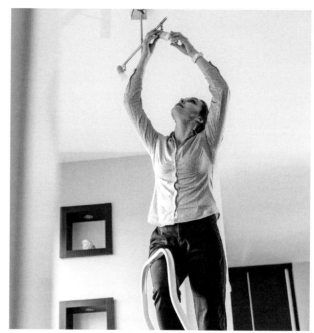

6.38 Home management. Which muscle(s) are most active for forearm supination when changing an overhead light bulb?

congruity and relying more on the joint capsule and collateral ligaments for dynamic stability. Locking in the extended position is possible even without active contraction of the triceps.

▶TRY IT

Sit on the floor with your elbows extended under the force of gravity (without triceps contraction) at your side. Now, with your wrists extended and palms flat on the ground, depress your scapulae (shoulder girdle), pushing weight through the extended elbows.

Did you notice your elbow passively "locking" in hyperextension? See if you can raise your body off the floor in this manner and scoot from side to side.

Were you successful? If so, you just demonstrated a modified technique used for bed mobility and transfers, referred to as a scapular depression transfer. This technique is commonly used by individuals with spinal cord injuries (SCIs) at the C6 level, who have lost active elbow extension but still have shoulder girdle control and can extend their wrists. Elbow bony congruity allows downward force to pass through the locked elbow in a closed-chain position to elevate the body, allowing for functional transfers (6.39).

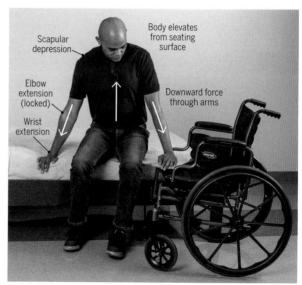

6.39 Scapular depression transfer. How can the scapula compensate for a loss of active elbow extension for bed mobility and transfers?

Cubital Tunnel Syndrome

Have you ever been texting in bed, holding a smartphone or tablet close to your face, and noticed numbness in your ring and small fingers? As you learned earlier, this is due to the increased pressure and tension on the ulnar nerve in the cubital tunnel with the elbow in a flexed position.

The tingling typically goes away after straightening the elbow for a few minutes. However, persistent symptoms may indicate cubital tunnel syndrome, which—if left untreated—may lead to more chronic symptoms or even muscle atrophy.

Modifying an individual's environment, habits and routines, or method for performing a specific activity in ways that minimize elbow flexion may decrease stress to the nerve and lessen symptoms as a result. Positions of sleep and rest, often maintained continuously for several hours, can also be improved with the use of a soft wrap or orthosis to discourage elbow flexion.

Ulnar Collateral Ligament Injury

Recall that the ulnar and radial collateral ligaments stabilize the elbow against medial and lateral forces. The elbow is anatomically positioned in mild valgus, so the UCL is thicker and relatively stronger than the RCL.

The UCL plays a major role in throwing technique for athletes such as baseball pitchers, particularly those with a sidearm style. As the arm accelerates forward with the shoulder externally rotated, the UCL endures extreme tensile stress, transmitting forces generated

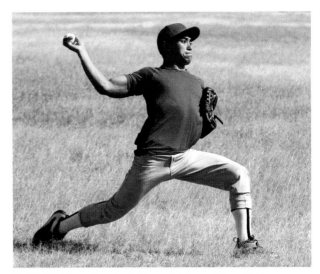

6.40 Pitching a baseball. How might repetitive pitching impact the elbow joint and its surrounding ligaments?

by the lower extremities, core, and shoulder to the forearm and hand to throw a fastball across the plate (**6.40**). Over time, repetitive forceful elongation of the UCL may lead to plastic deformation, resulting in instability and loss of velocity for throwing athletes.

General Stiffness and Flexion Contractures

The elbow has a high degree of bony congruity and strong reinforcing collateral ligaments, as well as neurovascular structures that pass through tight anatomical spaces. While beneficial, these features predispose the elbow to general stiffness after a fracture or dislocation.

Full elbow extension (the close-pack position) places considerable tension on its surrounding ligaments. After injury, the elbow often must be immobilized in some degree of flexion to allow for healing. Typically, patients prefer the flexed position, even when the elbow is not immobilized, to avoid painful tension on these supporting structures and pain receptors in the joint capsule.

Maintaining a flexed elbow for a time may be necessary to restore stability but may also lead to adaptive shortening of the surrounding soft tissues, particularly the UCL and joint capsule. Commonly, this leads to a **flexion contracture**, or limited active and passive extension due to soft tissue restrictions. Elbow flexion contractures are common after orthopedic immobilization.

Extension contractures, or a position of extension with limited flexion, are less common but do occur and can significantly impact function. Osteoarthritis (OA) may also develop after a traumatic elbow injury that

CLINICAL APPLICATION
Tommy John Surgery

Reconstructive surgery addressing UCL dysfunction was developed in the 1970s by Los Angeles Dodgers team physician Dr. Frank Jobe. Using a tendon transfer, Jobe reconstructed the injured UCL of pitcher Tommy John. The surgery was an overwhelming success: John continued pitching in the major leagues for twelve years after the surgery, with 164 of his 288 career wins coming after the surgery.[4] The technique is now widely used for collegiate and professional pitchers, many of whom return to full performance even after multiple procedures.

Research UCL injuries. In what other sports are they found? What additional functional activities might contribute to elongation and laxity of the UCL?

disrupts the precise alignment of the articular surfaces and joint mechanics.

Think about activities and occupations that might be difficult without full elbow extension. Patients frequently express difficulty with feeding themselves, washing their hair, and lifting and carrying, as well as using an ATM. How might you modify these types of activities for an individual with long-term, or even permanent, loss of elbow motion?

Overly aggressive treatment at the elbow should be avoided, as this may increase inflammation or damage surrounding soft tissues. Instead, experienced practitioners often focus on using low-load prolonged stress to restore soft tissue length and joint mobility. Static progressive orthoses apply low-load stress to encourage safe, incremental tissue elongation to restore functional motion for occupational performance (6.41).

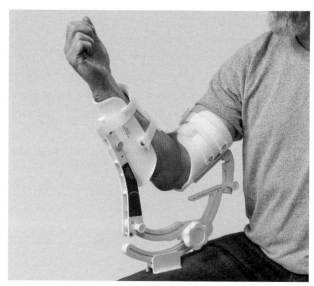

6.41 Mobilization orthosis. How could a static progressive orthosis be used as an intervention to support occupational performance?

Cumulative Trauma Disorders

Because the medial and lateral humeral epicondyles provide the origin for the flexor-pronator and extensor-supinator muscle groups, these locations are susceptible to **cumulative trauma disorders (CTDs)**.

Repetitive musculoskeletal forces, whether from rapid finger movements while typing or extended forceful grasp for a racket sport, can cause microtrauma to the related tendinous muscle origins. This in turn may lead to acute inflammation and eventual degeneration (wear and tear). Two common forms of CTDs at the elbow are **lateral epicondylosis** (tennis elbow) and **medial epicondylosis** (golfer's elbow). These diagnoses are commonly referred to as lateral and medial epicondylitis. However, the term epicondylosis is more accurate in describing the degenerative nature of the pathology.

A recent Nielsen survey found US adults spend more than eleven hours per day interacting with digital media in the form of laptop computers, tablets, or smartphones.[5] This trend represents thousands of repetitions of digital flexion and extension each hour, with prolonged cyclical tensioning of the opposing flexor and extensor tendons at their respective origins, along with the demands of other ADLs and IADLs.

Many muscles that originate at the elbow contribute to wrist and finger motion and strength. Gripping and object manipulation also involve the wrist flexor and extensor muscles to stabilize the wrist and transmit force to the fingers. Leisure or work occupations involving repetitive gripping, such as playing tennis or using manual tools, may also contribute to cumulative trauma (6.42).

You may be familiar with the Person-Environment-Occupation (PEO) Model by now, especially if you researched it for Jamie's case at the beginning of this chapter. This model is frequently used as a theoretical guide for ergonomic evaluation and intervention. Following this model, clinicians may introduce preventative measures such as warm-up activities, modify a workstation or tools to promote neutral joint angles, and modify

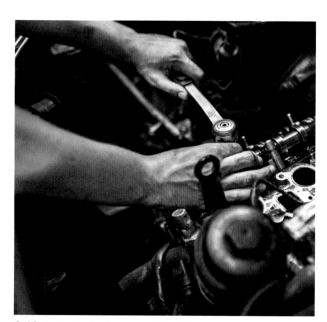

6.42 Auto mechanic. How might this work occupation contribute to cumulative trauma of the elbow, wrist, and hand?

the way a worker completes tasks in order to decrease tension on soft tissues, particularly tasks performed with the elbow extended.

The elbow and forearm contribute essential purposeful movement of the upper extremity to occupational performance. Along with shoulder motion, the elbow and forearm movements position the hand for manipulating objects, interacting with the environment, and communicating.

As we move distally into the complex anatomy of the hand, remember that the upper extremity functions as a unit, and fine motor control of the hand requires stable motion and positioning of the shoulder, elbow, and forearm.

APPLY AND REVIEW

Jamie Robbins

Jamie arrives at the clinic for her OT evaluation. After reviewing her occupational profile (refer to the beginning of the chapter), you ask some additional questions and complete a physical examination.

Jamie reports she has been experiencing pain of 8/10 on the visual analog scale (VAS) when using her left forearm and hand and pain of 4/10 at rest. The pain is of a sharp quality, localized to the elbow. She denies left neck and shoulder pain but does experience occasional numbness and tingling, mainly in her ring and small fingers.

She demonstrates full active range of motion throughout her neck and upper extremities, but movements of the left wrist and hand are painful. You decide not to perform MMT on her left elbow or wrist due to her pain level but note all movements of her right elbow, forearm, and wrist demonstrate 5/5 strength. She has 55 lb. of grip strength in her right hand, but again, you avoid grip strength testing in the left hand due to pain with grasp.

Palpation reveals tenderness on the tendon origins just distal to the medial and lateral epicondyles of her left elbow. Specific orthopedic tests—Maudsley's and Mill's—are both positive. She also experiences significant pain with passive wrist and digit extension. Do some research to see what these tests might indicate.

Think about all the components of Jamie's evaluation using a top-down approach: consider her occupational profile first, then analyze the performance skills and related anatomy to identify specific limitations to occupational performance. As you piece together

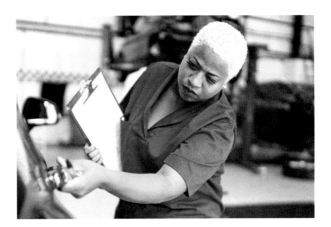

these various components using clinical reasoning, consider the following questions:

- What diagnosis (or diagnoses) do you suspect based on the information provided?
- How might Jamie's IADLs and work and leisure occupations be contributing to her symptoms? Are her performance patterns a factor?
- What modifications or adaptations would you recommend for the specific work and leisure occupations you identified from her occupational profile?
- Do some research on the diagnosis (or diagnoses) you suspect. What interventions does the research support as beneficial?
- If Jamie's company were to hire you as a consultant, what education or recommendations might you provide to prevent CTDs for a group of assembly line workers that perform similar repetitive work tasks?

Review Questions

1. Which articulation of the elbow is *primarily* responsible for elbow flexion and extension?
   a. humeroulnar joint
   b. humeroradial joint
   c. proximal radioulnar joint (PRUJ)
   d. radiocarpal joint

2. Which of the following ADLs would be significantly limited by a loss of elbow flexion in the dominant upper extremity?
   a. hygiene
   b. lower body dressing
   c. self-feeding
   d. both A and C

3. You are working with a patient with stiffness of the forearm that significantly limits their active forearm supination. Which of the following motions would compensate for this specific loss of forearm motion?
   a. shoulder abduction and internal rotation
   b. shoulder and elbow flexion
   c. shoulder adduction and external rotation
   d. contralateral trunk flexion and shoulder internal rotation

4. Which of the following structures provides the *most* medial stability to the elbow?
   a. ulnar collateral ligament
   b. annular ligament
   c. radial collateral ligament
   d. oblique cord

5. The humeroulnar joint is *best* described as what type of articulation?
   a. uniaxial pivot
   b. uniaxial hinge
   c. triaxial ball-and-socket
   d. biaxial pivot

6. For which of the following would the biceps brachii muscle be *most* active?
   a. unscrewing a light bulb overhead with your left hand
   b. using a screwdriver to tighten a screw with your right hand, with the arm at the side
   c. using a screwdriver to tighten a screw with your left hand, with the arm at the side
   d. unscrewing a light bulb overhead with your right hand

7. Which of the following would be *most* difficult for an individual who has a significant deficit in pronation of both forearms?
   a. lifting and carrying a large box
   b. self-feeding
   c. washing their hair
   d. typing on a standard keyboard

8. Laxity of the medial collateral ligament (MCL) of the elbow may contribute to which of the following?
   a. cubitus valgus
   b. cubitus varus
   c. elbow flexion contracture
   d. median nerve compression

9. Prolonged repetitive elbow flexion may contribute to tension and compression on the ulnar nerve at which elbow landmark?
   a. radial head
   b. olecranon
   c. cubital tunnel
   d. antecubital fossa

10. A fall on outstretched hands (FOOSH) with the elbow extended would *most* likely cause which of the following at the elbow?
    a. anterior dislocation
    b. olecranon fracture
    c. posterior dislocation
    d. radial head fracture

See Answer Key in back of book.

Notes

1. American Occupational Therapy Association, *Occupational Therapy Practice Framework: Domain and Process*, 4th ed. (Bethesda, MD: AOTA Press, 2020).

2. Carol A. Oatis, *Kinesiology: The Mechanics and Pathomechanics of Human Movement*, 3rd ed. (Philadelphia: Wolters Kluwer, 2017).

3. Oatis, *Kinesiology*.

4. Brandon J. Erickson et al., "Rate of Return to Pitching and Performance after Tommy John Surgery in Major League Baseball Pitchers," *American Journal of Sports Medicine* 42, no. 3 (March 2014): 536–43, https://doi.org/10.1177/0363546513510890.

5. Nielsen Company, "Time Flies: U.S. Adults Now Spend Nearly Half a Day Interacting with Media," Insights, July 31, 2018, http://www.nielsen.com/us/en/insights/news/2018/time-flies-us-adults-now-spend-nearly-half-a-day-interacting-with-media.html.

Bibliography

American Occupational Therapy Association. *Occupational Therapy Practice Framework: Domain and Process*. 4th ed. Bethesda, MD: AOTA Press, 2020.

Avers, Dale, and Marybeth Brown. *Daniels and Worthingham's Muscle Testing: Techniques of Manual Examination and Performance Testing*. 10th ed. St. Louis, MO: Saunders, 2019.

Biel, Andrew. *Trail Guide to Movement: Building the Body in Motion*. 2nd ed. Boulder, CO: Books of Discovery, 2019.

Biel, Andrew. *Trail Guide to the Body: A Hands-On Guide to Locating Muscles, Bones, and More*. 6th ed. Boulder, CO: Books of Discovery, 2019.

Clarkson, Hazel M. *Joint Motion, Muscle Length, and Function Assessment: A Research-Based Practical Guide*. 2nd ed. Philadelphia: Wolters Kluwer, 2020.

Erickson, Brandon J., Anil K. Gupta, Joshua D. Harris, Charles Bush-Joseph, Bernard R. Bach, Geoffrey D. Abrams, Angielyn M. San Juan, Brian J. Cole, and Anthony A. Romeo. "Rate of Return to Pitching and Performance after Tommy John Surgery in Major League Baseball Pitchers." *American Journal of Sports Medicine* 42, no. 3 (March 2014): 536–43. https://doi.org/10.1177/0363546513510890.

Greene, David Paul, and Susan L. Roberts. *Kinesiology: Movement in the Context of Activity*. 3rd ed. St. Louis, MO: Elsevier, 2017.

Keough, Jeremy L., Susan J. Sain, and Carolyn L. Roller. *Kinesiology for the Occupational Therapy Assistant: Essential Components of Function and Movement*. 2nd ed. Thorofare, NJ: SLACK, 2017.

Lundy-Ekman, Laurie. *Neuroscience: Fundamentals for Rehabilitation*. 5th ed. St. Louis, MO: Elsevier, 2018.

Nielsen Company. "Time Flies: U.S. Adults Now Spend Nearly Half a Day Interacting with Media." Insights, July 31, 2018. http://www.nielsen.com/us/en/insights/news/2018/time-flies-us-adults-now-spend-nearly-half-a-day-interacting-with-media.html.

Oatis, Carol A. *Kinesiology: The Mechanics and Pathomechanics of Human Movement*. 3rd ed. Philadelphia: Wolters Kluwer, 2017.

Pendleton, Heidi McHugh, and Winifred Schultz-Krohn. *Pedretti's Occupational Therapy: Practice Skills for Physical Dysfunction*. 8th ed. St. Louis, MO: Elsevier, 2017.

Standring, Susan. *Gray's Anatomy: The Anatomical Basis of Clinical Practice, International Edition*. 41st ed. Cambridge, UK: Elsevier, 2016.

CHAPTER 7

Wrist and Hand

Learning Objectives

- Describe the bones, joints, and muscles contributing to purposeful movement of the wrist and hand.

- Identify the primary purposeful movements of the wrist and hand within the context of occupational performance.

- Develop competency in goniometry and manual muscle testing (MMT) as clinical assessment techniques for the wrist and hand.

- Explain the connection between somatosensory input and motor output, including the impact of sensorimotor deficits on occupational performance.

- Use clinical reasoning to identify limitations of the wrist and hand that may affect occupational performance.

Key Concepts

boutonniere deformity

carpal tunnel syndrome (CTS)

claw hand

composite grasp

cylindrical grasp

dart thrower's motion

de Quervain's tenosynovitis

Dupuytren's contracture

extensor tendon injury

extrinsic muscle

flexor tendon injury

hand of benediction

hook grasp

intrinsic minus

intrinsic muscle

intrinsic plus

lateral (key) pinch

palmar arch

spherical grasp

swan-neck deformity

tenodesis

three-jaw chuck pinch

tip pinch

trigger finger

wrist drop

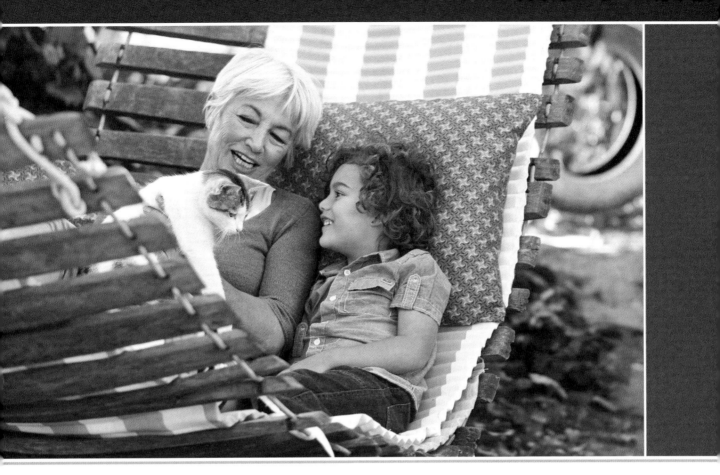

Occupational Profile: Audrey Purdum

AUDREY PURDUM is a sixty-seven-year-old female who recently retired after working for thirty-two years as a registered nurse. Audrey lives with her spouse of forty-two years, and they stay active. She has several cats, a garden, and many grandchildren who keep her busy.

A few weeks ago, as Audrey was walking down the steps to her driveway, she fell and sustained a fall-on-outstretched-hands (FOOSH) injury. Her spouse was not home, but fortunately a neighbor saw the incident and came to her aid. She was able to walk, though she had significant pain in her dominant right forearm.

We will revisit Audrey throughout this chapter. First, let's think about the fall that caused her injury. Falls are a leading cause of injury-related deaths in the older adult population, and many are preventable.[1] The wrist and hand, reflexively extended to break the fall, are often injured.

- What factors may have contributed to Audrey's fall?
- What role might occupational therapy play in preventing falls among the older adult population?
- What specific preventative measures might you implement to prevent a fall in the home environment for someone like Audrey?

Keep these questions in mind as you read about the underlying anatomy and movement of the wrist and hand.

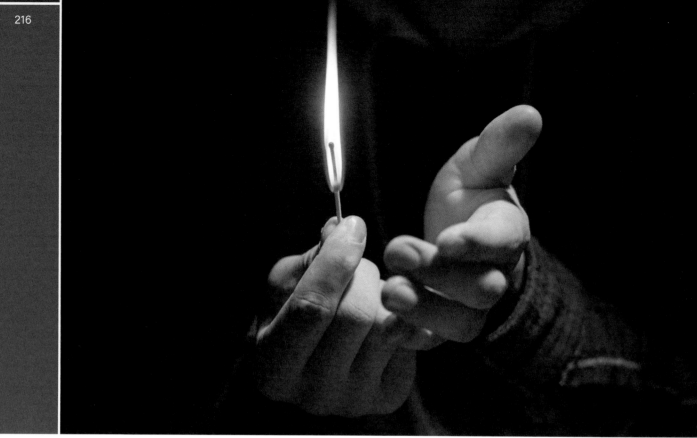

7.1 Hand function relies on complex sensorimotor interaction.

Wrist and Hand: Instruments of Precision

To illustrate the complex sensorimotor processes involved with purposeful activity of the wrist and hand, consider striking a match (**7.1**). Proprioception, or your sense of position in space, guides your fingers to pinch and press the match with just the right amount of force. Your wrist then rapidly moves from radial to ulnar deviation (side to side), generating enough friction to spark a flame. Meanwhile, receptors in your skin alert the brain to increasing heat sensation in your fingertips, reminding you to keep a safe distance to avoid injury. In this way, detailed sensory information from your hands guides your motor output. Any sensorimotor deficits would have a significant impact on this simple action and many other occupations.

The hand is the most biomechanically complex machine in human functional anatomy. While the shoulder and elbow supply gross positioning and stability, the wrist and hand give us the fine motor control and purposeful dexterity we need to interact with our external environment.

Whether we are tying our shoes, sending a text message, gripping a tool, or signing a check, the sensorimotor system of the hand adapts to exert just the right amount of force, guided by sensory input, to precisely manipulate objects using various grip and pinch patterns.

A thorough understanding of the anatomy and sensorimotor function of the wrist and hand will serve you and your future patients well as you implement assessments and interventions to restore occupational performance. For example, a patient with loss of active range of motion (AROM) due to osteoarthritis may benefit from built-up grips on tools that aid dexterity for a primary leisure occupation like needlework. A child with limited fine motor control may benefit from play-based occupations as interventions to practice pinch and grasp. Psychosocial factors affecting a patient's motivation can also limit occupational engagement with the hands, encouraging a client-centered, holistic approach.

This chapter describes the intricate anatomy supporting the vast purposeful ability of the hands. As instruments of precision, the wrist and hand feature special connective tissues, such as the palmar fascia and pulley systems, as well as unique sensorimotor, occupational, and clinical considerations. Spend time working with the highly detailed and specific assessments of the wrist and hand featured in the *OT Guide to Goniometry & MMT* eTextbook.

The wrist and hand present a unique and rewarding opportunity for the skilled occupational therapy practitioner to restore meaningful occupation for individuals like Audrey Purdum from the case study across the life span.

AUDREY PURDUM | Although we don't have a specific diagnosis for Audrey yet, we know the mechanism of her injury, or how it occurred: a FOOSH. We also know that, in general, bones become weaker as we age. Consider these factors as we examine the osteology of the wrist and hand. Think about what specific injury may have resulted from her fall.

Osteology: Bones of the Wrist and Hand

The bones of the wrist and hand are designed and arranged to support functional grasp and pinch, which are essential components of occupational performance (**7.2**). There are many landmarks you will want to familiarize yourself with by using the digital palpation resources that accompany this textbook. These are particularly important to know for detailed assessment and intervention as a future practitioner.

Distal Radius and Ulna

The relative position of the bones of the forearm, wrist, and hand changes significantly with motion. Let's begin our examination in the anatomical position (**7.3**). In this position, the radius and ulna remain parallel between the elbow and wrist. The ulna narrows as the radius widens, forming the primary articular surface for the wrist joint.

Bony Landmarks of the Distal Radius and Ulna

Several important bony landmarks of the distal radius and ulna, with palpation, help to guide physical assessment (**7.3**).

The **radial styloid** is on the radial aspect of the radius, and the **ulnar styloid** is found on the dorsal aspect of the lateral ulna.

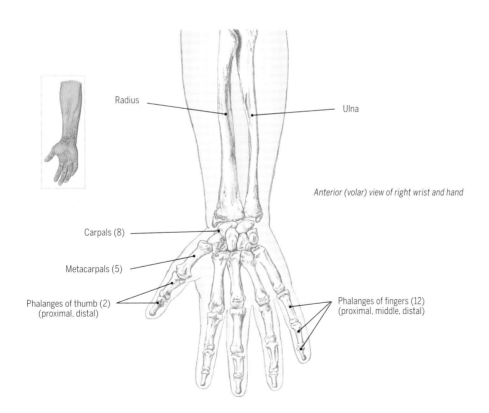

7.2 Bones and bony landmarks of the wrist and hand

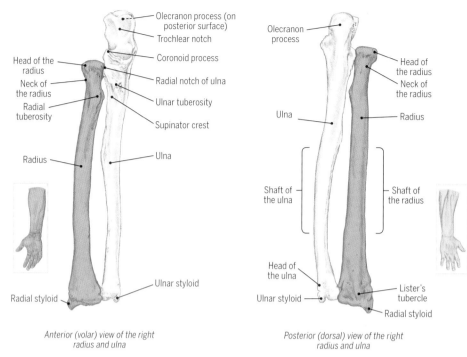

Anterior (volar) view of the right radius and ulna

Posterior (dorsal) view of the right radius and ulna

7.3 Distal radius and ulna

There is also a small, rounded tubercle on the dorsal aspect of the distal radius called **Lister's tubercle**. Lister's tubercle acts as a pulley for the extensor pollicis longus (EPL) tendon, presented later in the chapter, which wraps around its medial aspect to direct its force to extend the thumb.

AUDREY PURDUM | Audrey's neighbor drove her to the emergency room, and X-rays were taken. She was diagnosed with a Colles' fracture of the right distal radius. Audrey had surgery the following morning—open reduction internal fixation (ORIF)—to repair the fracture. She was discharged home the same day, with her spouse helping take care of her as she recovered.

The orthopedic surgeon gave her orders for outpatient occupational therapy services beginning one week post-op (after surgery). He also told her to keep her wrist immobilized in the splint that was put on after surgery.

- Do some research on Colles' fractures. How did Audrey's fall contribute to this type of wrist injury?
- Why was surgery required rather than immobilization in a cast?
- Take another look at Audrey's occupational profile. How will the temporary loss of function in her dominant right hand impact her occupational performance?

Carpals

The **carpals** are eight irregularly shaped bones (known collectively as the carpus) located between the distal radius and ulna and the metacarpals of the hand (**7.4**).

Of the seven carpal bones involved in wrist motion, three—scaphoid, lunate, and triquetrum—form the curved **proximal carpal row**. The bones of the proximal row articulate with each other, with the forearm bones, and with bones of the distal carpal row. The other four—trapezium, trapezoid, capitate, and hamate—form the

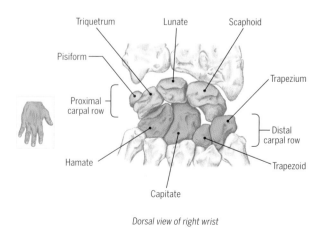

Dorsal view of right wrist

7.4 Carpals

distal carpal row. The bones of the distal row articulate with each other, with bones of the proximal row, and with the metacarpals.

Several mnemonic devices exist to remember the carpal bones in order. We'll use S̲traight L̲ine T̲o P̲inky H̲ere C̲omes T̲he T̲humb (scaphoid, lunate, triquetrum, pisiform, hamate, capitate, trapezoid, trapezium).

The carpal bones fit together like pieces of a three-dimensional puzzle, demonstrating some gliding in relation to one another and providing the structure for the proximal transverse arch of the palm (see **7.7**). Palpate the carpals at the base of the palm and you will feel a stable contour designed to contribute to grasp and object manipulation, allowing the hand to wrap around an object.

Bony Landmarks of the Carpals

Press the front of your palm down against a tabletop. Where do you feel the most pressure? There are two predominant bony landmarks at the base of the volar palm. On the ulnar aspect of the palm, just distal to the wrist crease, is the **pisiform**, the eighth carpal bone. This small sesamoid bone, attached to the triquetrum, is easily palpated (**7.5**). The pisiform is a distinct insertion for the flexor carpi ulnaris (FCU) tendon.

Opposite the pisiform, on the radial aspect of the volar palm, the anterior **scaphoid** can be palpated. Spanning the wrist between the scaphoid and pisiform is the flexor retinaculum, the ligament that forms the carpal tunnel.

Distal and radial to the pisiform lies the **hook of the hamate**, which forms a protective bony roof over the ulnar nerve as it passes through the palm.

▶TRY IT

Observe the palm of your hand while slowly flexing your fingers into a tight fist. How does the space between each finger change as they flex?

Did you notice the fingers naturally adduct toward the middle finger as they flex and abduct as they extend? The involuntary pattern creates a functional seal between the fingers to hold small objects like coins or beads in the hand. This natural convergence of the fingers is due in part to the variable oblique shape of each metacarpal head, directing individual finger flexion toward the center of the palm.

Moving to the dorsal aspect of the palm, an important anatomical landmark on the radial side is the **anatomical snuffbox**, a concave deepening formed by the tendons of the thumb (see **7.40**). The scaphoid forms the bony base of the anatomical snuffbox and can easily be palpated there.

Metacarpals and Phalanges

Metacarpals and phalanges are the individual bones of the fingers (**7.6**). The first segment of each finger is its **metacarpal**. Collectively, the metacarpals form the bony structure of the palm.

The proximal end of a metacarpal expands into a base that articulates with the distal carpal row. The distal end of a metacarpal expands to form a rounded head that articulates with the proximal phalanx of the digit.

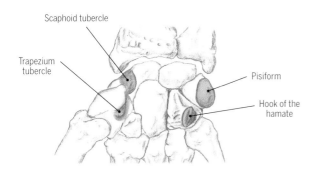

Scaphoid tubercle

Trapezium tubercle

Pisiform

Hook of the hamate

Volar view of right wrist

7.5 Anterior bony landmarks

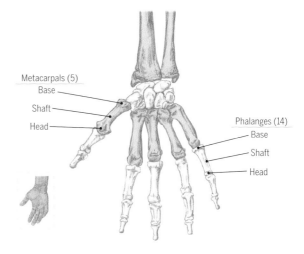

Metacarpals (5)
Base
Shaft
Head

Phalanges (14)
Base
Shaft
Head

Volar view of right wrist and hand

7.6 Metacarpals and phalanges

These rounded heads vary slightly, contributing to the convergence of the fingers when making a fist.

The metacarpals also give structure and length to the palm and supply bony origins for the intrinsic muscles of the hand (the muscles that lie within the palm). The metacarpal heads, stabilized by surrounding ligaments, form the **distal transverse arch**, complementing the **proximal transverse arch** to enhance grasp and object manipulation (**7.7**).

The **palmar arches** allow the palm to fold around objects, contouring to their unique size and shape to increase surface contact. Touch the tips of your small finger and thumb together. Do you notice the radial and ulnar aspects of the palm coming together? This position also accentuates the **longitudinal arch** that lies perpendicular to the transverse arches, passing through the palm proximal to distal.

The four metacarpals of the fingers are longer than the metacarpal of the thumb but comparably more slender. The bases of the digital metacarpals articulate not only with carpal bones but also with each other, while the metacarpal of the thumb is completely independent.

Each of the four fingers contains three **phalanges**: a **proximal phalanx**, a **middle phalanx**, and a **distal phalanx** (**7.6**). The thumb has a proximal and a distal phalanx only.

Each proximal phalanx has a concave surface at its proximal end (base) to articulate with the head of its corresponding convex metacarpal head. The distal end (head) articulates with the middle phalanx. The phalanges are key for occupational performance: not only do they provide structure for grasp and pinch, they also communicate and express emotion.

Bony Landmarks of the Digits

Metacarpals and phalanges are similar in shape, with condyles at each proximal end and a rounded head on the distal end forming the joint with the adjacent bone segment.

The metacarpals are easily palpated as they extend beyond the distal row of carpal bones, spreading into a fan shape to supply the structure for the expanse of the palm. The **metacarpal heads**, or knuckles, are palpable dorsally at the distal end of the bone when the hand is making a fist.

The **phalangeal (digital) condyles** are palpable on the medial and lateral aspects of the proximal interphalangeal

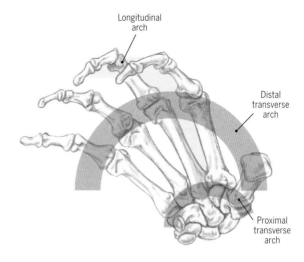

Longitudinal arch

Distal transverse arch

Proximal transverse arch

Volar view of right hand

7.7 Palmar arches of the hand

(PIP) and distal interphalangeal (DIP) joints, which we will explore later in the joints section. Similar to the metacarpals, the heads of the phalanges can also be palpated at their distal ends when the fingers are flexed.

CLINICAL APPLICATION
Finger Lingo

Clinically, the fingers are often referred to numerically as D1 (thumb), D2 (index), D3 (middle), D4 (ring), and D5 (small). Phalangeal segments are commonly called P1 (proximal phalanx), P2 (middle phalanx), and P3 (distal phalanx). To practice, make a fist but extend D1 and D5 (**7.8**).

If you received an order from a physician to "fabricate a custom orthosis (splint) to protect a fracture of D4 P3," what finger segment would you address?

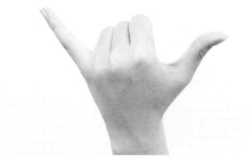

7.8 Extension of D1 (thumb) and D5 (small finger). Hang loose!

Joints

The shoulder and elbow each consist of a few joints that support movement to grossly position the arm. In contrast, the wrist and hand feature more than twenty joints that supply the coordinated precision to support occupational performance. Let's examine the unique design that lends function to each joint.

Distal Radioulnar Joint

Structural classification: pivot

Functional (mechanical) classification: uniaxial

Movements: pronation, supination

The medial surface of the distal radius contains a shallow articular depression, called the ulnar notch, for articulation with the head of the ulna. The medial aspect of the distal ulna (head of the ulna) articulates with the radius at the **distal radioulnar joint (DRUJ)**, facilitating rotation of the forearm (**7.9**).

The joint is supported by the **volar** and **dorsal radioulnar ligaments**. These ligaments provide stability as the radius rotates around the ulna in the distal forearm for pronation and supination (in cooperation with the proximal radioulnar joint, presented in Chapter 6).

Wrist (Radiocarpal Joint)

Structural classification: ellipsoid

Functional (mechanical) classification: biaxial

Movements: flexion, extension, radial deviation, ulnar deviation

Wrist, as a general term, is often used to describe the distal ends of the radius and ulna and adjacent carpal bones, a functional bridge that connects the hand and forearm. The proximal row of carpal bones (scaphoid, lunate, and triquetrum) forms a joint with the distal radius and the triangular fibrocartilage (TFC). The distal end of the radius expands to articulate directly with the scaphoid and lunate. This part of the wrist is known as the **radiocarpal joint**, and it sustains 80 percent of the force through the wrist with weight-bearing in a neutral position (**7.9**).

The remaining 20 percent of the force is absorbed by the **ulnocarpal complex**, formed by the distal ulna, lunate, and triquetrum, with the triangular fibrocartilage complex (TFCC) acting as a shock absorber between

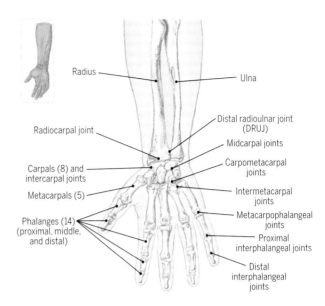

Anterior (volar) view of right forearm and hand

7.9 Joints of the wrist and hand

the bone surfaces.[2] Some sources describe this as the **ulnocarpal joint**, but it is important to note that the ulna does not articulate directly with the carpal bones (see **7.12**).

Compressive forces moving through the wrist, as when pushing down on the arms of a chair to stand up, are primarily absorbed at the radiocarpal joint by the radius and scaphoid. The ulnocarpal joint becomes more involved with more forceful grasp or weight-bearing. The open-pack position of the wrist as a whole is in neutral (not flexed or extended), and its close-pack position is in full extension.

The radiocarpal joint is the primary articulation between the distal forearm and proximal carpal bones. But global motion of the wrist involves movement between the carpal bones as well. Within each row, there are articulations between adjacent carpal bones referred to as **intercarpal joints**. The entire proximal row also articulates with the distal carpal row, referred to as the **midcarpal joint** (**7.10**).

Global movements of the wrist may seem simple when viewed externally, but they reflect complex arthrokinematic patterns of the radiocarpal, midcarpal, and intercarpal joints. Anatomists, kinesiologists, and clinicians have studied and attempted to describe the complex pattern of motion between individual carpal

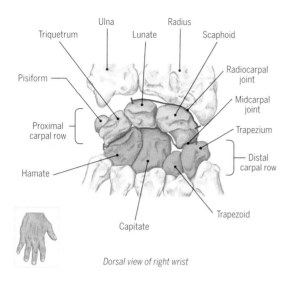

Dorsal view of right wrist

7.10 Radiocarpal and midcarpal joints

bones and the wrist as a whole. While disagreement about the precise mechanical patterns persists, several general concepts regarding wrist arthrokinematics guide clinical practice:[3]

- The axes of motion for both flexion and extension, as well as radial and ulnar deviation, appear to be located near the proximal capitate.
- All global wrist motions involve both the radiocarpal and midcarpal joints.
- The distal carpal row moves more as a single unit, while the proximal carpal bones demonstrate more independent movement.

Wrist and Carpal Ligaments

Numerous ligaments support the wrist and carpal joints and are typically named for the bones they connect (**7.12**).

CLINICAL APPLICATION
Joint Mobilization

Understanding the general concepts of wrist arthrokinematics is important in practice when you are passively moving, or mobilizing, the wrist to restore motion.

The radiocarpal joint, as the primary articulation of the wrist, is a convex-on-concave joint with the rounded scaphoid and lunate projecting into the recesses of the distal radius. As noted in Chapter 1, joints arranged this way rotate (roll) in one direction and translate (glide) in the opposite.

In general terms, this pattern holds true with the wrist. Flexion involves volar rolling and dorsal gliding of the carpals, while extension involves the opposite. Ulnar deviation involves rolling toward the ulna and gliding to-

ward the radius, while radial deviation involves the opposite (**7.11**).

This is a simplification of wrist arthrokinematics, but it informs clinical practice to a certain extent. For example, if an individual has stiffness after a healed distal radius fracture, this may restrict carpal gliding at the radiocarpal joint, limiting global motion of the wrist. Joint mobilization, a form of manual therapy, can help restore the volar and dorsal gliding needed for global extension and flexion of the wrist.

Suppose your goal for a patient is to improve wrist extension. Based on the arthrokinematic pattern of the wrist, in what direction would you manually glide the proximal carpal row?

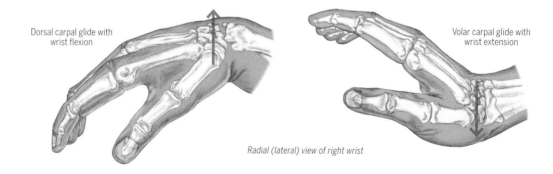

Dorsal carpal glide with wrist flexion

Volar carpal glide with wrist extension

Radial (lateral) view of right wrist

7.11 Arthrokinematic pattern of the wrist and carpals

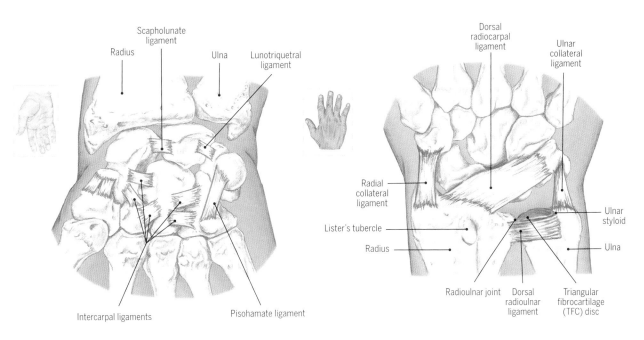

Volar view of right wrist,
showing ligaments of intercarpal joints

Dorsal view of right wrist,
showing ligaments of radiocarpal joints

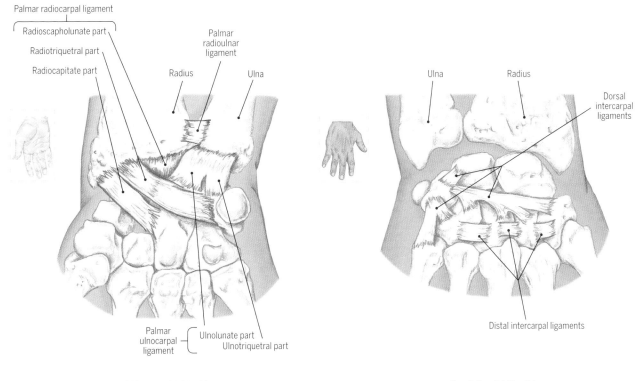

Volar view of right wrist,
showing ligaments of radiocarpal joints

Dorsal view of right wrist,
showing ligaments of intercarpal joints

7.12 Wrist and carpal ligaments

Extrinsic ligaments, such as the radioscapholunate ligament, bridge the distal radius or ulna and the carpal bones. Intrinsic ligaments, such as the pisohamate ligament, join carpal bones. These ligaments serve a dual purpose. They stabilize the wrist but also have imbedded mechanoreceptors that supply valuable proprioceptive sense to guide purposeful movement.

While all of the ligaments in this region contribute to stability to some degree, the scapholunate ligament, ulnotriquetral ligament, and TFCC supply critical stability and are more commonly injured.

The **triangular fibrocartilage complex (TFCC)** acts as a cushion between the distal ulna and carpals and also contributes to stability on the ulnar aspect of the wrist. It serves as a shock absorber for weight-bearing and is susceptible to injury with forceful rotation of the forearm. The TFCC is composed of the following (**7.12**):

- TFC disc
- palmar and dorsal radioulnar ligaments
- palmar ulnocarpal ligaments
- ulnar collateral ligament
- extensor carpi ulnaris tendon sheath

Injury to any one of these components can lead to considerable pain and limit the functional motion and strength of the wrist.

Carpometacarpal Joints of the Fingers

Structural/functional classification: gliding
Movements: primarily volar/dorsal gliding (ring and small more mobile)

The bases of the metacarpals of the digits articulate with the distal row of carpal bones—the **carpometacarpal (CMC) joints**—and with each other—the **intermetacarpal joints**.

The bases of the finger metacarpal bones are bound to each other and to the distal row of carpal bones by several ligaments (**7.13**). These ligaments and the structural configuration of the joints limit CMC joint mobility, but mobility of the ring and small finger CMC joints is greater than the index and middle finger.

Look at the back of your hand while making a tight fist. Take note of any motion at the CMCs of the fingers. Do you notice more mobility of the ring and small finger metacarpals compared to the index and middle finger metacarpals? The increased mobility of the ring and small finger CMC joints enhances the force generated by these fingers for forceful grasp (**7.13**). The stability of

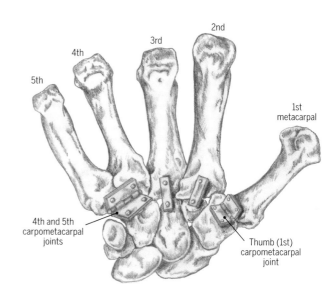

7.13 Variable mobility of the CMC joints contributes to hand function.

the index and middle finger CMC joints supports precise movements involving opposition of these fingers with the thumb, or pinch patterns. In general, the radial aspect of the hand (thumb, index and middle fingers) is designed for precision, while the ulnar aspect (ring and small fingers) is geared more toward forceful grip.

Metacarpophalangeal Joints

Structural classification: ellipsoid
Functional (mechanical) classification: biaxial
Movements: flexion, extension, abduction, adduction

The convex heads of the finger metacarpals articulate with the shallow concave bases of the proximal phalanges at the **metacarpophalangeal (MCP) joints** (**7.14**). These are condyloid joints that allow flexion, extension, abduction, and adduction.

The volar aspect of the fibrous capsule of an MCP joint thickens into a fibrocartilaginous plate called the **volar plate**, limiting hyperextension of the joint. The borders of each plate are connected to the adjacent plate by a thick transverse band of ligamentous fibers, the **deep transverse metacarpal ligament**. This ligament is taut (tight) when the MCP joints are flexed, limiting abduction and keeping the fingers together for functional grasp.

As concave-on-convex joints, the MCPs rotate (roll) and translate (glide) in the same direction. Flexion involves volar gliding, and extension involves dorsal gliding. In general, the collateral ligaments of the MCPs are taut in flexion (the close-pack position of the MCP) and relaxed with extension (the open-pack position of the MCP).

Interphalangeal Joints

Structural classification: hinge
Functional (mechanical) classification: uniaxial
Movements: flexion, extension

Two similar joints form the articulations between the phalanges: the **proximal interphalangeal (PIP)** and **distal interphalangeal (DIP) joints** (7.14).

The PIP joints of the fingers are extremely important for power grip. No adduction or abduction occurs at these hinge joints; only flexion and extension occur. A PIP joint is formed by an articulation of the head of the proximal phalanx and the base of the middle phalanx. These joints feature collateral ligaments as thickenings on either side of their joint capsules to limit medial and lateral movement. Similar to the MCP and DIP joints, the PIPs have volar plates to stabilize them anteriorly and prevent hyperextension.

A DIP joint is structurally very similar to the PIP, but it is smaller, with relatively less movement available. The interphalangeal (IP) joints, similar to the MCPs, have a concave-on-convex arrangement with an arthrokine-

matic pattern of rotation and translation in the same direction. The IP joints' open-pack position is in slight flexion, and their close-pack position is full extension. These joints feature simultaneous, coordinated flexion and extension for grasp and release of objects.

Carpometacarpal Joint of the Thumb

Structural classification: saddle
Functional (mechanical) classification: biaxial
Movements: flexion, extension, abduction, adduction

The CMC joint of the thumb is the articulation between the trapezium and 1st metacarpal, sometimes referred to as the **basilar joint** of the thumb. As a saddle joint, it has two concave surfaces, like a rider in a saddle (7.15).

This unique biaxial arrangement permits flexion, extension, abduction, and adduction. In addition, some rotation accompanies all of these movements, which contributes to thumb opposition to the fingers to facilitate pinch.

The significant mobility of the CMC, along with its relatively shallow joint surfaces, requires more ligamentous support than the other joints of the thumb to maintain stability. It is stabilized by its joint capsule as well as the **anterior oblique (beak)**, **posterior oblique**, **dorsoradial**, and **intermetacarpal ligaments** (7.15). The anterior oblique, or beak ligament, is a primary

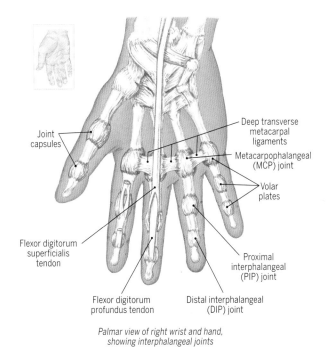

Palmar view of right wrist and hand, showing interphalangeal joints

7.14 Supporting ligaments of the MCP, PIP, and DIP joints

7.15 Saddle design of the CMC joint of the thumb

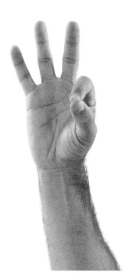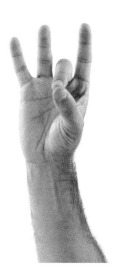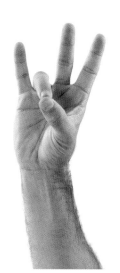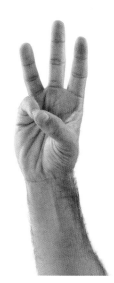

7.16 Thumb opposition

stabilizer against the significant dorsal forces that pinch imposes on the metacarpal, which acts as a rigid lever. Palpate the dorsal aspect of the CMC joint while completing a key pinch by pressing the pad of the thumb against the radial aspect of the index finger. Did you notice the metacarpal protruding dorsally against your fingertips?

The trapezium positions the thumb anterior to (in front of) the palm and digits, optimizing functional opposition. Opposition involves the tip of the thumb touching (opposing) the tip of a finger and includes rotation, turning the volar aspect of thumb toward the fingers (**7.16**).

 CLINICAL APPLICATION
CMC Joint Osteoarthritis

The CMC joint, or basilar joint, of the thumb is one of the most common sites of osteoarthritis in the hand due to the force demands on its unique saddle design over years of repetitive use (**7.17**). When the joint becomes unstable, the base of the metacarpal migrates dorsally due to the strong pull of the abductor pollicis longus (APL) and extensor pollicis brevis (EPB) tendons.

Conservative interventions include activity modification, adaptive grips, and orthoses to stabilize the joint and decrease pain with use. More advanced degeneration may require surgery to reconstruct the joint, known as a ligament reconstruction and tendon interposition (LRTI) procedure. The surgery removes arthritic bone on the joint surfaces and replaces it with a grafted tendon, or autograft, to prevent further wear and tear.

What compensatory or adaptive techniques might improve function and decrease pain for someone experiencing CMC osteoarthritis?

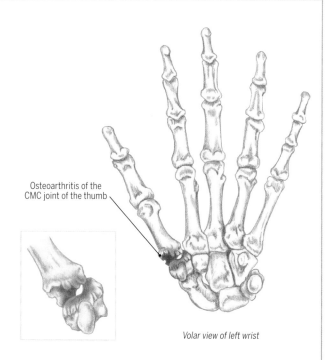

Osteoarthritis of the CMC joint of the thumb

Volar view of left wrist

7.17 Osteoarthritis of the CMC joint of the thumb

You can observe this by looking at the dorsal hand with your thumb extended away from the palm. In this position, only the back of the thumb (dorsal aspect) is visible. Now touch the tip of your thumb to the tip of the middle finger. Can you see the volar aspect (pad) of the thumb? This natural rotation is due in part to the arrangement of the ligaments of the CMC, which passively direct rotational force to the metacarpal of the thumb.

The MCP and IP joints of the thumb are essentially hinge joints, but they are less mobile than the IP hinges of the fingers. They feature similar stabilizing collateral ligaments and a volar plate.

Musculature and Movement

The muscles of the wrist and hand are complicated, often crossing and acting on multiple joints. For example, the flexor digitorum profundus (FDP) crosses the wrist, MCP, PIP, and DIP of each finger. The FDP can flex all of these joints but is the only muscle that can flex the DIP.

The muscles are broadly categorized as **extrinsic muscles** (originating proximal to the wrist) and **intrinsic muscles** (contained entirely within the hand). Functionally, the extrinsic muscles generate greater force, whereas the intrinsic muscles direct precise control of the fingers and thumb, supporting grip, pinch, and object manipulation.

Before reading about each muscle, you may find it helpful to remember a few general anatomical guidelines: The flexor and pronator muscles originate at the medial elbow and traverse the volar forearm. The extensor and supinator muscles originate at the lateral elbow and cross the dorsal forearm.

Because of the complexity of these different muscle forces, the muscles of the hand are presented proximal to distal in broad functional groups, such as flexors. This order also helps illustrate their functional significance.

After you have examined these muscles in detail, use the *OT Guide to Goniometry & MMT* eTextbook to practice your clinical assessment techniques for the wrist and hand. Think about the specific muscle(s) contributing to the functional motions as you assess them.

AUDREY PURDUM | Two days after surgery, Audrey is at home awaiting her first OT visit. She is taking prescribed pain medication, and her pain is manageable.

However, she is concerned about the swelling and stiffness in her wrist and hand. She notices that her hand is throbbing, and she cannot see the wrinkles around the joints on the back of her hand. Her fingers are free out of the postoperative splint, but she is hesitant to move them and feels they are becoming stiff.

Although she is trying to maintain her daily routine using her noninjured left hand, she is having difficulty with dressing, bathing, and taking care of things around the house. Her spouse is willing to help, but Audrey is very independent—and, she admits, a bit stubborn.

- Is there anything Audrey can do to safely decrease or prevent the swelling and stiffness in her fingers?
- What compensatory or adaptive techniques might be beneficial for her to maintain functional independence until she regains the use of her wrist and hand?

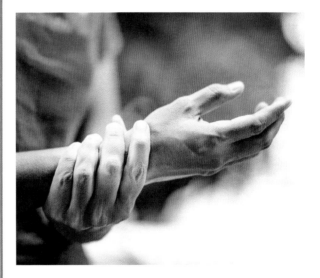

Extrinsic Flexor Muscles

Flexor carpi radialis (FCR)
Flexor carpi ulnaris (FCU)
Palmaris longus (PL)
Flexor digitorum superficialis (FDS)
Flexor digitorum profundus (FDP)
Flexor pollicis longus (FPL)

The muscles in this group generate force to flex the wrist, fingers, and thumb for grip and pinch (**7.18**).

Flexor Carpi Radialis and Flexor Carpi Ulnaris

Flexor carpi radialis (FCR) and **flexor carpi ulnaris (FCU)** are wrist flexors that originate at the common flexor origin at the medial epicondyle of the humerus and insert on opposite sides of the wrist (**7.19**). As a force couple, the FCR and FCU provide pure wrist flexion, exerting similar force at each side of the wrist, as when bouncing a ball.

They may also form a force couple for radial and ulnar deviation of the wrist, contracting with their counterpart ulnar (extensor carpi ulnaris) or radial (extensor carpi radialis longus and extensor carpi radialis brevis) wrist extensor muscle, as when hammering a nail.

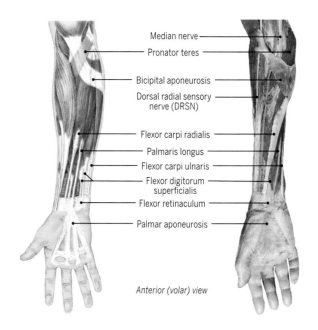

Median nerve
Pronator teres
Bicipital aponeurosis
Dorsal radial sensory nerve (DRSN)
Flexor carpi radialis
Palmaris longus
Flexor carpi ulnaris
Flexor digitorum superficialis
Flexor retinaculum
Palmar aponeurosis

Anterior (volar) view

7.18 Superficial extrinsic flexor muscles of the wrist and hand

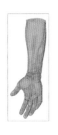
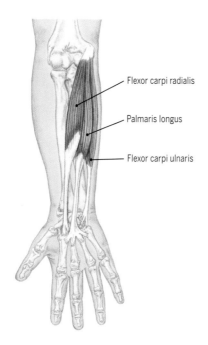

Flexor carpi radialis
Palmaris longus
Flexor carpi ulnaris

Anterior (volar) view of right forearm and wrist, showing superficial layer of flexors

7.19 Flexor muscles of the wrist

FLEXOR CARPI RADIALIS

Purposeful Activity	
P	Self-feeding, writing, sewing
A	**Flex** the wrist (radiocarpal joint) **Radially deviate** the wrist (radiocarpal joint) May assist to **flex** the elbow (humeroulnar joint)
O	Common flexor tendon from medial epicondyle of humerus
I	Bases of 2nd and 3rd metacarpals
N	Median C6 to C8

FLEXOR CARPI ULNARIS

Purposeful Activity	
P	**Hammering a nail, playing the piano, swiping on a tablet**
A	**Flex** the wrist (radiocarpal joint) **Ulnarly deviate** the wrist (radiocarpal joint) Assist to **flex** the elbow (humeroulnar joint)
O	Humeral head: Common flexor tendon from medial epicondyle of humerus Ulnar head: Posterior surface of proximal two-thirds of ulna
I	Pisiform, hook of the hamate, and base of 5th metacarpal
N	Ulnar C7 and C8, T1

Palmaris Longus

Palmaris longus (PL) is another superficial flexor muscle on the anterior forearm with a thin muscle belly attaching to the palmar aponeurosis (**7.20**). Around 10 percent of people do not have the PL. For those who do, it can be used for tendon transfer procedures, serving as a viable tendon for grafting without significant impact to the wrist or hand.

PALMARIS LONGUS	
Purposeful Activity	
P	Contributing to object grasp
A	**Tense** the palmar fascia **Flex** the wrist (radiocarpal joint) May assist to **flex** the elbow (humeroulnar joint)
O	Common flexor tendon from medial epicondyle of humerus
I	Flexor retinaculum and palmar aponeurosis
N	Median C6 to C8, T1

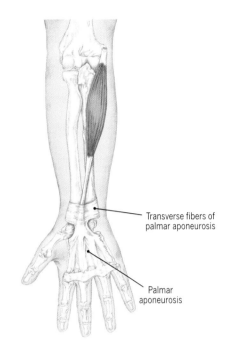

Transverse fibers of palmar aponeurosis

Palmar aponeurosis

Anterior (volar) view of right forearm and wrist

7.20 Palmaris longus

▶TRY IT

Do you have a palmaris longus? Let's find out. Touch the tip of your thumb and small finger together and flex your wrist. If you have a PL, you will notice a tendon popping out beneath the skin at your wrist (**7.21**).

The tendon is bowstringing with wrist flexion because it lies above the transverse carpal ligament (carpal tunnel). All of the other flexor tendons lie within the carpal tunnel, which acts as a pulley, keeping the tendons in place and directing their force to the wrist and digits.

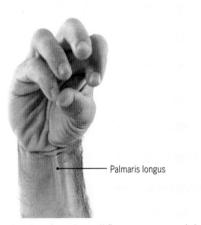

Palmaris longus

7.21 Opposing the thumb and small finger may reveal the palmaris longus at the wrist if you have it.

Flexor Digitorum Superficialis

The **flexor digitorum superficialis (FDS)** has a broad origin, with fibers from the medial epicondyle, coronoid process of the ulna, and proximal radius coming together to form a single muscle belly on the anterior forearm (**7.22**).

Just proximal to the wrist, the fibers divide into four individual tendons, passing through the carpal tunnel and inserting into the middle phalanx of each digit. At its insertion, the FDS tendon bifurcates (splits in two), allowing the FDP tendons to pass through the center and insert into the distal phalanx.

The FDS contributes to flexion at each joint it crosses, but it is the only muscle that can independently flex the PIP joints of the digits. To observe this unique action of the FDS, flex the PIP joints of your fingers while keeping the DIPs extended. This action generates forces involved with grasp and pinch.

FLEXOR DIGITORUM SUPERFICIALIS	
Purposeful Activity	
P	Brushing your teeth, combing your hair, carrying a briefcase (functional grasp and pinch)
A	**Flex** the 2nd through 5th fingers (metacarpophalangeal and proximal interphalangeal joints) **Flex** the wrist (radiocarpal joint)
O	Common flexor tendon from medial epicondyle of humerus, ulnar collateral ligament, coronoid process of ulna, interosseous membrane, and proximal shaft of radius
I	Sides of middle phalanges of 2nd through 5th fingers
N	Median C7 and C8, T1

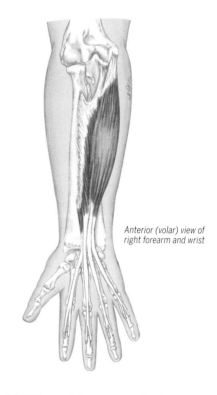

Anterior (volar) view of right forearm and wrist

7.22 Flexor digitorum superficialis

Flexor Digitorum Profundus

Flexor digitorum profundus (FDP) is a deep muscle of the anterior forearm, originating from the proximal ulna and interosseous membrane (**7.23**).

Similar to the FDS, individual tendons emerge from its muscle belly and pass through the carpal tunnel. It runs deep to the FDS tendons in the fingers and passes through the split tendon of the FDS, inserting into the distal phalanx of each digit (**7.24**).

The FDP contributes to flexion of all joints of the wrist and digits, and it is the only muscle that can flex the DIP joint. The DIP joint cannot independently flex without some flexion of the PIP joint, as the FDP crosses both joints. However, the FDP joint can be tested by blocking the PIP joint and attempting to flex the DIP in isolation.

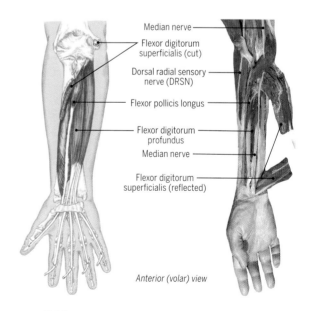

Median nerve

Flexor digitorum superficialis (cut)

Dorsal radial sensory nerve (DRSN)

Flexor pollicis longus

Flexor digitorum profundus

Median nerve

Flexor digitorum superficialis (reflected)

Anterior (volar) view

7.23 Deep flexor muscles of the fingers and thumb

FLEXOR DIGITORUM PROFUNDUS
Purposeful Activity

P   Playing racket sports, drawing, writing (functional grasp and pinch)

A   **Flex** the 2nd through 5th fingers (metacarpophalangeal and distal interphalangeal joints)
  Assist to **flex** the wrist (radiocarpal joint)

O   Anterior and medial surfaces of proximal three-quarters of ulna

I   Bases of distal phalanges, volar surface of 2nd through 5th fingers

N   2nd and 3rd fingers: Median C7 and C8, T1
  4th and 5th fingers: Ulnar C7 and C8, T1

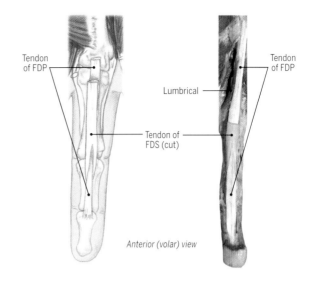

Anterior (volar) view

7.24 Insertions of FDP and FDS tendons

CLINICAL APPLICATION
Flexor Tendon Injuries

Flexor tendon injuries of the wrist, digits, and thumb are often a result of a laceration from a knife or other sharp object. Examples include a knife slipping while cutting out the pit of an avocado or separating frozen hamburger patties, a fall on the blade of an upturned ice skate while playing hockey, and, more seriously, a suicide attempt.

Injuries are classified based on the anatomical location, or zone, of injury. There are five distinct zones of injury, each with its unique anatomy and clinical challenges (**7.25**).

For example, a zone I injury is at the distal end of the finger and involves only the FDP tendon. A zone II injury is referred to as no-man's-land due to its clinical complexity. It includes the adjacent FDP and FDS, which are susceptible to adhesion due to postoperative scar tissue.

Protocol-guided rehabilitation includes a dorsal blocking orthosis to protect the repaired tendon. Some form of early motion is generally advised to promote tendon gliding and prevent adhesions between the healing tendons, which may significantly limit motion.

Though less common, **extensor tendon injuries** also occur, and their treatment is based on zones of injury and on the specific anatomical structures involved. Along with a protective custom orthosis and management of the healing tendon, occupation-based interventions include an adaptive one-hand technique during early-phase rehabili-

tation. In the later phase, the focus might shift to specific client-centered occupations with approval from the referring physician. What one-handed ADL techniques might be beneficial in the early phase of recovery?

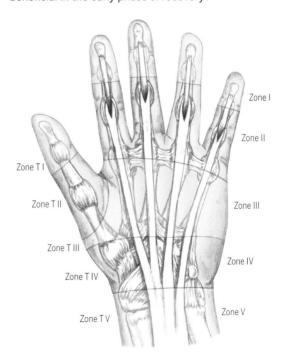

Volar view of the right hand with flexor tendon zones

7.25 Flexor tendon injuries are classified by zone.

The FDP and FDS are designed with precisely the right amount of length and tension for coordinated flexion of the PIP and DIP joints to grasp and manipulate objects.

The tendons are held in position on the digits by a pulley system arranged as annular (ring) and cruciate (cross) ligament fibers along the tendon pathway. Similar to eyelets on a fishing pole, the pulleys prevent the tendon from pulling away from the finger (bowstringing) during motion (**7.26**).

For any one finger, there are five annular (A1–A5) pulleys, designed as rings of parallel fibers around the tendon, and three cruciate (C1–C3) pulleys that form an X across the tendon.

The A2 (2nd annular) and A4 (4th annular) pulleys are most important for preventing bowstringing. They are susceptible to injury during activities like rock climbing, which may exert extreme force through the tendons in a flexed position (**7.27**).

The A1 (1st annular) pulley is frequently the source of a condition known as trigger finger, an inflammatory condition that can eventually lead to locking of the finger in the flexed position (**7.28**).

CLINICAL APPLICATION
Trigger Finger

Trigger finger, also known as stenosing tenosynovitis, is a condition in which a finger becomes lodged (usually temporarily) in a flexed position (**7.28**). The finger may then straighten with a snap, like a trigger being pulled and released.

Trigger finger occurs when inflammation narrows the space within the pulley through which the flexor tendons pass. If trigger finger is severe, the finger may become locked in a flexed position.

People whose work or hobbies involve repetitive gripping actions are at higher risk of developing trigger finger than those not involved in such activities. The condition is also more common for individuals with diabetes.

Treatment of trigger finger varies depending on the severity and may require a surgical release. Conservative interventions focus on decreasing repetitive gripping and preventing prolonged flexion of the finger. How might you maintain the finger in an extended position overnight to prevent triggering?

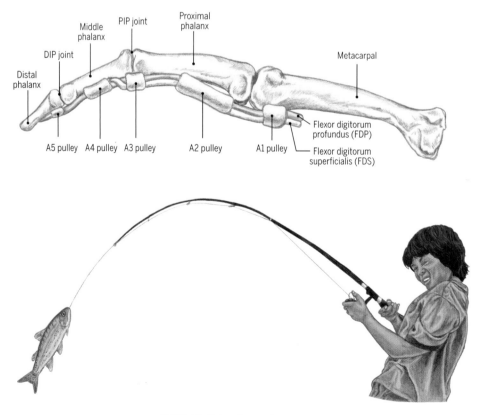

7.26 Digital pulley system

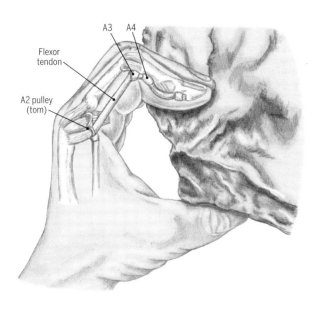

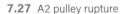

7.27 A2 pulley rupture

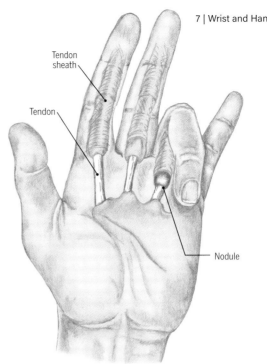

7.28 Trigger finger

Flexor Pollicis Longus

The **flexor pollicis longus (FPL)** is the thumb's version of the FDP, the only extrinsic flexor of the thumb (**7.29**). Originating from the proximal radius, the tendon of the FPL passes through the carpal tunnel with the other digital flexors prior to terminating in the distal phalanx of the thumb.

The FPL is able to flex all joints of the thumb. It is the only muscle that can flex the IP joint, generating force to oppose the tip of the thumb with the tips of the index and middle fingers for precise activities such as writing and needlework.

FLEXOR POLLICIS LONGUS	
Purposeful Activity	
P	Texting, sewing, doing beadwork (tip pinch)
A	**Flex** the thumb (interphalangeal joint) **Flex** the thumb (metacarpophalangeal and carpometacarpal joints) Assist to **flex** the wrist (radiocarpal joint)
O	Anterior surface of radius and interosseous membrane
I	Base of distal phalanx of thumb
N	Median C6 to C8, T1

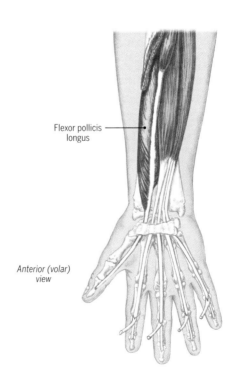

Anterior (volar) view

Flexor pollicis longus

7.29 Flexor pollicis longus

Extrinsic Extensor Muscles

Extensor carpi radialis longus (ECRL)

Extensor carpi radialis brevis (ECRB)

Extensor carpi ulnaris (ECU)

Extensor digitorum (ED)

Extensor indicis (EI)

Extensor digiti minimi (EDM)

Abductor pollicis longus (APL)

Extensor pollicis brevis (EPB)

Extensor pollicis longus (EPL)

The extrinsic extensor muscles of the wrist and hand originate primarily at the lateral epicondyle, traverse the dorsal forearm, and cross the wrist within six anatomical tunnels, or compartments (**7.30**).

The **extensor retinaculum** is a fibrous band that crosses over the compartments, holding the tendons in place at the wrist level. This arrangement forms a pulley system to direct the forces applied by the extensor tendons on the wrist, fingers, and thumb.

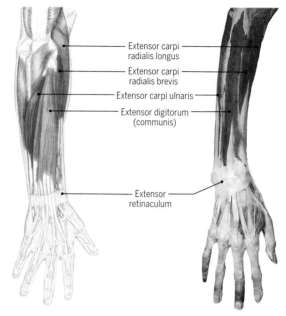

Posterior (dorsal) view

7.30 Extrinsic extensor muscles of the wrist and hand

Extensor Carpi Radialis Longus and Brevis

The **extensor carpi radialis longus (ECRL)** and **brevis (ECRB)** follow a similar pathway from the lateral elbow to the wrist, with the ECRL originating at the supracondylar ridge of the humerus and ECRB originating from the common extensor tendon at the lateral epicondyle (**7.31**).

EXTENSOR CARPI RADIALIS LONGUS AND BREVIS	
Purposeful Activity	
P	Playing pickleball or table tennis, painting a wall, stabilizing your wrist for strong grasp
A	**Extend** the wrist (radiocarpal joint) **Radially deviate** the wrist (radiocarpal joint) Assist to **flex** the elbow (humeroulnar joint)
O	Longus: Distal one-third of the lateral supracondylar ridge of humerus Brevis: Common extensor tendon from the lateral epicondyle of humerus
I	Longus: Base of 2nd metacarpal Brevis: Base of 3rd metacarpal
N	Longus: Radial C5 to C8 Brevis: Radial C6 to C8

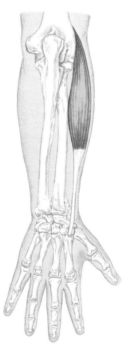
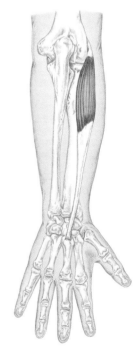

Extensor carpi radialis longus

Extensor carpi radialis brevis

Posterior (dorsal) views of right forearm and wrist

7.31 Radial extensor muscles of the wrist

Both muscles contribute to wrist extension as a force couple with the extensor carpi ulnaris (ECU), such as when painting. They also generate force for radial deviation, along with the FCR, as when you sip hot tea from a mug. The muscles have a small moment for elbow flexion as they cross both the elbow and wrist.

Both are commonly involved in lateral epicondylosis, discussed in Chapter 6.

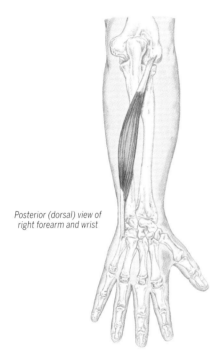

Posterior (dorsal) view of right forearm and wrist

7.32 Extensor carpi ulnaris

Extensor Carpi Ulnaris

The **extensor carpi ulnaris (ECU)** originates from the common extensor tendon at the lateral epicondyle, with some fibers from the proximal ulna (**7.32**).

In synergy with the ECRL and ECRB, this muscle contributes to extension of the wrist. It may also work in synergy with the FCU for ulnar deviation, as when casting a fishing line.

EXTENSOR CARPI ULNARIS	
Purposeful Activity	
P	Hammering, playing the violin, writing
A	**Extend** the wrist (radiocarpal joint) **Ulnarly deviate** the wrist (radiocarpal joint)
O	Common extensor tendon from the lateral epicondyle of humerus
I	Base of 5th metacarpal
N	Radial C6 to C8

▶TRY IT

Hold your hand out in front of you and make a tight fist. You will note that the wrist extends slightly. Now lay your hand flat on a tabletop and palpate the base of the 2nd (index) and 3rd (middle) metacarpals. Make a fist again. You just felt the tendons of the ECRL and ECRB contract. This highlights how the wrist extensors are important wrist stabilizers for this movement.

Remember that the finger flexors (FDS and FDP) both cross the wrist and exert flexion force at the wrist and digits when making a fist. The wrist extensors counteract this force, preventing the wrist from flexing and directing the forces of flexion to the fingers.

Slight wrist extension also increases tension on the finger flexors, generating more force for grip strength. This is why grip is strongest with the wrist in neutral or slightly extended.

Use a dynamometer (a device used to measure force) to test your grip strength with the wrist in neutral or slightly extended. Now try with the wrist flexed. What happens?

Did you notice a significant decrease in strength? With the wrist flexed, the finger flexors are on slack (relaxed), with decreased tension to apply force to the digits. A neutral to slightly extended wrist position when using tools is an important principle of ergonomics. This ensures optimal grip strength and balanced functional tension to the forearm flexors and extensors.

Extensor Digitorum (Communis)

The **extensor digitorum (ED)** (also called the extensor digitorum communis) originates from the common extensor tendon at the lateral epicondyle and splits into four distinct tendons in the distal forearm (**7.33**). This muscle is essential for simultaneous extension of the fingers, as when releasing an object in a trash can, as well as for individual finger extension, such as when typing.

The tendons are held centrally over the dorsal wrist within the 4th extensor compartment, which acts as a pulley to maintain tendon position and direct its line of pull. Past the wrist, the tendons diverge (spread out), with each tendon crossing the metacarpal head of each finger.

Look at the back of your hand while extending your wrist and fingers. Can you see the ED tendons contract beneath the skin? Now make a tight fist and notice how the tendons remain in place over the back of each meta-carpal head (knuckle). Unique ligament fibers called **sagittal bands** encircle the tendon at this level, forming the **extensor hood** to maintain the position of the ten-don on the dorsal metacarpal head (**7.34**).

As the ED tendon passes over the proximal phalanx, it trifurcates (splits into three), forming the **central slip** and **lateral bands**. The central slip remains aligned over the axis of the finger and inserts into the middle phalanx, providing force for PIP extension. The lateral

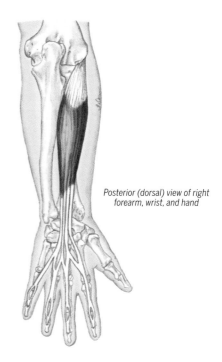

Posterior (dorsal) view of right forearm, wrist, and hand

7.33 Extensor digitorum

bands, as the name suggests, progress laterally on each side of the PIP joint, reconnecting to form the **terminal tendon**, which inserts into the distal phalanx for DIP extension.

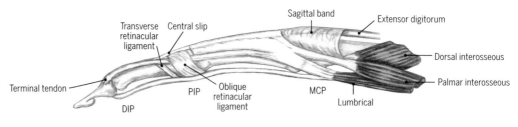

Lateral view

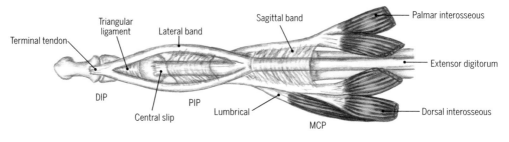

Dorsal view

7.34 Extensor tendon pathways in the finger

These segments of the ED are joined by fibers of the lumbricals and interossei (intrinsic muscles), which enhance the force of finger extension. This complex arrangement of tendons for digital extension is collectively referred to as the **extensor mechanism**.

The **oblique retinacular ligament (ORL)** is also a connection between the volar proximal phalanx and dorsal distal phalanx, reinforcing the link between the PIP and DIP joints (**7.34**).

EXTENSOR DIGITORUM

Purposeful Activity

P   Typing, swiping up on a smartphone

A   **Extend** the 2nd through 5th fingers (metacarpophalangeal and interphalangeal joints)
     Assist to **extend** the wrist (radiocarpal joint)

O   Common extensor tendon from the lateral epicondyle of humerus

I   Bases of middle and distal phalanges of 2nd through 5th fingers

N   Radial C6 to C8

▶TRY IT

You can see the ED in action on your own hand. Make a fist and extend the MCP joints only while keeping the PIP and DIP flexed in a fist. This is possible because the ED can act independently (separate from the PIP and DIP) at the MCP, with the FDS and FDP maintaining the PIP and DIP joints in the flexed position.

Now try to extend only the PIP joint, keeping the DIP joint flexed. Why do you think this is so difficult? Think about the lateral bands and how they act on the PIP and DIP joints.

CLINICAL APPLICATION
Boutonniere and Swan-Neck Deformities

Injuries to specific parts of the extensor tendon of the finger result in predictable patterns of deformity. Have you ever jammed your finger, maybe from a basketball or volleyball hitting the tip of the extended digit? Forceful flexion can result in a strain or rupture of the central slip or terminal tendon (**7.35**).

When the central slip is damaged, the PIP joint cannot fully extend, which also causes the lateral bands to shift anteriorly, hyperextending the DIP joint. This is referred to as a **boutonniere deformity** (PIP flexion with DIP hyperextension). Left untreated, it may result in a flexion contracture of the PIP joint and can significantly impair functional use of the hand.

A **swan-neck deformity** involves the opposite position: PIP hyperextension with DIP flexion. A lax PIP volar plate or damage to the terminal tendon can cause this deformity.

Orthoses may help to restore balance to these delicate structures and promote purposeful movement of the fingers. In what position would you want to splint the PIP joint to correct a mild swan-neck or boutonniere deformity?

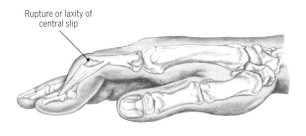

Rupture or laxity of central slip

Boutonniere deformity

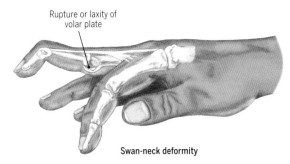

Rupture or laxity of volar plate

Swan-neck deformity

7.35 Boutonniere and swan-neck deformities of the finger

Extensor Indicis and Extensor Digiti Minimi

The index and small fingers sometimes have additional extensor tendons: the **extensor indicis (EI)** (**7.36**) and **extensor digiti minimi (EDM)** (not pictured), respectively.

These muscles originate on the distal forearm and merge with the extensor digitorum near the metacarpal head. They provide more independence of extension for the index and small fingers than for the ring and middle fingers.

These tendons are absent in some of the population. When present, they are often used for tendon transfers. There is no significant functional impact, though they come in handy at heavy metal concerts (**7.37**).

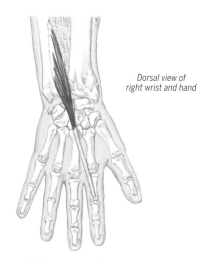

Dorsal view of right wrist and hand

7.36 Extensor indicis

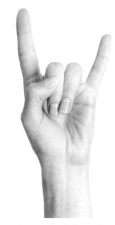

7.37 Action of the extensor indicis and extensor digiti minimi. Rock on!

EXTENSOR INDICIS	
Purposeful Activity	
P	Pointing at something, indicating you are number one
A	**Extend** the 2nd finger (metacarpophalangeal joint) **Adduct** the 2nd finger May assist to **extend** the wrist (radiocarpal joint)
O	Posterior surface of distal shaft of ulna and interosseous membrane
I	Tendon of the extensor digitorum at the level of the 2nd metacarpal
N	Radial C6 to C8

Extensors of the Thumb

Abductor pollicis longus (APL)
Extensor pollicis brevis (EPB)
Extensor pollicis longus (EPL)

There are three distinct extrinsic muscles that abduct and extend the thumb: the **abductor pollicis longus (APL)**, **extensor pollicis brevis (EPB)**, and **extensor pollicis longus (EPL)** (**7.38**, **7.39**).

The muscles originate from the dorsal mid to distal forearm, with insertions at the base of the thumb metacarpal (APL), proximal phalanx (EPB), and distal phalanx (EPL). The APL radially abducts and extends the CMC joint, the EBP extends the MCP joint, and the EPL extends the IP joint. As each crosses the wrist, collectively they contribute to radial abduction of the wrist as well.

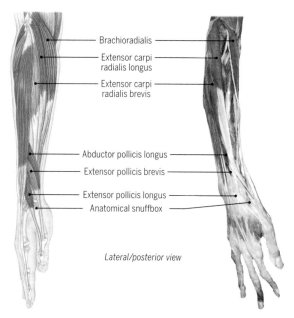

Brachioradialis
Extensor carpi radialis longus
Extensor carpi radialis brevis
Abductor pollicis longus
Extensor pollicis brevis
Extensor pollicis longus
Anatomical snuffbox

Lateral/posterior view

7.38 Extensor/abductor muscles of the thumb

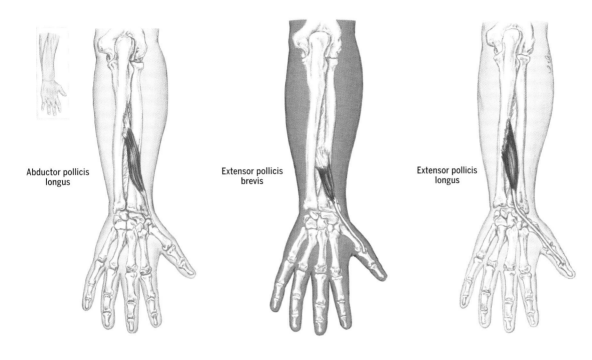

Posterior (dorsal) views of right forearm, wrist, and hand

7.39 Extensors of the thumb

ABDUCTOR POLLICIS LONGUS

Purposeful Activity

P Texting, picking up an infant

A **Radially abduct** the thumb (carpometacarpal joint)
Extend the thumb (carpometacarpal joint)
Radially deviate the wrist (radiocarpal joint)

O Posterior surface of radius and ulna, and interosseous membrane

I Base of 1st metacarpal

N Radial C6 to C8

EXTENSOR POLLICIS LONGUS AND BREVIS

Purposeful Activity

P Giving a thumbs-up, flipping a coin

A **Extend** the thumb (interphalangeal joint), EPL only
Extend the thumb (metacarpophalangeal and carpometacarpal joints)
Radially deviate the wrist (radiocarpal joint)

O Longus: Posterior surface of ulna and interosseous membrane
Brevis: Posterior surface of radius and interosseous membrane

I Longus: Base of distal phalanx of thumb
Brevis: Base of proximal phalanx of thumb

N Radial C6 to C8

CLINICAL APPLICATION
Anatomical Snuffbox

The extensor tendons of the thumb form a unique anatomical landmark. At the level of the wrist, the extrinsic abductor and extensor tendons of the thumb form the anatomical snuffbox (**7.40**).

Abduct your thumb away from the palm. You will notice three tendons emerge with a depression in between. The radial border of the snuffbox is formed by the APL and EBP tendons, while the ulnar border is formed by the EPL tendon.

Several musculoskeletal pathologies occur around the anatomical snuffbox. Understanding the anatomy helps to guide palpation for differential diagnosis. For example, palpating between the tendons (in the snuffbox) applies pressure to the scaphoid, a commonly fractured carpal bone.

The APL and EPB tendons, held in place within the 1st dorsal compartment, represent a common site of tendinitis known as de Quervain's. Also called "texting thumb," the condition occurs due to friction of these tendons within the 1st dorsal compartment with repetitive thumb or wrist motion (see **7.53**). What adaptive or compensatory strategies might limit the repetitive strain on these specific tendons?

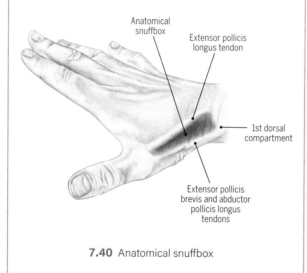

7.40 Anatomical snuffbox

Intrinsic Hand Muscles

Thenar muscles
Hypothenar muscles
Palmar interossei
Dorsal interossei
Adductor pollicis
Lumbricals

The intrinsic muscles, which originate and terminate distal to the wrist (contained completely within the hand), guide precise movement of the fingers and thumb as well as stabilize and balance forces within the hand (**7.41, 7.42**).

The fast-twitch fibers of the intrinsic muscles provide the high-velocity movement needed for fine motor activities such as typing, playing an instrument, or needlework. Take a look at the front of your palm. Do you notice two prominent muscle groups formed by muscle bellies on each side of the palm? The muscles at the base of the thumb make up the **thenar eminence**, and the muscles at the base of the small finger are known as the **hypothenar eminence**.

Another group of intrinsic muscles known as the palmar and dorsal interossei lie between the metacarpals of the digits and thumb. Additionally, the lumbricals arise from the tendon of the FDP and insert into the extensor mechanism of each finger. Though these muscles are complex, it helps to conceptualize them in these distinct groups as we discuss each in greater detail.

Thenar Muscles

Abductor pollicis brevis (APB)
Flexor pollicis brevis (FPB)
Opponens pollicis (OP)

The thenar muscles consist of **abductor pollicis brevis (APB)**, **flexor pollicis brevis (FPB)**, and **opponens pollicis (OP)** (**7.41, 7.42**). The ABP and FPB lie adjacent to each other just beneath the skin.

As a group, the thenar muscles abduct, flex, and medially rotate the thumb at the CMC joint to oppose the thumb and fingers. The APB has the best moment for abduction, the FPB for flexion, and the OP for medial rotation (opposition). These muscles are active with precise movements of the hand, such as when texting or playing video games.

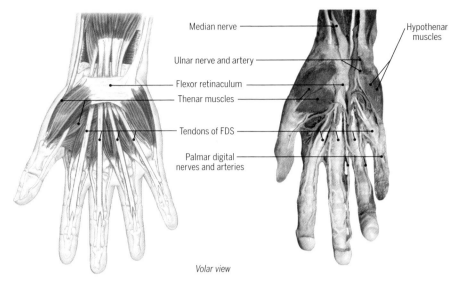

Volar view

7.41 Thenar and hypothenar muscle groups

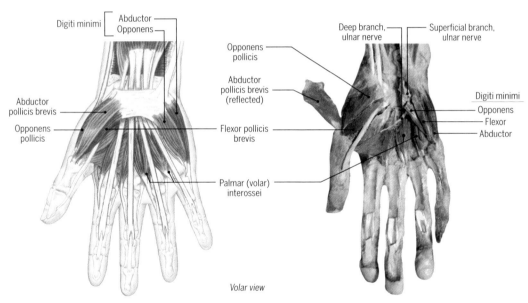

Volar view

7.42 Intrinsic muscles of the hand

ABDUCTOR POLLICIS BREVIS	FLEXOR POLLICIS BREVIS	OPPONENS POLLICIS
Purposeful Activity	**Purposeful Activity**	**Purposeful Activity**
P Texting, hitting the space bar when typing	**P** Writing, doing beadwork, putting change in a vending machine (functional pinch)	**P** Grasping spherical objects like a tennis ball or an orange
A **Abduct** the thumb (carpometacarpal and metacarpophalangeal joints) Assist in **opposition** of the thumb	**A** **Flex** the thumb (carpometacarpal and metacarpophalangeal joints) Assist in **opposition** of the thumb	**A** **Opposition** of the thumb at the carpometacarpal joint (bringing the pads of the thumb and 5th finger together)
O Flexor retinaculum, trapezium and scaphoid tubercles	**O** Superficial head: Flexor retinaculum Deep head: Trapezium, trapezoid, and capitate	**O** Flexor retinaculum and tubercle of the trapezium
I Base of proximal phalanx of thumb	**I** Base of proximal phalanx of thumb	**I** Entire length of 1st metacarpal bone, radial surface
N Median C6 to C8, T1	**N** Superficial head: Median C6 to C8, T1 Deep head: Ulnar C8 and T1	**N** Median C6 to C8, T1

Hypothenar Muscles

Abductor digiti minimi (ADM)
Flexor digiti minimi (FDM)
Opponens digiti minimi (ODM)

Similar to the thenar group, the hypothenar muscles consist of the **abductor digiti minimi (ADM), flexor digiti minimi (FDM)**, and **opponens digiti minimi (ODM)** (**7.41**, **7.42**). The muscle fibers of the ADM and FDM merge and insert into the ulnar base of the proximal phalanx of the small finger, providing independent abduction and flexion.

Together the thenar and hypothenar muscles open and close the palm, increasing the span of grasp for larger objects when abducted or opposing (coming together) to conform to a small object in the palm (**7.43**).

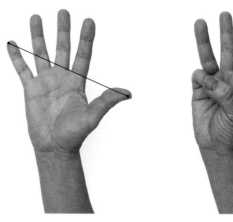

7.43 The thenar and hypothenar muscles open and close the palm.

ABDUCTOR DIGITI MINIMI	
Purposeful Activity	
P	Typing, playing the piano
A	**Abduct** the 5th finger (metacarpophalangeal joint) Assist in **opposition** of the 5th finger toward the thumb (metacarpophalangeal joint)
O	Pisiform and tendon of flexor carpi ulnaris
I	Base of proximal phalanx of 5th finger, ulnar surface
N	Ulnar C7 and C8, T1

FLEXOR DIGITI MINIMI	
Purposeful Activity	
P	Playing the trumpet, typing
A	**Flex** the 5th finger (metacarpophalangeal joint) Assist in **opposition** of the 5th finger toward the thumb
O	Hook of hamate and flexor retinaculum
I	Base of proximal phalanx of 5th finger, volar surface
N	Ulnar C7 and C8, T1

OPPONENS DIGITI MINIMI	
Purposeful Activity	
P	Holding a spherical object like a tennis ball or an orange
A	**Opposition** of the 5th finger at the carpometacarpal joint
O	Hook of hamate and flexor retinaculum
I	Shaft of 5th metacarpal, ulnar surface
N	Ulnar C7 and C8, T1

▶TRY IT

Take a look at the front of your palm with your thumb and fingers extended. Notice that the pad of the tip of the thumb is facing you.

Now slowly touch the thumb to the tips of the index and middle fingers (tripod pinch). This motion is produced by the thenar muscles. Did you notice that the pad of the thumb is now facing the digits? Not only does the thumb flex and adduct toward the palm during pinch, the metacarpal also rotates slightly, bringing the pads of the thumb and digit together.

Palmar Interossei

The **palmar interossei** lie between the metacarpals of the digits (*inter* = between; *osse* = bone) and adduct the digits toward the middle finger, which serves as the midline for adduction (**7.44**). Note the middle finger has no palmar interossei, as it cannot adduct to itself; it only abducts away from midline.

The palmar interossei of the index, ring, and small fingers are referred to as the 1st, 2nd, and 3rd palmar interosseous muscles, respectively. The palmar interossei adduct the digits at the MCP and extend the PIP and DIP joints, as when playing the piano.

PALMAR INTEROSSEI	
Purposeful Activity	
P	Holding a flat object like a book or sandwich (MCP flexion with PIP/DIP extension), playing the piano
A	**Adduct** the thumb, 2nd, 4th, and 5th fingers toward the 3rd finger Assist to **flex** the thumb, 2nd, 4th, and 5th fingers at the metacarpophalangeal joints Assist to **extend** the thumb, 2nd, 4th, and 5th fingers at the interphalangeal joints
O	Base of 1st, 2nd, 4th, and 5th metacarpals
I	Base of the proximal phalanx of the related finger and the extensor aponeurosis
N	Ulnar C8 and T1

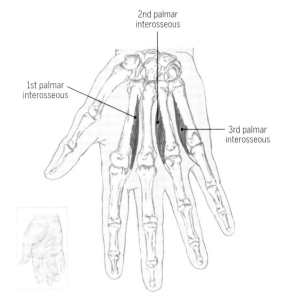

Volar view of right hand

7.44 Palmar interossei

Dorsal Interossei

The **dorsal interossei** are also positioned between the metacarpals of the digits but insert opposite to the palmar interossei, on the outside of the proximal phalanx relative to the middle finger, and abduct the digits at the MCP joint (**7.45**). They are larger and originate from adjacent metacarpal shafts but still insert at the extensor mechanism at the proximal phalanx. This allows the dorsal interossei to contribute to the force of PIP and DIP extension, in synergy with the palmar interossei.

The dorsal interossei, from radial to ulnar, are referred to as the 1st, 2nd, 3rd, and 4th dorsal interosseous muscles. The 1st dorsal interosseous is part of the thumb web space, or the muscles that span the space between the thumb and index finger.

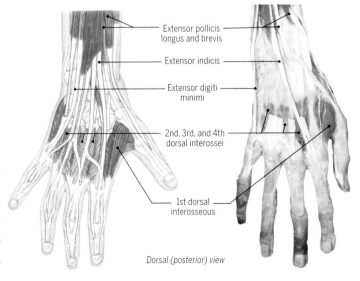

Dorsal (posterior) view

7.45 Dorsal interossei

Take a look at the figures of the dorsal and palmar interossei (**7.44**, **7.45**). Do you notice any other obvious differences? The small finger lacks a dorsal interosseous muscle, as it has the hypothenar abductor digiti minimi for abduction. Also, the middle finger has two dorsal interossei to allow abduction in either direction. Note, too, that all of the interossei (palmar and dorsal) are innervated by the ulnar nerve.

To remember the respective actions of the palmar and dorsal interossei, remember PAD (palmar adduct) and DAB (dorsal abduct).

DORSAL INTEROSSEI
Purposeful Activity

P	**Cutting with scissors (1st dorsal interosseous), typing, giving the Vulcan salute from *Star Trek***
A	**Abduct** the 2nd, 3rd, and 4th fingers at the metacarpophalangeal joints Assist to **flex** the 2nd, 3rd, and 4th fingers at the metacarpophalangeal joints Assist to **extend** the 2nd, 3rd, and 4th fingers at the interphalangeal joints
O	Adjacent sides of all metacarpals
I	Base of the proximal phalanx of the 2nd, 3rd, and 4th fingers and the extensor aponeurosis
N	Ulnar C8 and T1

Adductor Pollicis

Adductor pollicis (AP) is a deep triangular muscle in the radial aspect of the palm (**7.46**). This muscle plays an important role in lateral (key) pinch, adducting the thumb against the radial aspect of the index finger, described later in the chapter. Along with the 1st dorsal interosseous, the AP forms the web space of the thumb.

ADDUCTOR POLLICIS
Purposeful Activity

P	**Brushing your hair, turning a key, swiping a credit card (lateral pinch)**
A	**Adduct** the thumb (carpometacarpal and metacarpophalangeal joints) Assist to **flex** the thumb (metacarpophalangeal joint)
O	Capitate, 2nd and 3rd metacarpals
I	Base of proximal phalanx of thumb
N	Ulnar C8 and T1

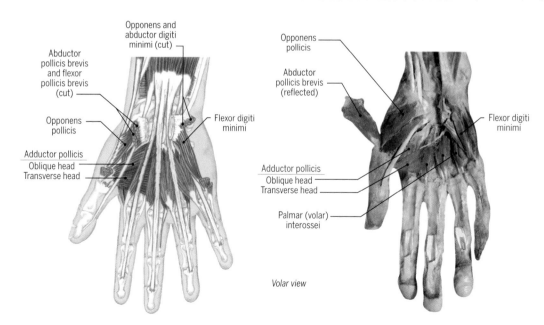

Volar view

7.46 Deep intrinsic muscles of the hand

Lumbricals

The **lumbricals** are unique wormlike muscles of the hand that help to balance flexion and extension forces within the fingers (**7.47**).

The lumbricals originate from the FDP tendon in the palm and terminate dorsally into the radial aspect of the extensor tendon near the metacarpal joint. This unique arrangement helps to balance the forces of the extrinsic flexor and extensor muscles of the hand. As the lumbricals contract, the FDP is pulled distally, relaxing the tendon and simultaneously extending the PIP and DIP joints by applying force through the extensor mechanism. As a group, along with the interossei, the lumbricals contribute to MCP joint flexion and extension of the PIP and DIP joints.

The role of the intrinsic and extrinsic muscles is discussed in greater detail in the next section.

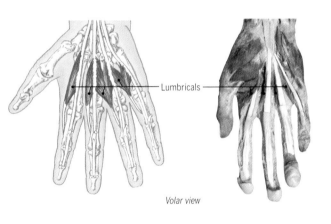

Volar view

7.47 Lumbricals

LUMBRICALS OF THE HAND

Purposeful Activity

P   Holding a flat object like a book or sandwich (MCP flexion with PIP/DIP extension)

A   **Extend** the 2nd through 5th fingers at the interphalangeal joints
Flex the 2nd through 5th fingers at the metacarpophalangeal joints

O   Surfaces of the flexor digitorum profundus tendons

I   Extensor aponeurosis on dorsal surface of phalanges

N   2nd and 3rd fingers: Median C6 to C8, T1
4th and 5th fingers: Ulnar C7 and C8, T1

CLINICAL APPLICATION
Ulnar Nerve Injury

Injuries to the individual nerves of the hand present with unique symptoms and affect occupational performance.

Ulnar nerve injuries may present with sensory and motor deficits, depending on severity. Motor loss includes all of the interossei muscles, the adductor pollicis, and lumbricals of the ring and small finger. What functional deficits would you anticipate with this pattern of motor loss?

You may notice muscle atrophy, or hollowing, between the metacarpals as well as weakness of finger abduction and adduction with loss of the interossei. The ring and small fingers may also begin to claw at the PIP and DIP joints due to imbalanced forces between the intrinsic and extrinsic muscles.

However, perhaps the most significant motor impairment is loss of lateral (key) pinch (see **7.80**) due to weakness of the adductor pollicis muscle. What tasks would become difficult with loss of key pinch?

AUDREY PURDUM | Think about the soft tissues (muscles, tendons, and ligaments) in Audrey's forearm, wrist, and hand. By the time of her OT evaluation, she will have been immobilized for a week.

- What effect do you think this immobilization will have on the surrounding soft tissues? How can soft tissues be safely mobilized without impacting the healing process of the fractured bone?
- Do some research on wrist fracture rehabilitation. What types of interventions are typically implemented in the early phase of recovery?

Special Connective Tissue of the Wrist and Hand

Numerous ligaments connect the carpal bones to one another, to the distal radius and ulna, and to the metacarpals. There are also special ligaments within the hand. The ligaments presented here are the most significant ones pertaining to OT clinical practice.

Transverse Carpal Ligament and the Carpal Tunnel

The **transverse carpal ligament**, or **flexor retinaculum**, passes from side to side across the volar surface of the carpus. On the ulnar side of the palm it attaches to the hamate and pisiform, and on the radial side it attaches to the trapezium and scaphoid. This arrangement creates an osseofibrous tunnel (a bony floor with a ligamentous roof) at the base of the volar palm. Through this **carpal tunnel** pass the extrinsic flexor tendons of the fingers and thumb and the median nerve.

The transverse carpal ligament prevents these tendons from bowstringing, or pulling away from the carpus during digital flexion. Within the carpal tunnel, the tendons are enveloped by synovial sheaths that allow them to glide smoothly within such a confined space.

Palmar Aponeurosis

A thick layer of fascia called the **palmar aponeurosis** spans the palm from the distal edge of the transverse carpal ligament to the proximal aspect of the fingers (**7.49**).

CLINICAL APPLICATION
Carpal Tunnel Syndrome

The limited space within the carpal tunnel contains nine tendons and the median nerve. **Carpal tunnel syndrome (CTS)** describes increased pressure within the carpal tunnel (often related to repetitive motion) reducing blood flow to the small arteries that supply the median nerve (**7.48**).

Refer back to Chapter 2. In what part of the hand would you expect numbness and tingling for someone experiencing carpal tunnel syndrome? Left untreated, symptoms may progress to weakness of the thenar muscles of the thumb. Formal sensory testing is used clinically to identify the pattern and severity of sensory impairment.

Conservative interventions include occupational performance modification, orthoses, and education to decrease compression at the carpal tunnel. A wrist cock-up orthosis and workstation modifications encourage a more neutral wrist with activity, as the flexed position increases pressure on the median nerve within the carpal tunnel.

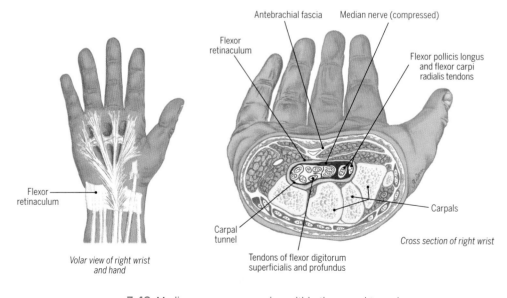

Volar view of right wrist and hand

Cross section of right wrist

Antebrachial fascia

Median nerve (compressed)

Flexor retinaculum

Flexor pollicis longus and flexor carpi radialis tendons

Flexor retinaculum

Carpals

Carpal tunnel

Tendons of flexor digitorum superficialis and profundus

7.48 Median nerve compression within the carpal tunnel causes numbness in the shaded part of the hand.

This thick fascial membrane provides protection to the neurovascular structures beneath and forms channels that maintain the position of the flexor tendons. After traversing the palm, the tendons enter the fingers and are held in place by the annular and cruciate pulleys, discussed earlier in the chapter.

Overlying the tendons and pulley system are **synovial sheaths**, which lubricate the tendons to reduce friction as the tendons move relative to one another. The tendons lie in a common synovial sheath in the wrist and palm with separate sheaths for each digit (**7.50**).

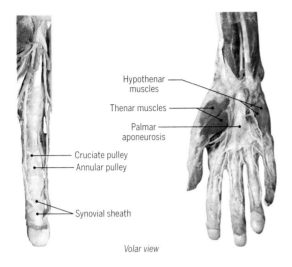

Hypothenar muscles

Thenar muscles

Palmar aponeurosis

Cruciate pulley
Annular pulley

Synovial sheath

Volar view

7.49 Special connective tissues of the hand

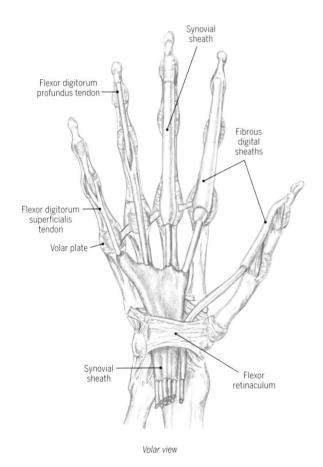

Synovial sheath

Flexor digitorum profundus tendon

Fibrous digital sheaths

Flexor digitorum superficialis tendon

Volar plate

Synovial sheath

Flexor retinaculum

Volar view

7.50 Synovial sheaths

CLINICAL APPLICATION
Dupuytren's Contracture

Dupuytren's contracture is the result of a disease process involving abnormal thickening of the palmar aponeurosis, typically leading to contracture of the ring and small fingers (**7.51**). The pathology usually begins with a nodule near the distal palmar crease and progresses to tight cords, which often leads to contracture of the fingers.

Conservative measures are generally ineffective for preventing the contracture from progressing. Surgical release (fasciotomy) or injection may be used to address the contracted fascia. Postoperative rehabilitation involves custom splinting to maintain digital extension as well as extensive scar management to maintain motion.

How would contractures of the ring and small fingers impact occupational performance?

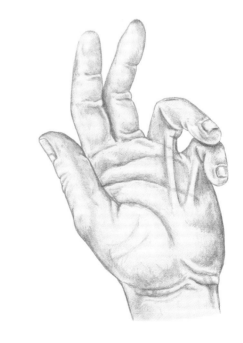

7.51 Dupuytren's contracture

Extensor Retinaculum

On the dorsal forearm at the level of the distal radius and ulna, transverse ligament fibers create a dense **extensor retinaculum**. The retinaculum separates the tendons into six distinct compartments, stabilizing and directing the force produced by the tendons in the appropriate direction (**7.52**).

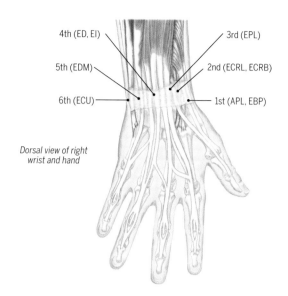

Dorsal view of right wrist and hand

7.52 Extensor retinaculum and compartments

CLINICAL APPLICATION
De Quervain's Tenosynovitis

Now also known as texting thumb, **de Quervain's tenosynovitis** was first described by Fritz de Quervain, a Swiss surgeon, in 1895 (**7.53**).

This cumulative trauma disorder (CTD) of the tendons of the 1st dorsal compartment (APL and EBP) has increased with the rise of mobile technology. Adults in the United States spend an average of 2.5 hours per day interfacing with such technology, with the wrist in ulnar deviation and the thumb rapidly moving, increasing friction within the 1st dorsal compartment as the tendons glide.[4]

De Quervain's is also a common pathology for new mothers. How would the role of a new mother potentially contribute to these symptoms? OT interventions often include activity modification, a thumb spica orthosis to rest inflamed tendons, and modalities for acute pain.

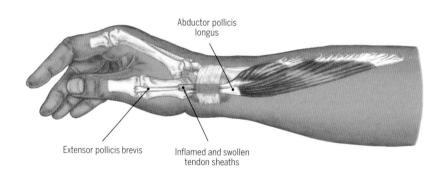

7.53 De Quervain's tenosynovitis

Purposeful Movement of the Wrist and Hand

Purposeful movement of the wrist and hand is intimately interconnected and often engages multiple muscle groups. Precise finger function for object manipulation and grasp requires proximal stability of the wrist. The extrinsic and intrinsic muscles function together to provide the delicate balance of stability and motion that is essential to occupational performance. Figures **7.54–7.67** feature various muscle groups of the wrist and hand presented in the context of occupational performance, with prime movers listed first. Asterisks indicate muscles not shown.

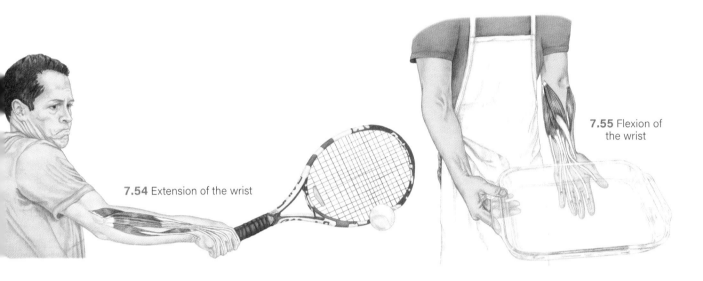

7.54 Extension of the wrist

7.55 Flexion of the wrist

Extension
(*antagonists on flexion*)
Extensor carpi radialis longus
Extensor carpi radialis brevis
Extensor carpi ulnaris
Extensor digitorum (assists)
Extensor indicis (assists)*

Flexion
(*antagonists on extension*)
Flexor carpi radialis
Flexor carpi ulnaris
Palmaris longus
Flexor digitorum superficialis
Flexor digitorum profundus (assists)
Flexor pollicis longus (assists)

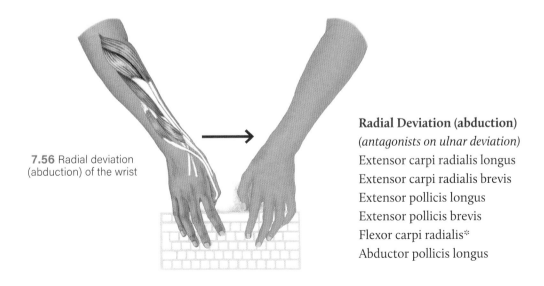

7.56 Radial deviation (abduction) of the wrist

Radial Deviation (abduction)
(*antagonists on ulnar deviation*)
Extensor carpi radialis longus
Extensor carpi radialis brevis
Extensor pollicis longus
Extensor pollicis brevis
Flexor carpi radialis*
Abductor pollicis longus

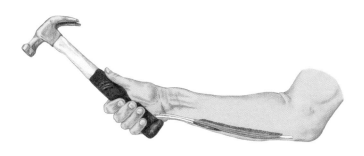

7.57 Ulnar deviation (adduction) of the wrist

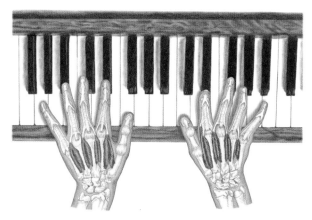

7.58 Abduction and adduction of fingers

Ulnar Deviation (adduction)
(*antagonists on radial deviation*)
Extensor carpi ulnaris
Flexor carpi ulnaris

Abduction and Adduction of Fingers (MCP joints)
Dorsal interossei (abduction)
Palmar interossei (adduction)

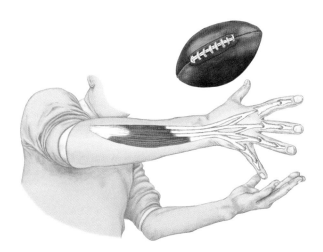

7.59 Extension of the 2nd through 5th fingers

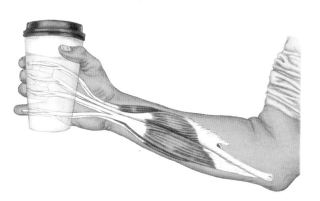

7.60 Composite flexion of the 2nd through 5th fingers

Extension of 2nd through 5th Fingers
(*antagonists on flexion*)
Extensor digitorum
Lumbricals*
Dorsal interossei (2nd–4th, assists)*
Palmar interossei (2nd, 4th, 5th, assists)*
Extensor indicis (2nd)*

Composite (all joints) Flexion of 2nd through 5th Fingers
(*antagonists on extension*)
Flexor digitorum superficialis (PIP, MCP, wrist flexion)
Flexor digitorum profundus (DIP, PIP, MCP, wrist flexion)
Flexor digiti minimi brevis (5th)*
Lumbricals*
Dorsal interossei (2nd–4th, assists)*
Palmar interossei (2nd, 4th, 5th, assists)*

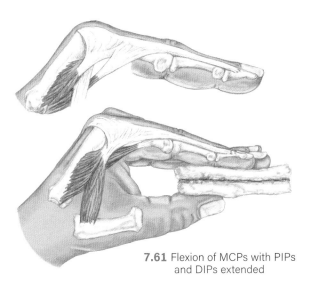

7.61 Flexion of MCPs with PIPs and DIPs extended

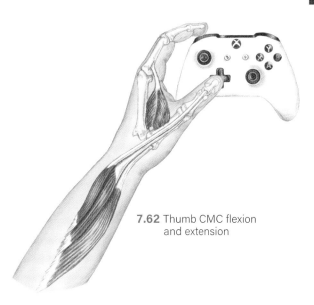

7.62 Thumb CMC flexion and extension

Flexion of MCPs with PIPs and DIPs Extended (intrinsic plus position)
Dorsal interossei
Palmar interossei*
Lumbricals*
Flexor digiti minimi (5th)*

Thumb CMC Flexion and Extension
Abductor pollicis longus (extension)
Extensor pollicis longus (extension)
Extensor pollicis brevis (extension)
Flexor pollicis longus (flexion)*
Flexor pollicis brevis (flexion)*
Adductor pollicis (flexion)*

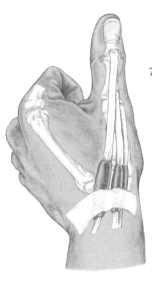

7.63 Thumb CMC radial abduction

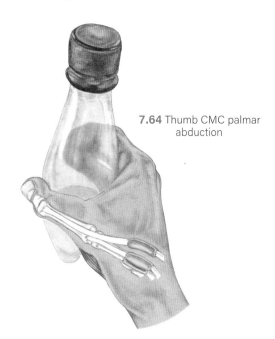

7.64 Thumb CMC palmar abduction

Thumb CMC Radial Abduction (abduction in frontal plane lateral to palm)
Abductor pollicis longus
Abductor pollicis brevis*
Extensor pollicis longus (assists)
Extensor pollicis brevis (extension)

Thumb CMC Palmar Abduction (abduction in sagittal plane anterior to palm)
Abductor pollicis brevis*
Abductor pollicis longus
Flexor pollicis longus (assists)*
Opponens pollicis (assists)*

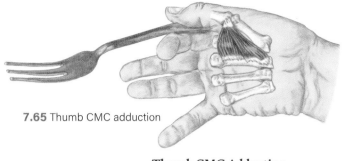

7.65 Thumb CMC adduction

Thumb CMC Adduction
Adductor pollicis
Flexor pollicis brevis*
Flexor pollicis longus (assists)*

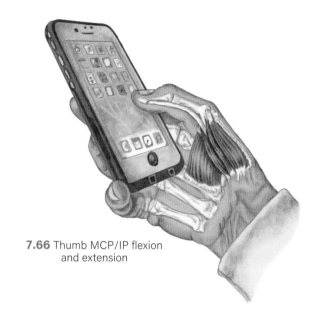

7.66 Thumb MCP/IP flexion and extension

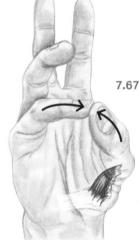

7.67 Opposition of the thumb

Opposition
Opponens pollicis
Flexor pollicis brevis (assists)*
Abductor pollicis brevis (assists)*

Thumb MCP/IP Flexion and Extension
Flexor pollicis longus (IP)
Flexor pollicis brevis (MCP)
Adductor pollicis (assists MCP)
Palmar interossei (1st, assists MCP)*

OT Guide to Goniometry & MMT: Wrist and Hand

The musculoskeletal structures that animate the hand are complicated. It takes time and clinical experience to develop familiarity, and there is always something new to learn. To build on the foundational knowledge you have developed, let's practice goniometry and MMT of the wrist, fingers, and thumb using the *OT Guide to Goniometry & MMT* eTextbook. These joints are much smaller and require a higher level of precision to obtain accurate measurements.

Also consider the length-tension relationship we discussed in Chapter 1. It is important to keep the joints that are proximal to the one being measured in a neutral position to prevent passive or active insufficiency from limiting joint motion.

Sometimes a quick approximate measurement of hand motion is needed. In these instances, measuring the distance from the fingertips or thumb to specific landmarks on the palm may be the best option. In other scenarios, using a goniometer is important to measure the exact motion of each individual joint.

Assessing the strength of individual joints of the hand using MMT is also necessary. Sometimes a specific pattern of weakness indicates a particular injury. Overall grip and pinch strength are essential components of object manipulation and grasp. Occupational therapists, along with other health care practitioners, use **dynamometry** to measure grip and pinch strength. A **dynamometer** is a device that measures force production and can be used to assess various grasp and pinch patterns. Similar to range-of-motion measurements, grip and pinch strength values can be compared to the nonaffected hand or with norms for age groups among males and females to identify baseline strength, set goals, and assess progress. The *OT Guide to Goniometry & MMT* eTextbook features detailed descriptions of assessment techniques for the wrist and hand, including dynamometry. Practice these techniques on a variety of individuals—females, males, children, adults, older adults—and note the differences in motion and strength.

Also make it a habit to narrate the underlying anatomy and functional purpose for various motions. Describe the extrinsic and intrinsic forces as well as the patterns of weakness that might be present with a specific nerve injury. Think about the motion and strength required for different occupations. Describing the anatomical and functional perspectives will help solidify your knowledge on multiple levels and get you thinking like an OT or OTA. For example, you might measure PIP flexion and describe the FDS and FDP muscles as contributing to the movement and strength at this joint as a contribution to gripping a steering wheel when driving.

Occupational and Clinical Perspectives

Continue to review the underlying functional anatomy of the wrist and hand. It takes time to master, and there is always more to learn. It is equally important to frame these structures through the lens of occupation and clinical practice. The rest of this chapter emphasizes the unique contribution of the wrist and hand to occupational performance as well as common clinical application.

Sensorimotor Function of the Hands

Purposeful use of the hands begins with sensory input from the median, ulnar, and radial nerves (see Chapter 2). Vision, touch, and proprioception guide the placement of our hands within our surrounding environment as well as fine movements of the fingers for object manipulation. Our hands can also function without visual input, guided solely by touch and proprioception. It's how you can type without looking at the keys or button the top button of your shirt (**7.68**).

A concert pianist illustrates the sensorimotor capability of hands that have been finely tuned to respond to subtle changes in sensory input, adjusting the speed and force of motion to produce the perfect pitch and volume. The hands play a similar role in ADLs and IADLs, so even a minor injury may significantly limit basic functional tasks.

It may be helpful to think of the hand in terms of precision and gross grasp. The radial aspect of the hand—the thumb and index and middle fingers—is designed for fine motor control, like threading a needle (**7.69**). Various pinch patterns, discussed later in this chapter, aid in manipulating very small objects, as when sewing or tying your shoes.

The ulnar aspect of the hand, with the more mobile CMC joints of the ring and small fingers, can generate more forceful grasp for an activity like carrying a heavy garbage bag. Make a tight fist and you will appreciate the difference in flexion and force on the radial and ulnar aspects of the hand.

Grasp and pinch of the hand are further stabilized and enhanced by the arches of the palm, which conform to and stabilize objects in the hand for manipulation by the fingers and thumb.

Biomechanics of the Wrist and Hand

Due to the complexity of the anatomy and forces acting on the wrist and hand, we will spend a little more time in this section describing biomechanical concepts from a functional perspective. With thirty-four distinct muscles acting on twenty-nine bones, the wrist and hand have complex biomechanics for activities like playing the guitar or opening a tight jar. While entire books have been written on wrist and hand biomechanics, here we will focus on the essentials related to occupation.

Think about your routine this morning. If it was like mine, it began with your hand relying on tactile sensation to feel its way to a smartphone to turn off an alarm in the dark. After remembering it was a workday, I took a shower, brushed my teeth, shaved, and got dressed, taking for granted the enormous volume of sensory input guiding motor output to avoid cutting myself with the razor or applying too much force on delicate gums with a toothbrush. After breakfast and a drive into work, I have been at my workstation writing this chapter,

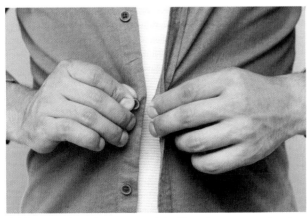

7.68 Buttoning a button on a shirt. How does sensory input guide hand function without visual input?

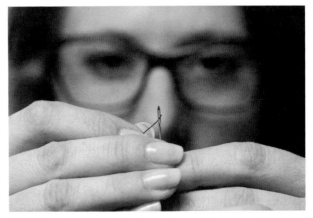

7.69 Threading a needle. How is the radial aspect of the hand designed uniquely for precision?

with thousands of repetitions of my fingers hitting a keyboard, again relying on muscle memory and proprioception (**7.70**).

Recall that the wrist, with its convex-on-concave arrangement, generally features rotation of the proximal carpals in one direction with gliding in the opposite direction. Joint stiffness or capsular tightness after immobilization may limit carpal gliding and overall wrist motion as a result.

As the wrist flexes and extends, it also changes the length and tension of the extrinsic flexor and extensor muscles acting on the hand. Remember, a muscle is strongest in a midrange position, which has the most sarcomere overlap and potential for gliding (contraction).

Composite motions of the wrist and hand—flexing or extending the wrist and fingers simultaneously—can be limited by active insufficiency if the agonist muscle (or muscles) has contracted as far as it can, or passive insufficiency if the antagonist muscle (or muscles) is tight and cannot elongate further. So maintaining the length and balanced tension of the opposing flexor and extensor muscles is important for occupational performance. A musculoskeletal or neurological injury can affect this length-tension relationship.

Keep your fingers relaxed and extend your wrist. Did you notice your fingers passively flex into a weak fist? This phenomenon is called **tenodesis** (**7.71**). The fist is created not by active finger flexion but rather by passive tension on the finger flexor muscles as the wrist actively extends.

Tenodesis can provide a functional grip for an individual with paralysis of the finger flexors but intact wrist extension, such as a person with a spinal cord injury at neurological level C6. In this case, passive insufficiency (tightness) of the extrinsic flexor muscles is desirable to facilitate a stronger tenodesis grip pattern with active wrist extension.

Many functional activities involve diagonal patterns of wrist motion, which combine flexion and ulnar deviation or extension and radial deviation, referred to as **dart thrower's motion** (**7.72**). This arthrokinematic pattern has been described as the most stable motion of the wrist, limiting stress on the carpals.[5]

A strong **composite grasp**, with all the fingers forcefully contracting together, such as when wringing out a washcloth, requires cooperation of the muscles of the wrist and fingers (**7.73**).

For the fingers to forcefully flex, the wrist must remain still (static), allowing the force of the extrinsic finger flexors (FDS and FDP) to flex the fingers into a fist without flexing the wrist. This cooperative effort is achieved by the wrist extensors (ECU, ECRB, and ECRL) activating simultaneously with the finger flexors.

▶**TRY IT**

Palpate the flexor and extensor muscles at your proximal forearm while making a fist. What do you feel?

Did you notice both muscle groups contracting? Did you also notice slight wrist extension as you made a fist? As the wrist extensors contract, the wrist is pulled into slight extension and stabilized while the fingers flex. Wrist extension increases the tension on the finger flexors, increasing the force of contraction as well as overall grip strength.

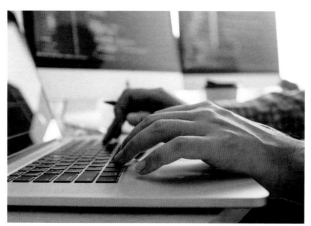

7.70 Describe the sensorimotor patterns involved with a repetitive activity like typing.

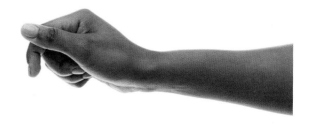

7.71 Tenodesis grip. How might active wrist extension compensate for loss of an active grip for an individual with paralysis of the finger flexors?

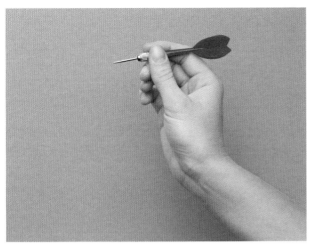

7.72 Describe the motion of the wrist when throwing a dart.

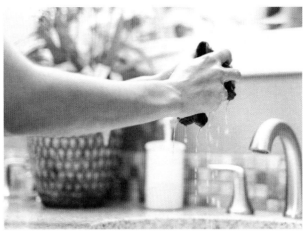

7.73 Wringing out a washcloth. How do the extensor muscles of the wrist contribute to grasp?

Extrinsic and Intrinsic Forces in the Hand

The forces acting on the fingers are complex. The extrinsic and intrinsic muscles respond to sensory feedback, providing the functional balance of forces needed for object manipulation, grasp, and release (**7.74**).

For finger flexion, the extrinsic muscles (FDS and FDP) flex the PIP and DIP, respectively, while also exerting force on the wrist and MCP joints. Simultaneously, the interossei and lumbricals, by way of their dorsal attachments on the proximal phalanges, enhance the force of

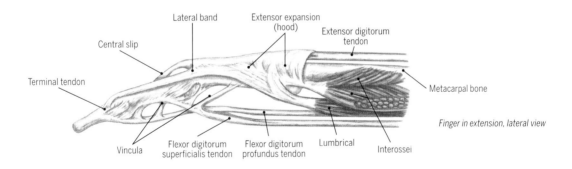

Finger in extension, lateral view

Central slip · Lateral band · Extensor expansion (hood) · Extensor digitorum tendon · Terminal tendon · Metacarpal bone · Vincula · Flexor digitorum superficialis tendon · Flexor digitorum profundus tendon · Lumbrical · Interossei

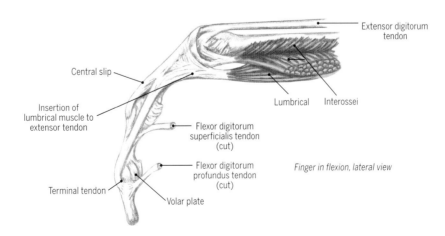

Finger in flexion, lateral view

Central slip · Insertion of lumbrical muscle to extensor tendon · Flexor digitorum superficialis tendon (cut) · Flexor digitorum profundus tendon (cut) · Terminal tendon · Volar plate · Lumbrical · Interossei · Extensor digitorum tendon

7.74 Tendon attachment sites in the fingers. Note the attachments of the interossei and lumbricals to the extensor mechanism. How does this arrangement enable these muscles to extend the IP joints (PIPs and DIPs)?

flexion at the MCP joints. Although small with limited excursion, the interossei muscles alone contribute an estimated 40 percent of the force of composite grasp.[6]

Functional objects vary in shape and size. A toothbrush, spatula, coffee mug, and pencil require different patterns of motion for functional use. The palmar arches allow the palm to fold inward, enveloping the unique shape of an object and increasing surface contact to enhance object manipulation (7.75). Independent motion of the fingers, sometimes referred to as **fractionation**, allows the fingers to adapt and conform to a wide variety of shapes and sizes.

Similar to flexion, functional extension uses a combination of extrinsic (ED, EI, EDM) and intrinsic muscles, such as when you are releasing an object or pointing with the index finger. The extensor digitorum extends all three joints of the finger via the central slip at the proximal phalanx and the terminal tendon at the distal phalanx. Simultaneously, the interossei and lumbricals enhance the force of extension, applying force through their similar attachments at the extensor hood.

Along with generating force for grip, the intrinsic muscles of the hand contribute to specific pinch patterns, described in the next section. The thenar and hypothenar muscle groups facilitate precise movements of the thumb and small finger. Another intrinsic muscle, the adductor pollicis, brings the thumb toward the palm, supplying the primary force for lateral (key) pinch against the radial aspect of the index finger.

As the name implies, the palmar and dorsal interossei lie between the metacarpal bones, supplying medial and lateral forces for abduction and adduction of the fingers. As the interossei insert into the extensor hood, they also have a moment to both flex the MCP and extend the interphalangeal (PIP and DIP) joints. These muscles are active for activities that involve placing the fingers in different positions relative to one another, such as when playing a stringed instrument (7.76).

The last and perhaps most unique intrinsic muscles are the lumbricals, the only muscles in the body to both originate and terminate in soft tissue. Originating from the radial aspect of the FDP of each digit, the lumbricals cross the radial aspect of the volar MCP joint to insert into the extensor hood. Similar to the interossei, the lumbricals serve to flex the MCP joint and extend the IP joints of each digit. The lumbricals also play an important role in balancing the intrinsic and extrinsic forces acting on the digits. As the digits extend, the lumbricals

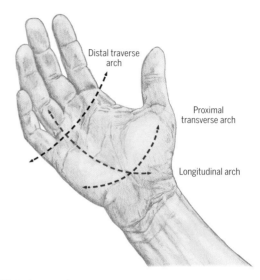

7.75 Palmar arches. How do the arches of the hand contribute to functional grasp?

pull the FDP distally, preventing flexor force on the distal digit, effectively inhibiting its own antagonist.

Flexion of the MCP joints with extension of the PIP and DIP joints describes the **intrinsic plus** position of the hand (7.77). This position elongates the interossei and lumbricals and maintains some tension on the collateral ligaments of the MCP and IP joints by keeping them in their respective close-pack positions.

An **intrinsic minus** position features clawing of the fingers, which posture in MCP hyperextension and IP flexion. This dysfunctional pattern is often present with an ulnar or combined median and ulnar nerve injury, which we'll look at in more detail a little later. When splinting the hand to immobilize after an injury or surgery, this position is often preferred to prevent adaptive shortening and contractures of the joints of the fingers.

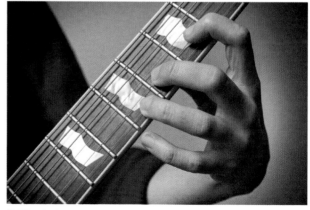

7.76 Playing the guitar. How do the interossei muscles contribute to playing a stringed instrument?

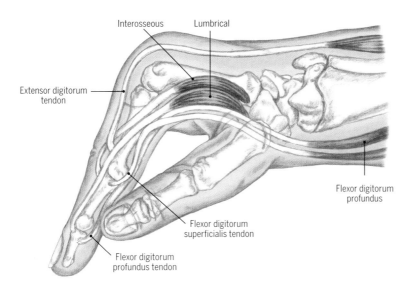

7.77 Intrinsic plus position. How does the intrinsic plus position of the hand maintain tension on the intrinsic muscles?

▶TRY IT

Recall that the fingers naturally come together toward the middle finger when we make a fist. The collateral ligaments of the MCP joints tighten in full flexion (their close-pack position), stabilizing the fingers in this position.

Abduct your fingers while they are extended and try to abduct them in a flexed fist position. Can you tell the difference?

These built-in biomechanics facilitate and stabilize functional grasp, preventing small objects from slipping through the fingers.

The variable shape of the metacarpal heads contributes to involuntary adduction of the fingers and convergence toward the scaphoid with flexion. The collateral ligaments of the metacarpophalangeal joints are also taut in flexion, limiting abduction of the digits in this position.

Prehensile Patterns (Grasp and Pinch)

As an occupation-based clinician, you'll want to keep in mind that biomechanics are not simply forces acting on joints. Rather, they are the physical means by which people exert their will and do the things they want to do. Occupations using the hands—dressing, driving, and painting, to name a few—feature different positions of the hand, or prehensile patterns, for purposeful use of objects.

Grasp is the term used to describe use of the entire hand to hold an object, whereas *pinch* involves varying use of the thumb and index and middle fingers for precise object manipulation (**7.78**).

In a broad sense, the radial aspect of the hand (thumb, index and middle fingers) facilitates precision for fine motor function of the hand, whereas the ulnar digits (ring and small fingers) are more involved with gross grasp. Grasp patterns include the following:

- **Cylindrical grasp** is midrange flexion of the digits around a tube-shaped object, such as when turning the steering wheel of a vehicle or swinging a golf club (**7.79**).
- **Spherical grasp** is varied flexion of the digits around a rounded object, such as when holding the underside of a bowling ball with the nondominant hand in preparation for bowling a strike.

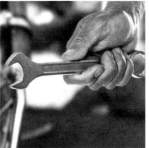
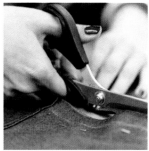

7.78 Describe the prehensile patterns involved with using a wrench or pair of scissors.

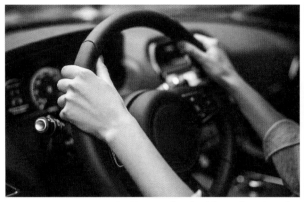
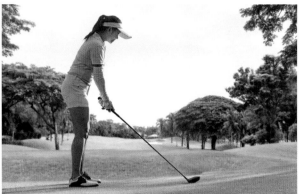

7.79 Describe the bilateral prehensile patterns involved with driving or golfing.

- **Hook grasp** is simultaneous flexion of the PIPs and DIPs with extension of the MCPs, such as when carrying a bucket or briefcase by the handle.
- **Composite grasp** uses maximal flexion of all digits to generate force for actions like squeezing water out of a towel. Perhaps surprisingly, the shorter ring and small fingers generate more force than the radial digits, as the CMC joints of these fingers flex for tighter composite flexion. You can see this when making a tight fist: the ring and small fingers noticeably flex at the CMC joint, while the index and middle CMCs remain relatively static. These cooperative motions facilitate cupping of the hand, bringing the small finger toward the thumb with the palm up.

Pinch patterns include the following:

- **Tip pinch** is used for precise movements such as threading a needle and involves the coordinated movements of the distal tips of the thumb and index finger.
- **Three-jaw chuck pinch**, also called tripod pinch, involves the tip of the thumb pressed against the tips of the index and middle fingers. You use this pinch when writing with a pen or pencil.
- **Lateral (key) pinch** involves the pad of the thumb pressed against the radial side of the index finger. As the name implies, this pinch is used to turn a key to unlock a door and is also handy for holding a fork (**7.80**) or, more delicately, for turning the pages of a book.

For many tasks, the digits remain in a static position of pinch opposition, whereas the wrist provides the functional motion needed for the task. Simply signing your name demonstrates this functional cooperation,

as the thumb and digits remain compressed statically around the pen, while the wrist provides smooth, fluid pen strokes.

Grip and pinch rely on the stabilizing muscles of the wrist as well as the extrinsic and intrinsic muscles of the fingers and thumb. Interventions aimed at improving functional grip or pinch might target these contributing muscle groups through exercises or activities to promote occupational performance.

There are many sources that describe typical grip and pinch strength based on age and sex, providing an estimate of normal grip strength. A patient's noninjured hand may also serve as a valid baseline measurement. Occupational therapy goals related to improving grip or pinch strength to improve performance of specific occupations are common in many practice settings.

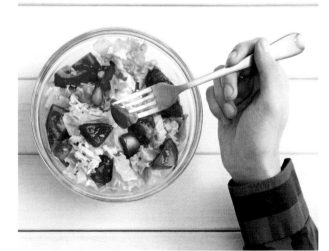

7.80 Using eating utensils. What pinch pattern is involved with the use of a fork for self-feeding?

▶TRY IT

How much grip and pinch strength is needed for basic function? Grip and pinch strength needs vary depending on the patient's functional needs. For example, an older adult who completes basic ADLs at home and knits as a leisure occupation likely does not require the same level of strength as a college athlete.

Research suggests that for most ADLs—bathing, dressing, toileting—approximately 20 lb. of grip strength is needed.[7] Grip strength peaks between 20 and 40 years of age and may also be a biomarker of aging.[8]

Using the *OT Guide to Goniometry & MMT* eTextbook, measure your own grip and pinch strength and compare the values to what is typical for your age and sex. How might you use grip and pinch strength to assess and set goals for your future patients?

Distal Radius Fracture

Fractures of the distal radius account for 25 percent of all pediatric fractures and 18 percent of all fractures in the older adult population.[9] Often the injury occurs as a result of a FOOSH as the hand comes into contact with the ground surface.

A fracture with a dorsal displacement of the distal bone segment is called a **Colles' fracture**, and a volarly displaced fracture is referred to as a **Smith's fracture** (**7.81**). Distal radius fractures can be simple extra-articular (outside the joint) injuries or more complex intra-articular (inside the joint) fractures.

Secondary complications associated with distal radius fractures include edema (swelling), scar tissue, nerve compression, and unresolved joint stiffness in the wrist and fingers. The severity of injury guides orthopedic intervention, rehabilitation timeline, and functional prognosis.

Early postoperative occupational therapy interventions include edema management, scar management, ADL modifications, and maintaining adjacent joint mobility to prevent the long-term impact of secondary complications. Additional OT intervention may involve balance assessment and fall prevention, particularly important for the older adult population.

Osteoarthritis

Osteoarthritis (OA), or wear-and-tear arthritis, can occur anywhere in the body where there is friction between bones, which is primarily in the joints. OA can be extremely painful and debilitating, depending on its location and severity.

Because the hands are so active, OA is common there, particularly in the joints of the fingers and thumb. The most common site in the hand for OA is the CMC joint of the thumb, as it sustains forces through its unique saddle design with grasp and pinch (see **7.17**). The angulation of the trapezium, anterior to the frontal plane, provides positional advantage for functional opposition of the thumb but also creates a focal point for mechanical force.

OA may also occur after a traumatic injury, such as a distal radius fracture in which the relative position of the bones has been altered, resulting in increased friction.

Conservative management of OA in the hands includes supporting orthoses, physical agent modalities (such as paraffin treatments), activity modification, or adaptive equipment (such as built-up grips) to decrease forces through affected joints. Advanced OA may require surgical intervention in the form of a joint replacement (arthroplasty) to restore functional motion or fusion (arthrodesis), sacrificing motion but typically eliminating pain.

Cumulative Trauma Disorders

Every machine has a degree of wear and tear, and the wrist and hands are no exception. Cumulative trauma disorders (CTDs) are pathologies that develop over time due to microtrauma to the body's tissues from repetitive

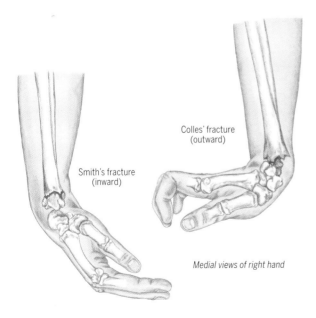

Colles' fracture (outward)

Smith's fracture (inward)

Medial views of right hand

7.81 Smith's and Colles' fractures. What might increase the risk of a distal radius fracture in the older adult population?

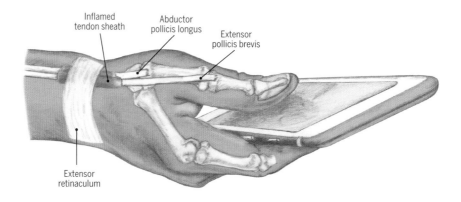

Inflamed tendon sheath

Abductor pollicis longus

Extensor pollicis brevis

Extensor retinaculum

7.82 Mobile device use. How might you address the person, environment, and occupation to prevent CTDs like de Quervain's tenosynovitis?

use. The rise of technology and associated repetitive motion of the hands may be a contributing factor to these types of disorders.

For example, texting thumb (de Quervain's tenosynovitis), discussed earlier in the chapter (see **7.53**), is inflammation of the synovial sheath and tendons of the 1st dorsal compartment due to friction from repetitive motion associated with mobile device use (**7.82**). Trigger finger (see **7.28**) and carpal tunnel syndrome (see **7.48**) are also common pathologies arising from tissue friction in tight anatomical spaces. Soft tissue inflammation may occur wherever focal, repetitive stresses are present.

Peripheral Nerve Injuries

Purposeful use of the hands requires discriminative touch, or specific, localized sensory input, to guide functional output. Using your hands without visual input, such as when buttoning the top button of a shirt or finding a dime in your pocket among other change, illustrates the specificity and necessity of guiding somatosensation (**7.83**).

Stereognosis refers to the ability to identify an object based on somatosensation alone, without visual input. While many of us use this sensory ability regularly without much conscious thought, such as when reaching for a smartphone to turn off the alarm in the dark, individuals with visual impairment rely more heavily on stereognosis and discriminative touch for function. Braille was developed specifically for individuals with blindness to compensate for visual loss by using touch to read, interpreting the precise patterns of raised dots with the fingertips.

Somatosensation also plays an important protective role for the hands. Distinct sensory receptors discern not only material shape and quality but also temperature, pain, or the threat of injury. Inadvertently placing your hand on a hot stovetop or against a sharp edge elicits a withdrawal reflex at the spinal cord level, with reflexive removal of the hand from the offending stimulus, often before the pain is perceived in the brain.

Peripheral nerve injuries contribute to distinct patterns of sensory and motor loss in the hand and digits. Symptoms range from transient numbness to complete paralysis, depending on the severity of the injury. Prolonged compression or tension on a nerve—related to pathologies like carpal tunnel and cubital tunnel

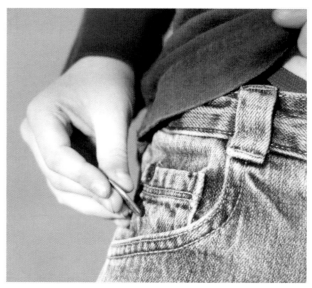

7.83 Describe the functional importance of discriminative touch and stereognosis.

syndromes—often manifests initially with numbness and tingling. However, if unaddressed, the symptoms may progress over time to include motor weakness. Traumatic injuries or the complete severance, or separation, of a nerve generally results in immediate sensory loss and paralysis.

Motor impairment of the radial, ulnar, or median nerve presents with distinct patterns of atrophy and loss of purposeful movement (**7.84**).

Compressive or traction injuries to the nerve may resolve over time, whereas traumatic severance will require surgical repair of the nerve itself or surgical tendon transfer to address motor deficits. Conservatively, compensatory strategies using custom orthoses, modified technique, or adaptive equipment serve to promote occupational performance. Additionally, stretching and splinting may help maintain soft tissue length or position while awaiting neural regeneration.

Radial nerve motor impairment leads to loss of wrist, digit, and thumb extension, more commonly known as **wrist drop**. This limits activities that require a neutral or extended position of the wrist, such as forceful gripping, typing, and dressing. Radial nerve sensory loss is isolated to the radial aspect of the dorsal wrist, fingers, and thumb, which means it has less effect on function as compared to ulnar or median sensory impairment.

A dynamic orthosis provides compensatory digital extension while maintaining the wrist in a functional extended position for functional grasp (**7.85**). A static

AUDREY PURDUM | Audrey is now noticing some numbness and tingling in her right hand. It does not seem to affect her entire hand; rather it mainly affects the volar side of the thumb, index finger, and middle finger. Her hand feels like it is asleep, which is keeping her awake at night. Audrey is looking forward to her first occupational therapy visit tomorrow to begin the rehabilitation process and get some answers.

- What do you think might be contributing to these symptoms?
- How is this related to her original injury (distal radius fracture)?

orthosis may be used at rest to prevent overstretch of the extensor muscles of the wrist and digits.

Ulnar motor impairment leads to **claw hand**, with classic hyperextension of the MCPs and loss of IP extension in the ring and small fingers. As the ulnar nerve innervates the palmar and dorsal interossei, as well as the lumbricals of the ring and small fingers, these digits present with an imbalance of force between the intrinsic and extrinsic muscles, contributing to the deformity. Additionally, loss of DIP flexion occurs due to ulnar innervation of the FDP to the ring and small fingers. Considerable weakness of lateral (key) pinch is common as well with denervation of the adductor pollicis.

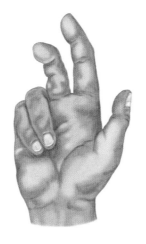
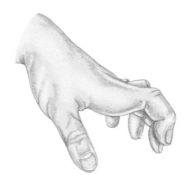
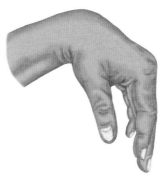

Hand of benediction
High median nerve injury

Claw hand
Ulnar or combined median/
ulnar nerve injury

Wrist drop
Radial nerve injury

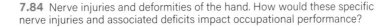

7.84 Nerve injuries and deformities of the hand. How would these specific nerve injuries and associated deficits impact occupational performance?

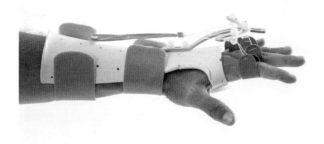

7.85 Dynamic digital extension orthosis. How might this orthosis compensate for loss of radial nerve to promote hand function?

Sensory loss is focused on the ulnar aspect of the palm and ring finger as well as the entire small finger.

Orthotic interventions involve positioning the MCPs in flexion to avoid contracture developing in the IP joints (**7.86**). A high ulnar nerve injury (proximal forearm) demonstrates less severe clawing because the extrinsic FDP is also impaired, whereas a low injury (distal forearm) will be more pronounced because extrinsic force is spared.

Median motor and sensory impairment, perhaps the most functionally limiting impairment, may be high (proximal forearm) or low (distal forearm), with varying deficits depending on the site of injury.

A high median nerve injury compromises the extrinsic long flexors of the index and middle fingers and thumb as well as the thenar muscle group. This leads to a deformity known as **hand of benediction**, the inability to flex the thumb and index and middle fingers as well as the loss of the web space of the thumb. This pattern of motor loss significantly limits fine motor and pinch,

as the thumb is unable to oppose the digits, which also have limited ability to flex.

Maintaining the web space of the thumb is vital while awaiting neural regeneration, as atrophy of the thenar muscles may lead to contracture of the web space and long-term impairment. A static opponens orthosis may be used to maintain the web space and position the thumb and digits in functional opposition (**7.87**).

A low median nerve injury results in solely intrinsic muscle paralysis, sparing the long flexors for digital and thumb flexion while compromising the web space due to thenar muscle loss.

Both high and low median nerve injuries impair sensation to the thumb, index and middle fingers, and radial aspect of the ring finger. A high median nerve injury will also impact sensation to the radial aspect of the palm. Sensory input in this area is essential to guide fine motor control of the hand.

As the hand provides the interface with the material world, it is also subject to acute traumatic injury in the form of bone fractures, soft tissue strains, tendon lacerations, burns, and wounds. Approximately one-third of all acute injuries seen in the emergency room involve injury to the upper extremity and hand. Anatomical complexity creates unique challenges for OTs working with hand injuries, and detailed communication with the referring provider is critical, particularly after surgical intervention.

As a generalist OT or OTA, you should be prepared to address wrist and hand limitations as an essential component of occupational performance. OTs may also specialize as a certified hand therapist (CHT) to address more complex upper extremity and hand dysfunction.

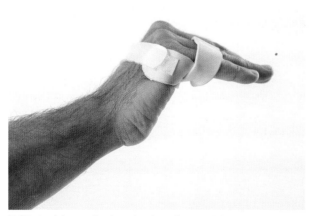

7.86 Anticlaw orthosis. What benefit would this orthosis provide an individual with an ulnar nerve injury?

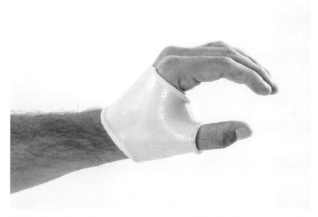

7.87 Short thumb opponens orthosis. What is the purpose of this orthosis for an individual with a median nerve injury?

APPLY AND REVIEW

Audrey Purdum

Audrey comes in for her occupational therapy evaluation one week after surgery. Her physician order states, "OT evaluation and treatment—conservative AROM of the forearm and wrist. No motion restrictions to the fingers or thumb. Avoid PROM and strengthening. Address edema and pain. Continue relative immobilization until physician follow-up at four weeks post-op."

She is eager to begin and has a lot of questions. Before you can begin her evaluation, she wants to know the following:

- How long will it take me to get back to normal?
- Why is my hand swelling and when will this go away? It's keeping me up at night!
- Is this numbness and tingling normal?
- When can I take this brace off?

After answering her questions, you review her occupational profile, as shown at the beginning of this chapter, and medical history. Her chart notes that she has osteoporosis. You begin a physical examination, taking comprehensive goniometry measurements of her injured right forearm and wrist and noninjured left side to establish a baseline for her normal motion. Her forearm and wrist AROM is as follows:

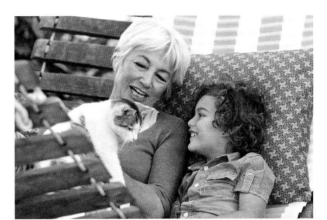

	RIGHT	LEFT
Forearm supination	10°	82°
Forearm pronation	15°	75°
Wrist flexion	10°	70°
Wrist extension	8°	75°
Wrist ulnar deviation	6°	18°
Wrist radial deviation	7°	15°

A gross visual assessment of her fingers and thumb reveals approximately 50 percent active composite (full) flexion with mild loss of extension of the fingers at the PIP and DIP joints.

You also take circumferential measurements at the wrist crease, midpalmar crease, MCPs, PIPs, and DIPs of the right hand and compare these to the same measurements on the left hand. You notice that the measurements for the right hand are approximately two centimeters greater than those for the left. What does this indicate?

You also assess the sensation in her right hand using monofilament testing and note decreased light touch through the volar thumb, index and middle fingers, and radial aspect of the ring finger. The back of her hand and the small finger appear to have normal sensation. What might this indicate?

Based on your review of Audrey's occupational profile and her evaluation, consider the following:

- Audrey's medical history specifies she has osteoporosis. How might this have contributed to her injury? What impact will it have on the rehabilitation process?
- What compensatory or adaptive techniques could you use to facilitate Audrey's occupational performance during the early phase of recovery (without functional use of the right hand)?
- How might you address and prevent further complications due to edema and loss of sensation?
- Based on your initial goniometry measurements, set one long-term (four to six weeks) and three short-term (two to three weeks) occupation-based goals to measure Audrey's progress with occupational therapy. Use the *OT Guide to Goniometry & MMT* eTextbook to find some suggestions for the wrist and hand.

Review Questions

1. What portion of the extensor digitorum extends the proximal interphalangeal (PIP) joints of the fingers?
   a. sagittal bands
   b. terminal tendon
   c. central slip
   d. extensor carpi radialis

2. What muscle bifurcates and inserts on the middle phalanx of each finger to flex the proximal interphalangeal (PIP) joint?
   a. flexor digitorum profundus
   b. flexor digitorum superficialis
   c. palmaris longus
   d. flexor pollicis longus

3. Which aspect of your hand would be *most* effective to use when wringing out a washcloth for bathing?
   a. ulnar aspect (ring and small fingers)
   b. distal fingertips and thumb
   c. central aspect (middle and ring fingers)
   d. radial aspect (thumb and index and middle fingers)

4. Which of the following pinch patterns would be *most* affected by an injury to the ulnar nerve?
   a. tip pinch
   b. lateral (key) pinch
   c. three-jaw chuck pinch
   d. composite grasp

5. Simultaneous contraction of the extensor carpi ulnaris (ECU) and the flexor carpi ulnaris (FCU) would produce what movement at the wrist?
   a. extension
   b. flexion
   c. radial deviation
   d. ulnar deviation

6. What is the only muscle that can flex the distal interphalangeal (DIP) joint?
   a. palmaris longus
   b. flexor digitorum profundus
   c. flexor digitorum superficialis
   d. flexor carpi ulnaris

7. Place the tip of your right index finger on the letter J of a computer keyboard in QWERTY format. Without moving your wrist, move the tip of your finger to the letter H. Which of the following muscles enables this functional motion?
   a. flexor digitorum profundus
   b. extensor digitorum
   c. 1st palmar interosseous
   d. 1st dorsal interosseous

8. The majority of the motion at the wrist occurs between which of the following bones?
   a. ulna, lunate, and triquetrum
   b. radius, scaphoid, and lunate
   c. ulna, scaphoid, and lunate
   d. radius, trapezium, and lunate

9. Which of the following pairs of muscles is essential for the motions of the thumb and index finger for tip pinch, as when threading a needle?
   a. flexor digitorum superficialis and flexor pollicis brevis
   b. flexor digitorum profundus and abductor pollicis longus
   c. adductor pollicis and flexor digitorum superficialis
   d. flexor digitorum profundus and flexor pollicis longus

10. Collectively, the interossei muscles of the hand contribute to all of the following movements *except*
    a. abduction of the fingers.
    b. adduction of the fingers.
    c. flexion of the distal interphalangeal (DIP) joints.
    d. flexion of the metacarpophalangeal (MCP) joints.

See Answer Key in back of book.

Notes

1. Centers for Disease Control and Prevention, National Center for Injury Prevention and Control, "Deaths from Older Adult Falls," CDC Injury Center, last reviewed July 9, 2020, https://www.cdc.gov/homeandrecreationalsafety/falls/data/deaths-from-falls.html.

2. Richard A. Berger, "The Anatomy and Basic Biomechanics of the Wrist Joint," *Journal of Hand Therapy* 9, no. 2 (April–June 1996): 92, https://doi.org/10.1016/S0894-1130(96)80066-4.

3. Carol A. Oatis, *Kinesiology: The Mechanics and Pathomechanics of Human Movement*, 3rd ed. (Philadelphia: Wolters Kluwer, 2017).

4. Nathan Short et al., "Defining Mobile Tech Posture: Prevalence and Position among Millennials," *Open Journal of Occupational Therapy* 8, no. 1 (2020): 1–10, https://doi.org/10.15453/2168-6408.1640.

5. Oatis, *Kinesiology*.

6. Scott H. Kozin et al., "The Contribution of the Intrinsic Muscles to Grip and Pinch Strength," *Journal of Hand Surgery* 24, no. 1 (January 1999): 64–72, https://doi.org/10.1053/jhsu.1999.jhsu24a0064.

7. Richard W. Bohannon et al., "Average Grip Strength: A Meta-Analysis of Data Obtained with a Jamar Dynamometer from Individuals 75 Years or More of Age," *Journal of Geriatric Physical Therapy* 30, no. 1 (2007): 28–30, https://www.ncbi.nlm.nih.gov/pubmed/19839178.

8. Avan Aihie Sayer and Thomas B. L. Kirkwood, "Grip Strength and Mortality: A Biomarker of Ageing?" *Lancet* 386, no. 9990 (July 18, 2015): 226–27, https://doi.org/10.1016/S0140-6736(14)62349-7.

9. Kate W. Nellans, Evan Kowalski, and Kevin C. Chung, "The Epidemiology of Distal Radius Fractures," *Hand Clinics* 28, no. 2 (May 2012): 113–25, https://doi.org/10.1016/j.hcl.2012.02.001.

Bibliography

Berger, Richard A. "The Anatomy and Basic Biomechanics of the Wrist Joint." *Journal of Hand Therapy* 9, no. 2 (April–June 1996): 84–93. https://doi.org/10.1016/S0894-1130(96)80066-4.

Biel, Andrew. *Trail Guide to Movement: Building the Body in Motion*. 2nd ed. Boulder, CO: Books of Discovery, 2019.

Biel, Andrew. *Trail Guide to the Body: A Hands-On Guide to Locating Muscles, Bones, and More*. 6th ed. Boulder, CO: Books of Discovery, 2019.

Bohannon, Richard W., Jane Bear-Lehman, Johanne Desrosiers, Nicola Massy-Westropp, and Virgil Mathiowetz. "Average Grip Strength: A Meta-Analysis of Data Obtained with a Jamar Dynamometer from Individuals 75 Years or More of Age." *Journal of Geriatric Physical Therapy* 30, no. 1 (2007): 28–30. https://www.ncbi.nlm.nih.gov/pubmed/19839178.

Centers for Disease Control and Prevention, National Center for Injury Prevention and Control. "Deaths from Older Adult Falls." CDC Injury Center. Last reviewed July 9, 2020. https://www.cdc.gov/homeandrecreationalsafety/falls/data/deaths-from-falls.html.

Greene, David Paul, and Susan L. Roberts. *Kinesiology: Movement in the Context of Activity*. 3rd ed. St. Louis, MO: Elsevier, 2017.

Kozin, Scott H., Scott Porter, Perrin Clark, and Joseph J. Thoder. "The Contribution of the Intrinsic Muscles to Grip and Pinch Strength." *Journal of Hand Surgery* 24, no. 1 (January 1999): 64–72. https://doi.org/10.1053/jhsu.1999.jhsu24a0064.

Lundy-Ekman, Laurie. *Neuroscience: Fundamentals for Rehabilitation*. 5th ed. St. Louis, MO: Elsevier, 2018.

Nellans, Kate W., Evan Kowalski, and Kevin C. Chung. "The Epidemiology of Distal Radius Fractures." *Hand Clinics* 28, no. 2 (May 2012): 113–25. https://doi.org/10.1016/j.hcl.2012.02.001.

Oatis, Carol A. *Kinesiology: The Mechanics and Pathomechanics of Human Movement*. 3rd ed. Philadelphia: Wolters Kluwer, 2017.

Pendleton, Heidi McHugh, and Winifred Schultz-Krohn. *Pedretti's Occupational Therapy: Practice Skills for Physical Dysfunction*. 8th ed. St. Louis, MO: Elsevier, 2017.

Sayer, Avan Aihie, and Thomas B. L. Kirkwood. "Grip Strength and Mortality: A Biomarker of Ageing?" *Lancet* 386, no. 9990 (July 18, 2015): 226–27. https://doi.org/10.1016/S0140-6736(14)62349-7.

Short, Nathan, Michell Mays, Alex Cool, Ariana Delay, Ali Lannom, Laryn O'Donnell, and Ruth Stuber. "Defining Mobile Tech Posture: Prevalence and Position among Millennials." *Open Journal of Occupational Therapy* 8, no. 1 (2020): 1–10. https://doi.org/10.15453/2168-6408.1640.

Standring, Susan. *Gray's Anatomy: The Anatomical Basis of Clinical Practice, International Edition*. 41st ed. Cambridge, UK: Elsevier, 2016.

PART IV

Lower Extremity

CHAPTER 8

Pelvis and Hip

Learning Objectives

- Describe the bones, joints, and muscles contributing to purposeful movement of the pelvis and hip.

- Identify the primary purposeful movements of the pelvis and hip within the context of occupational performance.

- Develop competency in goniometry and manual muscle testing (MMT) as clinical assessment techniques for the hip.

- Use clinical reasoning to identify limitations of the pelvis and hip that may affect occupational performance.

Key Concepts

angle of inclination

ankylosing spondylitis

anterior pelvic tilt

head, arms, and trunk (HAT)

hemiarthroplasty

hip fracture

hip precautions

iliotibial (IT) band syndrome

incontinence

pelvic floor (diaphragm)

pelvic obliquity

pelvic organ prolapse

pelvic rotation

pelvic tilt

posterior pelvic tilt

sciatica

total hip arthroplasty (THA)

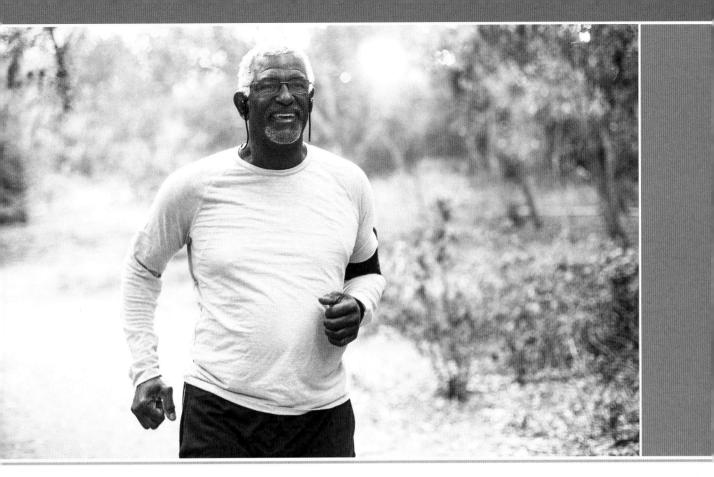

 Occupational Profile: Brian Kelton

BRIAN KELTON is an active sixty-eight-year-old man, recently retired as a high school principal, who enjoys playing tennis, swimming, cycling, and traveling with his spouse of more than forty years. An avid sportsman, he frequently competes in the National Senior Games and has advanced to regional competitions in several events over the past few years. He is also engaged in his local community, serving on several committees as well as the school board.

A few days ago, Brian was hiking with some friends, which he does every Saturday morning, rain or shine, and he fell, injuring his dominant right hip.

- Do some research on hip injuries. What types of injuries are common for older adults who sustain a fall?
- Consider the **Model of Human Occupation (MOHO)** and its emphasis on volition, habituation, environment, and performance skills. How might this theory guide your approach to working with someone like Brian?

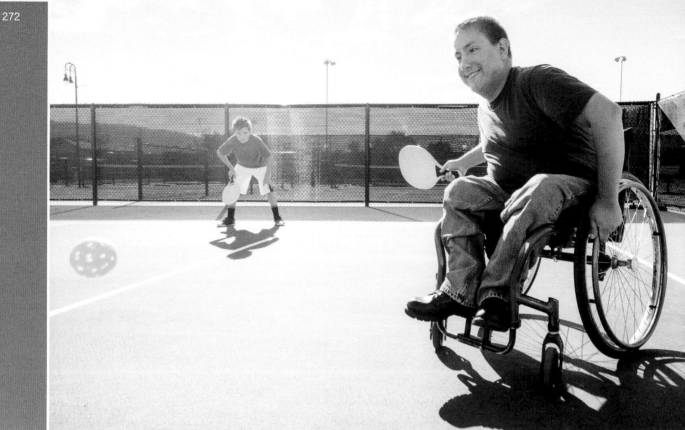

8.1 The pelvis and hip serve as a stable base for the head, arms, and trunk (HAT) to support occupational performance.

Pelvis and Hip: A Stable Base

Are you sitting upright while reading this book? Think about what supports the weight of your upper body in this position. The pelvis and hip create a stable base of support for the **head, arms, and trunk (HAT)**, supplying the proximal stability needed for distal mobility and function (**8.1**).

The pelvis is the interface between the lower extremities and spine. It absorbs the descending force of the weight of gravity on the upper body, as well as the ground reaction forces ascending from the lower extremities.

As the central point of the skeletal architecture of the body, the pelvis requires balance to maintain symmetry of the entire body. Unevenness in the pelvis translates to asymmetry of the spine and extremities. This can cause musculoskeletal imbalance and asynchrony of movement.

Because of this central role in movement, the pelvis is often the starting point for a practitioner's assessment when addressing an individual's positioning and mobility.

The pelvis is the proximal articulation for the hip joint, its link to the lower extremity. It supports the body during standing or movement. The hip also positions the lower

extremity—similar to how the shoulder positions the upper extremity—for targeted weight-bearing through the foot for functional mobility.

This chapter describes the bones, joints, and muscles that stabilize and move this central region of the body. As you process the material and apply it using the recurring resources and features integrated throughout the chapter, consider the broader impact of the pelvis and hip on occupational performance.

Osteology: Bones of the Pelvis and Hip

The pelvis is the skeletal floor of the body's trunk. Its position and movement are intimately related to the adjacent spine and hip (**8.2**). As you examine the bones that provide structure to this region, use the digital palpation resources provided to identify key surface landmarks. Many of these landmarks will be revisited later in the chapter as sites of muscle attachment or landmarks to guide clinical assessment using the *OT Guide to Goniometry & MMT eTextbook*.

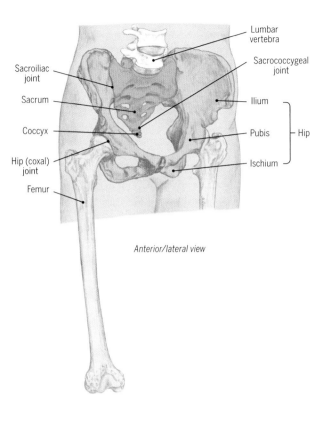

Anterior/lateral view

8.2 Bones of the pelvis and hip

Sacrum

The **sacrum** is a triangle-shaped bone located between the fifth lumbar vertebra and the **coccyx** (tailbone) (**8.3**, **8.4**). The sacrum is composed of five **sacral vertebrae** that fuse by early adulthood and form the posterior pelvic wall, which stabilizes and strengthens the pelvis.

As the most posterior portion of the lower vertebral column, the sacrum is a focal point of pressure when sitting or lying down. The first three sacral vertebrae are specialized to articulate with the ilia of the pelvis, which together make up the sacroiliac joint.

Bony Landmarks of the Sacrum

The bony landmarks of the sacrum serve as attachment sites for ligaments and muscles that support and stabilize the pelvis and lumbar spine.

The sacral **ala** is a bony triangular surface that is positioned lateral to the first sacral vertebra on either side of the sacrum. It is continuous with the iliac fossa of the anterior pelvis.

The axial borders of the sacrum are formed by the **sacral promontory**, its plateau-like superior surface, and the **sacral apex**, its inferior border articulating with the coccyx (**8.4**). The sacrum has sixteen openings,

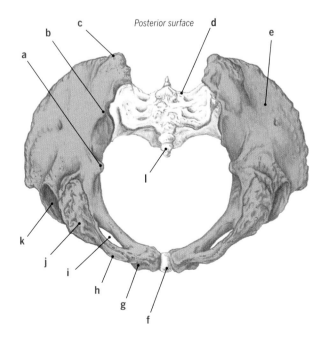

Inferior view

a. Ischial spine
b. Posterior inferior iliac spine (PIIS)
c. Posterior superior iliac spine (PSIS)
d. Sacrum
e. Gluteal surface of ilium
f. Pubic symphysis
g. Inferior ramus of the pubis
h. Ramus of ischium
i. Obturator foramen
j. Ischial tuberosity
k. Acetabulum
l. Coccyx

Black letters indicate bones; **red** letters indicate bony landmarks or other structures.

8.3 Sacrum, inferior view

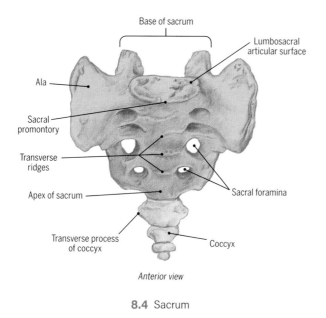

Base of sacrum

Lumbosacral
articular surface

Ala

Sacral
promontory

Transverse
ridges

Sacral foramina

Apex of sacrum

Transverse process
of coccyx

Coccyx

Anterior view

8.4 Sacrum

called **sacral foramina**, which serve as passageways for the anterior and posterior branches of the sacral nerves.

Pelvis

The **pelvis (pelvic girdle)** is formed by two **hip (coxal) bones** that are each composed of three distinct portions: the **ilium**, **pubis**, and **ischium** (**8.5**).

The hip bones attach to either side of the sacrum posteriorly and have a direct anterior connection via the **pubic symphysis**, a fibrocartilaginous disc (see **8.3**). The arrangement makes a three-dimensional bony bowl, tilted slightly anterior, as the functional link between the upper body and lower body. The female pelvis is wider than the male's; this larger pelvic bowl increases the area for carrying and delivering a child.

The ilium, pubis, and ischium meet at the **acetabulum**, which creates the socket for the head of the femur. The pubis and ischium encircle an opening called the **obturator foramen**, a protective passageway for nerves and blood vessels of the leg (**8.6**).

Bony Landmarks of the Pelvis

The bony landmarks of the pelvis provide attachment sites for structures that stabilize it against the converging forces generated by the upper body and lower body. The rounded edge of the superior border of the ilium is called the **iliac crest** (**8.6**, **8.7**). It is easily palpated by moving your hands down either side of your trunk. The most anterior point of the iliac crest is the **anterior superior**

iliac spine (ASIS), and its most posterior point is the **posterior superior iliac spine (PSIS)**. These are important palpable landmarks for assessing pelvic symmetry, discussed later in this chapter.

The broad span of bone beneath the iliac crest is the **iliac blade**. The anterior iliac blade is concave and is referred to as the **iliac fossa**, an attachment site for the muscles that flex the hip.

The posterior iliac blade features the rough L-shaped **auricular surface** for articulation with the sacrum. Just above this area is the **iliac tubercle**, the bony attachment site for the stabilizing sacroiliac ligaments. The posterior iliac blade also features **gluteal lines (anterior, posterior, inferior)** that delineate sites of attachment for the gluteal muscles.

The ilium narrows inferiorly beneath the **anterior inferior iliac spine (AIIS)** and **posterior inferior iliac spine (PIIS)** to form the posterior aspect of the acetabulum. A nearly 90° angle is formed beneath the PSIS, creating the **greater sciatic notch**. Many nerves and blood vessels of the lower extremity pass through this opening.

The **ischial body** forms the posterior portion of the acetabulum. It then curves inferiorly and connects to the pubis, encircling the obturator foramen, which is the pathway for the obturator artery, nerve, and vein.

The **ischial spine** projects posteriorly, creating the lesser sciatic notch beneath. The lower half of the ischial body is the **ischial tuberosity**, often the primary point

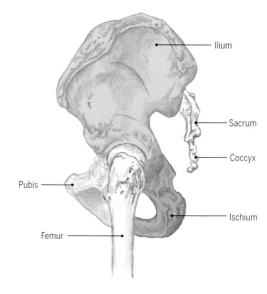

Ilium

Sacrum

Coccyx

Pubis

Ischium

Femur

Lateral view of left pelvis and hip

8.5 Pelvis

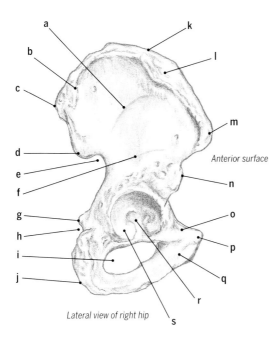

a. Anterior gluteal line
b. Posterior gluteal line
c. Posterior superior iliac spine (PSIS)
d. Posterior inferior iliac spine (PIIS)
e. Greater sciatic notch
f. Inferior gluteal line
g. Ischial spine
h. Lesser sciatic notch
i. Obturator foramen
j. Ischial tuberosity
k. Iliac crest
l. Iliac tubercle
m. Anterior superior iliac spine (ASIS)
n. Anterior inferior iliac spine (AIIS)
o. Superior ramus of the pubis
p. Pubic tubercle
q. Inferior ramus of the pubis
r. Acetabulum
s. Lunate surface of acetabulum

Anterior surface

Lateral view of right hip

8.6 Bony landmarks of the pelvis

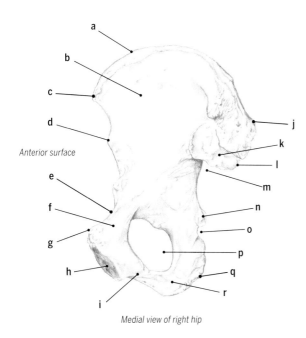

a. Iliac crest
b. Iliac fossa
c. Anterior superior iliac spine (ASIS)
d. Anterior inferior iliac spine (AIIS)
e. Pectineal line
f. Superior ramus of the pubis
g. Pubic tubercle
h. Symphyseal surface
i. Inferior ramus of the pubis
j. Posterior superior iliac spine (PSIS)
k. Auricular surface
l. Posterior inferior iliac spine (PIIS)
m. Greater sciatic notch
n. Ischial spine
o. Lesser sciatic notch
p. Obturator foramen
q. Ischial tuberosity
r. Ramus of the ischium

Anterior surface

Medial view of right hip

8.7 Bony landmarks of the pelvis

of pelvic contact with a seating surface—and a potential site for a pressure sore.

The **pubic body** of each hip bone is connected by fibrocartilage, forming the pubic symphysis. Superiorly, the pubis forms the anterior portion of the acetabulum.

Inferiorly, it rounds posteriorly, connecting to the ischium. The **pubic tubercle** lies on the anterior body of the pubis. It serves as an attachment for the **inguinal ligament**, which forms a ligamentous barrier between the trunk and lower extremity.

Femur

The **femur** is the longest bone in the body and the sole bone of the thigh (**8.8**). Proximally, it features a hemispheric, smooth **femoral head** that articulates with the acetabulum. The femoral head is composed of cancellous (spongy) bone, allowing for some bony flexibility to absorb the descending forces of the upper body through the hip.

The head of the femur is attached to the femoral shaft by the long **femoral neck**, angled at 120° to 130° to the axis of the shaft (females, on the average, have a slightly larger angle than males). This **angle of inclination** is greater at birth but decreases over time due to the loading stress of weight-bearing when walking. Functionally, the angle positions the femur medial (relative to the pelvis), placing the feet beneath the body to support standing and walking. The long shaft of the femur widens distally, forming the proximal aspect of the knee joint.

The femoral neck is typically oriented anterior to the femoral condyles, a position referred to as **femoral anteversion**. An excessive anterior angulation may result in intoeing, or a tendency for the foot to point medially. A decreased anterior angle of the femoral neck relative to its condyles or posterior angulation is called **femoral retroversion** and may contribute to out-toeing, or a lateral pointing of the feet.

Bony Landmarks of the Femur

Many of the bony landmarks of the femur serve as attachment sites for the powerful muscles that act on the hip and knee. Several landmarks will also be noted in the *OT Guide to Goniometry & MMT* eTextbook as reference points for performing clinical assessments.

The **greater trochanter** projects laterally from the proximal femur, providing an attachment for the muscles that abduct and externally (laterally) rotate the hip (**8.8**). The **lesser trochanter** lies inferior to the greater trochanter and projects medially as an attachment for the muscles that flex the hip. The trochanters are separated by the **intertrochanteric line** and **intertrochanteric crest**.

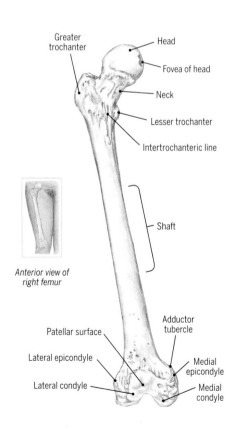

Greater trochanter
Head
Fovea of head
Neck
Lesser trochanter
Intertrochanteric line
Shaft

Anterior view of right femur

Patellar surface
Lateral epicondyle
Lateral condyle
Adductor tubercle
Medial epicondyle
Medial condyle

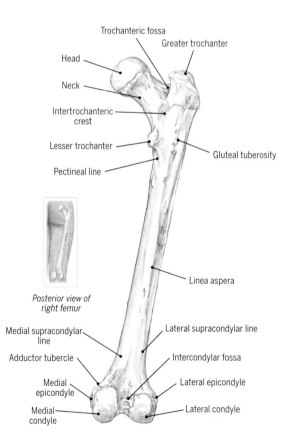

Trochanteric fossa
Greater trochanter
Head
Neck
Intertrochanteric crest
Lesser trochanter
Gluteal tuberosity
Pectineal line
Linea aspera

Posterior view of right femur

Medial supracondylar line
Adductor tubercle
Medial epicondyle
Medial condyle
Lateral supracondylar line
Intercondylar fossa
Lateral epicondyle
Lateral condyle

8.8 Femur

The posterior femur features the **linea aspera**, a bony ridge that serves as the attachment for muscles that adduct the hip.

Now that we know the skeletal structures of the pelvis and hip, we'll examine the joints of the pelvis and hip that contribute to purposeful movement.

Joints

The joints of the pelvis and hip are designed to absorb and transfer the converging forces from the weight of the body above and the lower extremities beneath. Powerful forces generated by the trunk and legs are transmitted through these joints to facilitate walking, running, serving a tennis ball, and other similar activities.

Sacroiliac Joint

The **sacroiliac (SI) joint** serves as a biomechanical link, transmitting ascending and descending forces, between the upper and lower body (**8.9**). There is considerable debate regarding the classification of and movement available at the SI joint. Most sources suggest the joint demonstrates a small amount of rotation and translation that may increase with pregnancy and decrease with age.[1]

Because the sacrum and ilium are oriented medial to lateral, significant shear forces are generated from the weight of the body above and ground reaction forces beneath. The SI joint is designed to stabilize the pelvis under the considerable strain of these opposing forces.

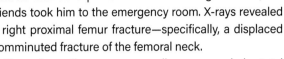

BRIAN KELTON | After Brian fell during his hike, his friends took him to the emergency room. X-rays revealed a right proximal femur fracture—specifically, a displaced comminuted fracture of the femoral neck.

The orthopedic surgeon on call recommended a total hip arthroplasty (THA). Brian was admitted to the hospital and scheduled for surgery that afternoon.

Do some research on this type of fracture and THA. Then answer the following questions:

- Why do you think the surgeon recommended a joint replacement instead of surgically repairing the fracture?
- How will a THA impact Brian's occupational performance over the short term and long term?

The rough articulating (auricular) surfaces between the ilia and sacrum are covered by cartilage and form a true synovial joint. As a result, these surfaces permit very little motion. Movement is resisted by the **posterior** and **anterior sacroiliac ligaments** that connect the sacrum and iliac tuberosity. Upward motion of the lower sacral segments and coccyx is prevented by the **sacrotuberous** and **sacrospinous ligaments** that stabilize the SI joint.

Degenerative changes in the SI joint may contribute to significant low back pain and are common in the older adult population.

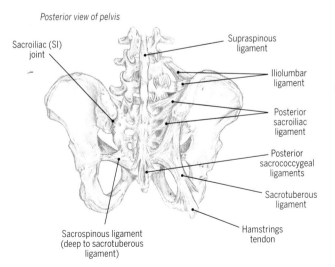

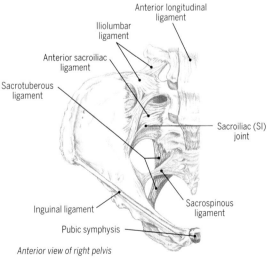

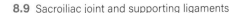

8.9 Sacroiliac joint and supporting ligaments

Hip Joint

Structural classification: ball-and-socket

Functional (mechanical) classification: triaxial

Movements: flexion, extension, abduction, adduction, external (lateral) rotation, internal (medial) rotation

The joint formed by the head of the femur and the acetabulum is the **hip joint (8.10)**.

The hip joint has some similarity in design to the glenohumeral joint—a ball-and-socket joint allowing for wide mobility with six distinct motions. However, the acetabulum demonstrates greater depth than the glenoid fossa, giving the hip greater surface contact and stability than the shoulder.

The depth of the acetabulum and the joint's bony congruity limit translation. The surrounding ligaments stabilize the femoral head in the acetabulum with movement. The open-pack position of the hip is in some flexion, abduction, and external rotation. Its close-pack position, with maximal ligament tension, is full extension with some internal rotation.

The hip joint's deep socket is supported by a strong joint capsule, limiting extremes of motion in all directions. The capsule is reinforced by the **iliofemoral**, **ischiofemoral**, and **pubofemoral ligaments**, which span the inferior pelvis and proximal femur. These ligaments encircle the head of the femur, stabilizing the joint from all directions and limiting excessive abduction and extension.

CLINICAL APPLICATION
Ankylosing Spondylitis

Conditions that impair mobility of the spine often have a significant impact on occupational performance.

Ankylosing spondylitis is an inflammatory condition in the spine that can lead to fusion of its skeletal structures. It often begins in the SI joint and may progress into the vertebrae. The fusion of these adjacent structures leads to significant limitations in mobility of the entire spine as well as significant pain.

There is currently no cure for the disorder. However, medication and rehabilitation may help to manage the symptoms, promote overall mobility and strength, or provide compensatory and adaptive strategies to maintain function.

What compensatory or adaptive techniques do you think might improve occupational performance for someone with pain and limited mobility due to ankylosing spondylitis in their SI joints and low back?

Internally, the hip joint is further stabilized by the **round ligament (ligamentum capitis femoris)**, a direct support between the acetabulum and femoral head. This unique ligament also contains an artery that provides blood supply to the femoral head. If the hip is dislocated, this structure may be damaged, leading to avascular necrosis (loss of blood supply) to the femoral head.

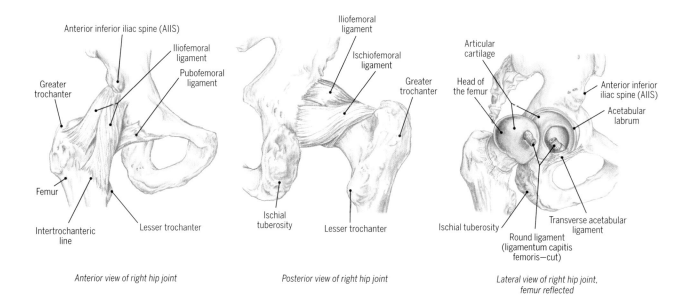

Anterior view of right hip joint

Posterior view of right hip joint

Lateral view of right hip joint, femur reflected

8.10 Hip (coxal) joint

Musculature and Movement

Similar to the shoulder, the hip, as the most proximal joint in the lower extremity, has an effect on the movement and position of the entire leg. Muscles of the pelvis and hip serve occupational performance beyond movement. They also supply the muscular boundary of the lower abdomen and facilitate bowel and bladder control.

Pelvic Floor (Diaphragm)

The **pelvic floor (diaphragm)** is the inferior muscular wall of the pelvic cavity (**8.11**). It is formed by layers of muscles that span the inferior pelvic bowl, primarily the **levator ani** and **coccygeus**.

The pelvic floor has openings for structures to pass from the pelvic cavity into the **perineum** (area between the legs). The most anterior opening of the pelvic floor is called the urogenital hiatus, the pathway for the

BRIAN KELTON | Think again about Brian's surgery and what you have learned about a total hip replacement (arthroplasty). What components of the hip joint does the prosthetic implant replace? Do individuals who have this procedure regain full motion and function? Why or why not?

urethra (males) and **vagina** (females). Just posterior to this opening is the **anorectal hiatus**, the passage for the rectum.

The surrounding muscle fibers of the levator ani play an important role in continence. The muscles contract to prevent defecation and urination and relax to allow excretion of waste. Pelvic floor dysfunction is discussed later in the chapter.

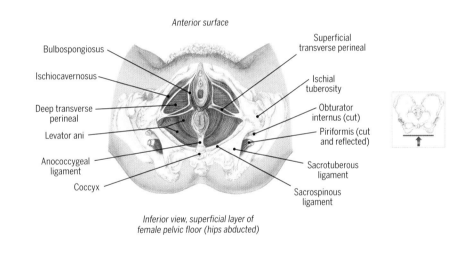

Inferior view, superficial layer of female pelvic floor (hips abducted)

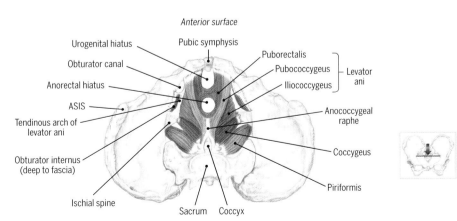

Superior view, superficial layer of female pelvic floor

8.11 Pelvic floor

Flexors of the Hip

Psoas major

Iliacus

This muscle group serves to advance the leg by flexing the hip to bring the foot off of the ground for functional mobility.

Psoas Major and Iliacus

The **psoas major** and **iliacus**, together known as the iliopsoas muscles, are the primary muscles that flex the hip (**8.12**).

The psoas major originates from the transverse processes of the lumbar vertebrae, and the iliacus originates from the iliac fossa. Both insert into the lesser trochanter.

The psoas minor is present in around only half the population. It has a similar pathway as the psoas major, but it inserts into the pubis as opposed to the iliac crest. What effect would contraction of the psoas minor have on the pelvis?

When the trunk and pelvis are stable, the muscles work together to flex the hip, moving the leg forward for ambulation (walking). Conversely, if the femur is stable in neutral, as when lying supine, these muscles may

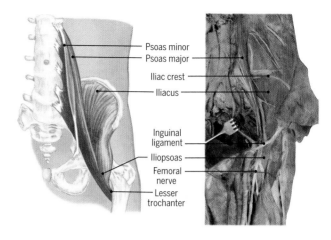

Anterior view

8.12 Flexors of the hip

also flex the trunk or tilt the pelvis anteriorly. Tightness of the iliopsoas may contribute to flexion of the trunk when standing upright or to anterior pelvic tilt.

The rectus femoris, a two-joint muscle that traverses the hip and knee, also has some ability to flex the hip (it is presented in Chapter 9).

PSOAS MAJOR	
Purposeful Activity	
P	Hiking, ascending stairs
A	*With the origin fixed:* **Flex** the hip (coxal joint) **Externally (laterally) rotate** the hip (coxal joint) *With the insertion fixed:* **Flex** the trunk toward the thigh **Tilt** pelvis anteriorly *Unilaterally:* Assist to **laterally flex** the lumbar spine
O	Bodies and transverse processes of lumbar vertebrae
I	Lesser trochanter
N	Lumbar plexus L1 to L4

ILIACUS	
Purposeful Activity	
P	Climbing a ladder, cycling
A	*With the origin fixed:* **Flex** the hip (coxal joint) **Externally (laterally) rotate** the hip (coxal joint) *With the insertion fixed:* **Flex** the trunk toward the thigh **Tilt** pelvis anteriorly
O	Iliac fossa
I	Lesser trochanter
N	Femoral L1 to L4

Extensors of the Hip

Gluteus maximus

Hamstrings

The extensors of the hip support bringing the hip to neutral from a flexed position, as when standing from a seated position, and moving the leg behind the body, as when walking.

Gluteus Maximus

The **gluteus maximus** is the largest (hence the name) and most superior of the gluteal muscles (**8.13**). Its broad proximal attachment includes the sacrum, coccyx, and posterior iliac crest. Its fibers are oblique, spanning the posterior pelvis and femur to attach at the iliotibial tract (upper fibers) and gluteal tuberosity (lower fibers).

The lower fibers are powerful hip extensors and are recruited with high force demands, as when running or climbing. The upper fibers, with their more lateral insertion, act to abduct and externally rotate the hip.

Hamstrings

The **hamstring muscles** are two-joint muscles crossing the hip and knee. As a result, they also significantly contribute to extension of the hip. (The hamstrings are covered in Chapter 9.)

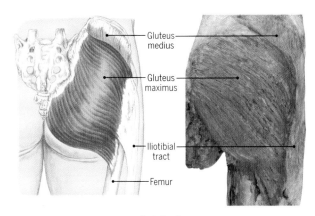

Posterior view

8.13 Gluteus maximus

GLUTEUS MAXIMUS	
Purposeful Activity	
P	**Ballroom dancing, doing gymnastics**
A	*All fibers:*
	Extend the hip (coxal joint)
	Externally (laterally) rotate the hip (coxal joint)
	Abduct the hip (coxal joint)
	Lower fibers:
	Adduct the hip (coxal joint)
O	Coccyx, edge of sacrum, posterior iliac crest, sacrotuberous and sacroiliac ligaments
I	Iliotibial tract (upper fibers) and gluteal tuberosity (lower fibers)
N	Inferior gluteal L5, S1 and S2

Abductors of the Hip

Gluteus medius and minimus

Tensor fasciae latae (TFL)

This muscle group contributes to movements of the leg laterally away from the body, such as when moving from side to side while playing pickleball or tennis.

Gluteus Medius and Minimus

The **gluteus medius** and **gluteus minimus** are often grouped together as the lesser gluteal muscles (**8.14**, **8.15**). The gluteus medius originates from the upper aspect of the ilium, and the gluteus minimus originates on the inferior aspect, with their fibers converging to insert at the greater trochanter.

Together the muscles act to abduct the hip. Individually, each muscle has some unique actions.

The lesser gluteal muscles also play an important role in stabilizing the pelvis and hip during ambulation. When you bring one leg off the ground to take a step, that side of the body is no longer supported. On the side of the stance leg, the gluteus medius and minimus contract to keep the pelvis on the opposite side from dropping. Additionally, the muscles prevent the stance leg from adducting. This action creates a stable balance between the pelvis and hip during ambulation.

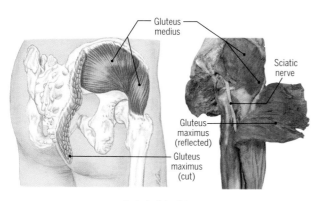

Posterior/lateral view

8.14 Gluteus medius

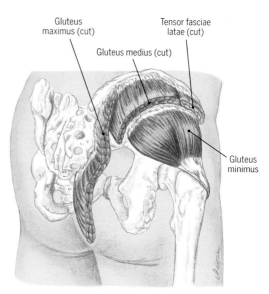

Posterior/lateral view of right buttock

8.15 Gluteus minimus and tensor fasciae latae

GLUTEUS MEDIUS

Purposeful Activity

P   Walking (stabilizes pelvis), doing yoga

A   *All fibers:*
   Abduct the hip (coxal joint)

   Anterior fibers:
   Flex the hip (coxal joint)
   Internally (medially) rotate the hip (coxal joint)

   Posterior fibers:
   Extend the hip (coxal joint)
   Externally (laterally) rotate the hip (coxal joint)

O   Gluteal surface of ilium, between posterior and anterior gluteal lines, just below the iliac crest

I   Lateral aspect of greater trochanter

N   Superior gluteal L4 and L5, S1

GLUTEUS MINIMUS

Purposeful Activity

P   **Doing tai chi, ice skating**

A   **Abduct** the hip (coxal joint)
   Internally (medially) rotate the hip (coxal joint)
   Flex the hip (coxal joint)

O   Gluteal surface of the ilium between the anterior and inferior gluteal lines

I   Anterior aspect of greater trochanter

N   Superior gluteal L4 and L5, S1

 CLINICAL APPLICATION
IT Band Syndrome

Iliotibial (IT) band syndrome is an overuse condition from repetitive strain of the IT band in athletes such as long-distance runners and cyclists. As the hip and knee flex and extend, the distal portion of the band moves back and forth across the femoral epicondyles of the knee. The friction between the connective tissue and these bony prominences can eventually cause pain and inflammation.

Some individuals may be predisposed to IT band syndrome because of an anatomical imbalance, such as a leg length discrepancy or an asymmetrical pelvis. Conservative interventions include rest, activity modification, stretching, or anti-inflammatory medications.

Weakness of the lesser gluteal muscles, particularly the gluteus medius, may result in contralateral dropping of the pelvis during ambulation, a pattern known as **Trendelenburg gait**. This atypical gait pattern and others are presented in Chapter 10.

Tensor Fasciae Latae

The **tensor fasciae latae (TFL)** originates at the iliac crest and its fibers span the lateral thigh to insert into the **iliotibial tract** (IT band), a supportive layer of fascia on the lateral thigh (**8.16**).

TENSOR FASCIAE LATAE AND ILIOTIBIAL TRACT
Purposeful Activity

P   **Running, cycling**

A   **Flex** the hip (coxal joint)
Internally (medially) rotate the hip (coxal joint)
Abduct the hip (coxal joint)

O   Iliac crest, posterior to the ASIS

I   Iliotibial tract

N   Superior gluteal L4 and L5, S1

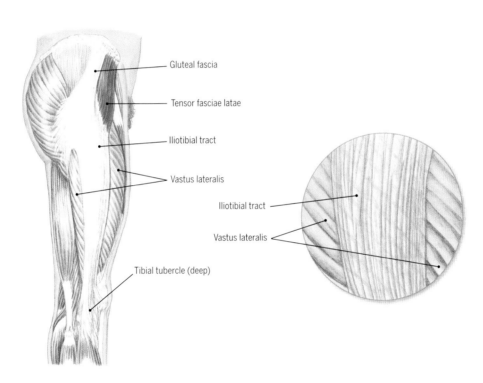

Gluteal fascia

Tensor fasciae latae

Iliotibial tract

Vastus lateralis

Iliotibial tract

Vastus lateralis

Tibial tubercle (deep)

Lateral view of right hip and thigh

8.16 Tensor fasciae latae

Adductors of the Hip

Adductor magnus

Adductor longus

Adductor brevis

Pectineus

Gracilis

The adductors of the hip act in the opposite direction of the abductors, bringing the leg medially toward the body, as when walking a straight line on a balance beam.

The **adductor muscles** span the inferior aspect of the pelvis and medial femur, an arrangement that provides each with the ability to adduct and internally (medially) rotate the hip (**8.17**). The muscles share a similar pathway but have unique attachment sites as well as contributions to other motions (**8.18**, **8.19**).

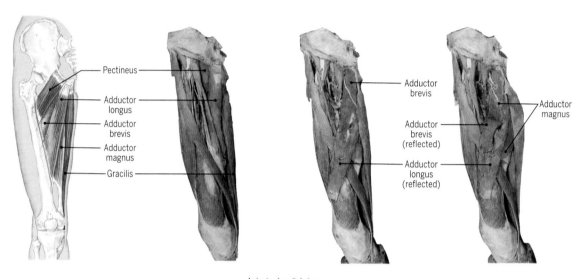

Anterior/medial view

8.17 Adductors of the hip

ADDUCTOR MAGNUS	
Purposeful Activity	
P	Doing gymnastics, wrestling
A	Adduct the hip (coxal joint) **Internally (medially) rotate** the hip (coxal joint) Assist to flex the hip (coxal joint) **Internally (medially) rotate** the flexed knee (tibiofemoral joint) ***Posterior fibers:*** **Extend** the hip (coxal joint)
O	Inferior ramus of the pubis, ramus of ischium, and ischial tuberosity
I	Medial lip of linea aspera and adductor tubercle
N	Obturator L2 to L4 and sciatic L4 and L5, S1

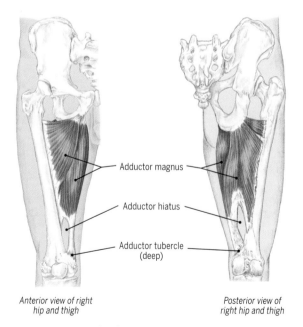

Anterior view of right hip and thigh

Posterior view of right hip and thigh

8.18 Adductor magnus

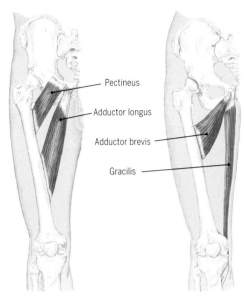

Pectineus
Adductor longus
Adductor brevis
Gracilis

Anterior views of right hip and thigh

8.19 Adductor longus and brevis, pectineus, and gracilis

ADDUCTOR LONGUS
Purposeful Activity

P Doing gymnastics, wrestling

A **Adduct** the hip (coxal joint)
Internally (medially) rotate the hip (coxal joint)
Assist to **flex** the hip (coxal joint)
Internally (medially) rotate the flexed knee (tibiofemoral joint)

O Pubic tubercle

I Pectineal line and medial lip of linea aspera

N Obturator L2 to L4

ADDUCTOR BREVIS
Purposeful Activity

P Doing gymnastics, wrestling

A **Adduct** the hip (coxal joint)
Internally (medially) rotate the hip (coxal joint)
Assist to **flex** the hip (coxal joint)
Internally (medially) rotate the flexed knee (tibiofemoral joint)

O Inferior ramus of pubis

I Pectineal line and medial lip of linea aspera

N Obturator L2 to L4

PECTINEUS
Purposeful Activity

P Doing gymnastics, wrestling

A **Adduct** the hip (coxal joint)
Internally (medially) rotate the hip (coxal joint)
Assist to **flex** the hip (coxal joint)
Internally (medially) rotate the flexed knee (tibiofemoral joint)

O Superior ramus of pubis

I Pectineal line of femur

N Femoral and obturator L2 to L4

GRACILIS
Purposeful Activity

P Doing gymnastics, wrestling

A **Adduct** the hip (coxal joint)
Internally (medially) rotate the hip (coxal joint)
Flex the knee (tibiofemoral joint)
Internally (medially) rotate the flexed knee (tibiofemoral joint)

O Inferior ramus of pubis

I Proximal, medial shaft of tibia at pes anserinus tendon

N Obturator L2 to L4

Rotators of the Hip

Piriformis
Quadratus femoris
Obturator internus
Obturator externus
Gemellus superior
Gemellus inferior

These muscles serve to rotate the hip and leg, pointing the toe inward or outward, for example, to help turn the body when walking or running.

The one-joint lateral rotators of the hip lie deep to the gluteus maximus and are sometimes referred to as the "deep six" muscles (**8.20**). As a group, they span the posterior sacrum and hip to the greater trochanter on the lateral femur. This arrangement resembles, to some degree, the posterior rotator cuff of the shoulder, positioned posteriorly for external rotation.

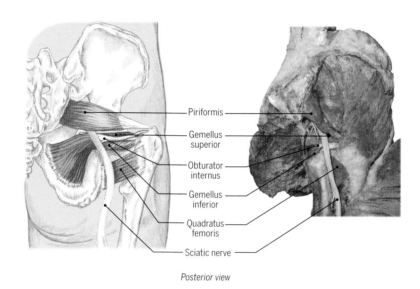

Posterior view

8.20 Rotators of the hip

PIRIFORMIS	
Purposeful Activity	
P	Getting out of a vehicle, hip-hop dancing
A	**Externally (laterally) rotate** the hip (coxal joint) **Abduct** the hip when the hip is flexed
O	Anterior surface of sacrum
I	Superior aspect of greater trochanter
N	Sacral plexus L5, S1 and S2

QUADRATUS FEMORIS	
Purposeful Activity	
P	Getting out of a vehicle, hip-hop dancing
A	**Externally (laterally) rotate** the hip (coxal joint)
O	Lateral border of ischial tuberosity
I	Intertrochanteric crest, between the greater and lesser trochanters
N	Sacral plexus L4 and L5, S1 and S2

OBTURATOR INTERNUS
Purposeful Activity

P Getting out of a vehicle, hip-hop dancing

A Externally (laterally) rotate the hip (coxal joint)

O Obturator membrane and inferior surface of obturator foramen

I Medial surface of greater trochanter

N Sacral plexus L5, S1 and S2

OBTURATOR EXTERNUS
Purposeful Activity

P Getting out of a vehicle, hip-hop dancing

A Externally (laterally) rotate the hip (coxal joint)

O Rami of pubis and ischium, obturator membrane

I Trochanteric fossa of femur

N Obturator L3 and L4

GEMELLUS SUPERIOR
Purposeful Activity

P Getting out of a vehicle, hip-hop dancing

A Externally (laterally) rotate the hip (coxal joint)

O Ischial spine

I Medial surface of greater trochanter

N Sacral plexus L5, S1 and S2

GEMELLUS INFERIOR
Purposeful Activity

P Getting out of a vehicle, hip-hop dancing

A Externally (laterally) rotate the hip (coxal joint)

O Ischial tuberosity

I Medial surface of greater trochanter

N Sacral plexus L4 and L5, S1 and S2

CLINICAL APPLICATION
Sciatica

Take a close look at the cadaver figure of the hip rotators (8.20). Do you notice the large nerve emerging from beneath the piriformis?

This is the **sciatic nerve**, which contributes to sensorimotor innervation of the lower leg. Tightness of the piriformis, or pressure on the back of the leg when seated, can compress the sciatic nerve. This condition is called **sciatica** and may result in pain and paresthesia (numbness and tingling) in the legs.

Conservative interventions may involve targeted stretching of the piriformis, as well as workstation and activity modification to remove any undue stress on the nerve. How might the height of the seat of a chair be a factor with this condition?

BRIAN KELTON | Brian was quite shaken by his injury, but he is recovering well after surgery on the general orthopedics floor of the acute care (hospital) facility.

As the occupational therapist covering the orthopedics floor, you receive physician orders to work with Brian and notice he has orders for physical therapy as well.

Prior to completing Brian's initial evaluation, you review his medical record and operative report. Brian's past medical history (PMHx) includes high blood pressure (hypertension) and a right rotator cuff repair. The operative report specifies Brian had a THA with an anterolateral approach.

Do some research on the anterior surgical approach for THA and answer the following questions:
- What specific anatomical structures are impacted?
- How long does it take to rehabilitate after this type of surgery?

Purposeful Movement of the Hip

Now let's look at the primary motions of the hip in the context of occupational performance. As you examine the specific movements, think about their impact on the position and movement of the rest of the body.

Figures **8.21–8.26** feature muscle groups of the hip in a functional context, with prime movers listed first. Asterisks indicate muscles not shown.

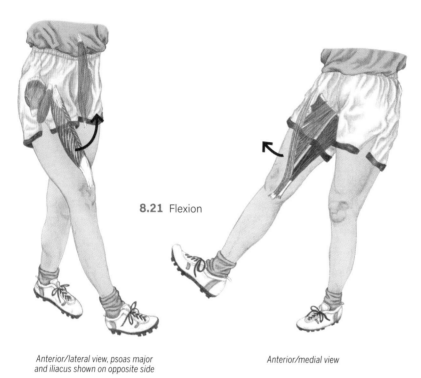

8.21 Flexion

Anterior/lateral view, psoas major and iliacus shown on opposite side

Anterior/medial view

Flexion

(antagonists on extension)

Psoas major

Iliacus

Tensor fasciae latae

Sartorius

Rectus femoris

Gluteus medius (anterior fibers)

Gluteus minimus*

Adductor longus (assists)

Pectineus (assists)

Adductor brevis (assists)

Adductor magnus (assists)

Extension

(antagonists on flexion)

Gluteus maximus (all fibers)

Biceps femoris (long head)

Semitendinosus

Semimembranosus

Adductor magnus (posterior fibers)*

Gluteus medius (posterior fibers)

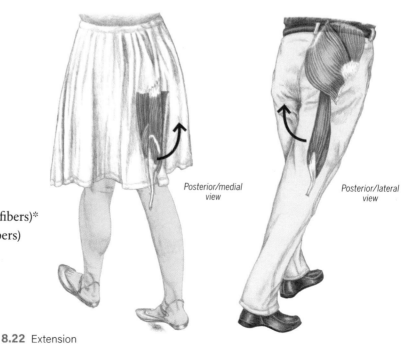

Posterior/medial view

Posterior/lateral view

8.22 Extension

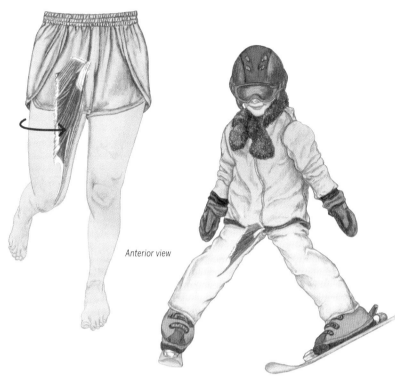

Anterior view

Internal Rotation (medial rotation)
(antagonists on external rotation)
Gluteus medius (anterior fibers)*
Gluteus minimus*
Tensor fasciae latae*
Adductor magnus
Adductor longus
Adductor brevis
Pectineus
Gracilis*
Semitendinosus (assists)*
Semimembranosus (assists)*

8.23 Internal rotation (medial rotation)

External Rotation (lateral rotation)
(antagonists on internal rotation)
Gluteus maximus (all fibers)
Piriformis
Quadratus femoris
Obturator internus
Obturator externus
Gemellus superior
Gemellus inferior
Gluteus medius (posterior fibers)
Psoas major
Iliacus
Sartorius
Biceps femoris (assists, long head)

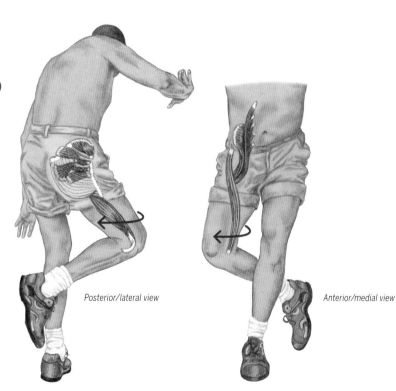

Posterior/lateral view

Anterior/medial view

8.24 External rotation (lateral rotation)

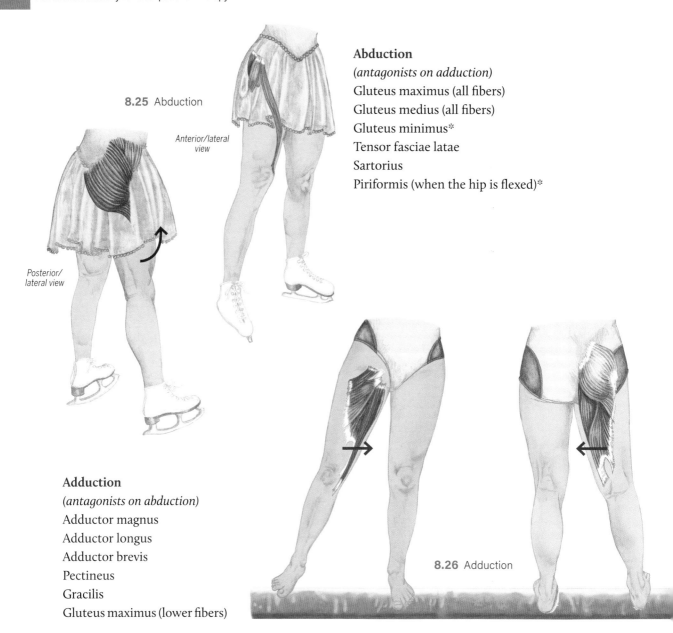

8.25 Abduction

Anterior/lateral view

Posterior/ lateral view

8.26 Adduction

Abduction
(*antagonists on adduction*)
Gluteus maximus (all fibers)
Gluteus medius (all fibers)
Gluteus minimus*
Tensor fasciae latae
Sartorius
Piriformis (when the hip is flexed)*

Adduction
(*antagonists on abduction*)
Adductor magnus
Adductor longus
Adductor brevis
Pectineus
Gracilis
Gluteus maximus (lower fibers)

OT Guide to Goniometry & MMT: Hip

Now that you are familiar with the bones, joints, and muscles that contribute to purposeful movement of the hip, let's practice clinical assessment techniques using the *OT Guide to Goniometry & MMT* eTextbook.

The hip has many two-joint muscles acting on it. You will need to pay particular attention to the position of the individual's hip and knee to prevent passive insufficiency and maximize joint motion when performing goniometry.

Many large and powerful muscle groups also act on the hip, and the way the patient and therapist are positioned affect the leverage and force on the joint for MMT. Be sure to pay attention to detail regarding the positions that are rec-

ommended for the patient and practitioner in the *OT Guide to Goniometry & MMT* eTextbook. They are recommended for safety and optimal measurement.

As you complete these assessments on the hip, practice palpating the recommended bony landmarks and think about the specific muscle groups acting on the joint. Also, consider the functional range of motion required for actions like walking, ascending or descending stairs, sitting on a toilet, or lifting while keeping the spine in a neutral position. Think about specific occupation-based goals that you might set for an individual with a limitation in movement or strength of the hip.

Occupational and Clinical Perspectives

As the skeletal support of the head, arms, and trunk (HAT), as well as the link between the core and lower extremities, the pelvis and hip play a central role in occupational performance. Dysfunction in this region can affect the motor performance skills of the entire body. In the following sections, we explore some common occupational and clinical considerations related to occupational performance.

Pelvic Alignment and Positioning

As a skeletal link, the pelvis transfers forces between the lower extremities and trunk to facilitate movement and function. A stable, neutral pelvis supports symmetrical and balanced static posture as well as dynamic movement throughout the body. Likewise, malalignment of the pelvis has a ripple effect on the core and extremities. When a practitioner assesses a patient's posture and functional mobility, it is beneficial to begin centrally, at the pelvis.

Think again of the pelvis as a three-dimensional bowl that is tilted slightly forward (anterior), so the back rim of the bowl is visible when the body is in anatomical position (**8.27**).

This pelvic bowl leans forward or backward (tilt), slants side to side (obliquity), and revolves clockwise or counterclockwise (rotation) to facilitate movements of the body. While a certain amount of pelvic movement is typical and facilitates functional mobility, excessive pelvic

BRIAN KELTON | Brian's physician orders for occupational therapy specify, "Evaluate and treat—address bed mobility, safe transfers, lower body dressing, and functional mobility. **Hip precautions**: avoid external rotation, extension, and adduction of the surgical hip. Weight-bearing as tolerated (WBAT) for transfers and mobility with respect to pain."

Before working with Brian, answer the following questions:

- Why do you think these hip precautions are in place after this specific surgical procedure?
- How will you work on bed mobility, transfers, and functional mobility while respecting the hip precautions specified in the order? It may be helpful to visualize and describe how you could work with a patient in this scenario to optimize safety and respect precautions, particularly when working with a patient in an acute care setting.
- Will Brian require a mobility device like a walker, crutches, or a cane?

mobility or asymmetry may indicate an underlying musculoskeletal imbalance or pathology.

Posterior pelvic tilt is a backward rotation of the pelvis, flattening the lumbar spine and typically increasing thoracic flexion, orienting the upper body downward. This position often occurs after prolonged sitting with fatigue of the core muscles. It usually involves tightness of the abdominal muscles, gluteals, and hamstrings with elongation of the hip flexors (**8.28**).

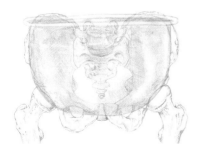
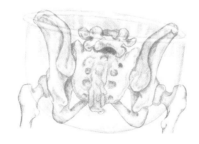
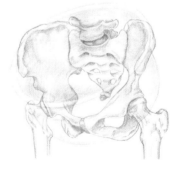

8.27 Pelvic tilt, obliquity, and rotation. How would these asymmetrical positions of the pelvis affect the rest of the body?

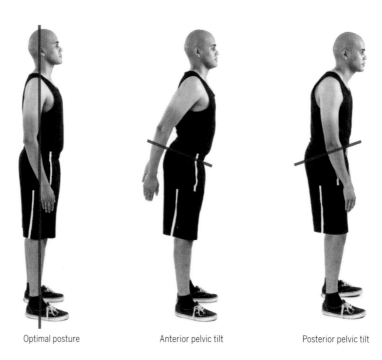

Optimal posture   Anterior pelvic tilt   Posterior pelvic tilt

8.28 Describe the position of the pelvis in optimal posture, anterior tilt, and posterior tilt. What muscle groups are elongated or tight?

In contrast, **anterior pelvic tilt** is forward rotation of the pelvis with the opposite effect, increasing lumbar lordosis and extension of the upper trunk. For example, think of a military officer standing at attention. The pelvis can also demonstrate asymmetrical rotation (forward relative to the opposite side) or obliquity (depressed relative to the opposite side), affecting the position of the core and extremities.

Assessment of the pelvis is often the first step for ergonomic evaluations or when fitting an individual for a wheelchair. Once the pelvis is stabilized and neutral, further adjustments can be made to optimize the position of the trunk and extremities.

A helpful starting point is to assess the position of the pelvis when the patient is supine, standing, or sitting (**8.29**).

 BRIAN KELTON | Addressing functional range of motion of the hip for various activities may also help in setting long-term goals for a patient. Consider an active older adult like Brian. He will likely want to achieve as much range of motion and strength as possible to resume his leisure activities. How much hip range of motion is realistic after a THA? Do some research on the outcomes for hip motion after this procedure.

The following are clinical definitions of the relevant positions, along with anatomical landmarks, used for assessment:

- **Pelvic tilt**—sagittal plane position. Entire pelvis tilts anterior or posterior. Observe alignment of the PSIS and ASIS in the transverse plane.
- **Pelvic rotation**—transverse plane position. Rotation of one side of the pelvis is anterior or posterior

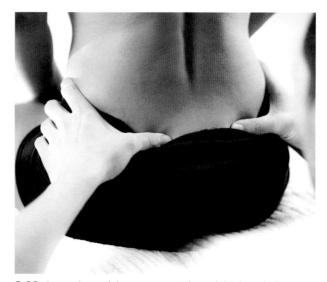

8.29 Assessing pelvic symmetry. What might the relative position of the PSIS tell you about the position of the pelvis?

in relation to the opposite side. Observe alignment of the ASIS or PSIS relative to the same landmark on the opposite side in the frontal plane.

- **Pelvic obliquity**—frontal plane position. One side of the pelvis is superior (higher) or inferior (lower) in relation to the other. Observe alignment of the ASIS or PSIS relative to the opposite side in the transverse plane.

Optimal standing posture involves slight anterior tilt, which supports the natural curvature of the spine to keep the body upright. This position vertically aligns the spinal vertebrae and weight-bearing joints of the legs, decreasing the amount of muscle force required to remain standing.

Seated posture typically involves hip and knee flexion, a position that creates an unequal balance of forces on the pelvis and trunk (**8.30**). This requires more of the core muscles—the erector spinae and abdominals—to maintain an upright position. As the core muscles begin to fatigue after prolonged sitting, the pelvis has a tendency to tilt posteriorly, increasing trunk flexion and orienting the upper body downward.

Over time, posterior pelvic tilt and its tendency to increase trunk flexion will tighten and shorten the abdominal and pectoral muscles, elongating and weakening the erector spinae and scapular stabilizers. This pattern of postural compromise can affect occupational performance in several ways. The upper body and head are oriented downward, limiting the visual field and environmental interaction. Because the scapula is poorly positioned, overhead movement of the shoulder

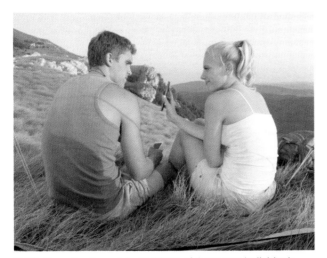

8.30 Describe the pelvic positions of these two individuals. How do the positions affect the posture of their entire bodies?

▶ TRY IT

Stand in front of a mirror with your hands on the highest point of your pelvis: the iliac crests on the sides of your lower trunk. Tilt your pelvis posteriorly. How does this change the pressure on your feet and the position of your hips and knees? What does it do to your upper body and the position of your head and neck?

Now tilt your pelvis forward. How does this change your overall posture?

Lastly, elevate one side of your pelvis and lower the other. Do you notice the asymmetry in your arms and legs?

How might these different pelvic positions affect an individual's functional mobility and interaction with the surrounding environment? How would they impact someone who uses a wheelchair for functional mobility?

orients the glenoid fossa downward. Breathing may also be impaired as the position limits chest expansion. Wheelchair users and individuals sitting at computer workstations are particularly susceptible to posterior pelvic tilt and the resulting postural compromise.

Functional Mobility

The pelvis and hip serve a primary role in **functional mobility**, transitioning the entire body from one place to another. This includes transferring from one surface to another—for example, from the bed to a wheelchair—as well as navigating an environment by using a wheelchair, walking, or running.

When a person ambulates (walks or runs), the pelvis features alternating rotation, obliquity, and tilt for reciprocal motion of the lower extremities. As the foot lifts off the ground, the ipsilateral pelvis rotates forward and drops slightly to facilitate advancement of the leg.

BRIAN KELTON | Think about Brian as he begins to stand. When bearing weight through his dominant right leg after surgery, he will experience some pain. If he is hesitant to shift his weight onto this leg due to the pain, what impact could that have on the position of his pelvis? How do you think this might affect the posture of his entire body? (If you'd like more information, look ahead to Chapter 10, especially the section on antalgic gait.)

As the foot comes into contact with the ground surface, ascending forces through the leg elevate the pelvis as it rotates posteriorly to facilitate hip extension. A small degree of alternating anterior and posterior tilt occurs as each leg advances and returns to neutral. We'll revisit this functional pattern in more detail in Chapter 10.

Many people—more than 3.6 million in the United States alone—rely on a wheeled mobility device (wheelchair or scooter) for functional mobility.[2] According to the American Occupational Therapy Association, occupational therapy is the only profession that uses a "client/environment/occupation perspective … to determine what equipment will be most beneficial in all the person's environments."[3] This client-centered, holistic approach restores much more than mobility; it may enable a child to attend school, an adult to continue to drive and work, or an older adult to continue to live safely in their home environment.

Occupational therapy practitioners often provide seating and mobility services, including fitting and modification of wheelchairs when needed, to facilitate an individual's functional mobility. Using a top-down approach, the practitioner considers a person's occupations and environmental needs to identify the right type of seating system.

Positioning and support of the pelvis and hip are essential components of a safe, effective seating system (**8.31**). Remember, the position of the pelvis will impact the entire body and should be addressed first.

Specific landmarks of the pelvis and hip can guide accurate measurements to ensure an appropriate fit, optimizing body position to promote occupational performance. Measuring the distance between the greater trochanters and adding one to two inches gives an idea of the necessary seat width. The distance from the PSIS to the back of the knee, minus one to two inches, is a common way to measure seat depth. Abnormal muscle tone, postural abnormality, or joint contracture may require customized supports to maintain a stable pelvis and core.

Recall that the sacrum and ischial tuberosities are common sites of skin pressure when seated or lying down. These areas and other bony landmarks must be carefully considered when developing a seating system. Individuals who have lost sensation on their back or buttocks, such as due to a spinal cord injury (SCI), may not feel discomfort related to building pressure. These individuals may require specialized pressure relief systems, like a ROHO® cushion (**8.32**). Wheelchair users

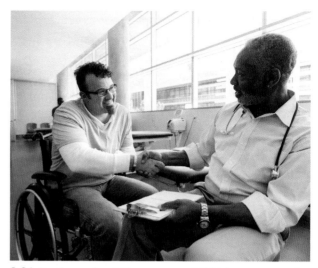

8.31 Seating and mobility assessment. Which measurements of the hip would be most important to determine appropriate dimensions for a wheelchair?

should also be encouraged to frequently shift their weight or the wheelchair position, if possible, to avoid continuous pressure over the same area, which may result in a pressure sore.

A more comprehensive perspective on functional mobility, including the role of the pelvis, is presented in Chapter 10.

Bowel, Bladder, and Sexual Function

As explained earlier, the pelvis forms a skeletal ring from which the muscles of the pelvic floor are suspended. These muscles form a continuous membrane with openings—the urethra, vagina, and anus—that are

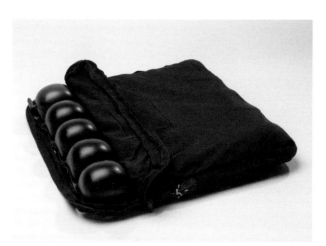

8.32 Specialty wheelchair cushion. How would this ROHO® cushion decrease pressure on bony landmarks of the pelvis and hip?

controlled by surrounding sphincter muscles, which regulate urination and defecation.

The pelvic floor muscles may weaken with age or, in women, may be torn or overstretched during childbirth. For men, prostate surgery often contributes to traumatic damage to the pelvic floor. When the pelvic floor becomes weak, this impairs the ability to control urination and defecation as well as to support the visceral structures of the lower abdomen. Pelvic floor weakness may also compromise the structural integrity of the vagina and, some sources suggest, reduce the ability to maintain an erection, affecting intimacy and sexual intercourse.[4]

Incontinence is a general term that refers to a loss of control of either the bowels (**fecal incontinence**) or the bladder (**urinary incontinence**). Incontinence is often a result of pelvic floor weakness.

Stress incontinence occurs when abdominal pressure increases from a bodily function, such as sneezing, coughing, laughing, or exercise, causing urine or feces to involuntarily leak. **Urge incontinence** describes the inability to control the bladder or bowels until an appropriate time to urinate or defecate (**8.33**).

For females, the pelvic floor also acts as a muscular hammock to support the pelvic organs lying superior to the vagina. With pelvic floor weakness, any of these structures—the uterus, rectum, or bladder—may herniate into the vagina. While not considered life threatening, **pelvic organ prolapse** may cause a great deal of discomfort and stress.

The types of prolapse are as follows:

- cystocele—when the bladder falls down into the vagina
- uterine prolapse—when the womb drops down into the vagina
- vaginal vault prolapse—when the vagina itself falls down
- enterocele—when the small bowel pushes against the vagina, causing a bulge
- rectocele—when the rectum falls

Many different factors may increase the risk of developing pelvic organ prolapse, such as number of vaginal deliveries; family history of prolapse; menopause; heavy lifting; obesity; chronic coughing from smoking, asthma, or chronic bronchitis; neurologic diseases; or ethnicity/race.

Physical symptoms include

- bulging or pressure from the vagina
- a sense that something is falling out
- pelvic pressure
- urine leakage, increased frequency of urination, chronic urinary tract infections, or difficulty urinating
- difficult bowel movements or trapping of stool
- lower backache
- painful sexual intercourse (dyspareunia) because of a bulge or protrusion

Women with pelvic organ prolapse can experience all, some, or none of these symptoms.

Conservative interventions include exercises to strengthen the pelvic floor. Sometimes called Kegel exercises, specific muscles of the pelvic floor are targeted to improve bowel and bladder control. In order to target these muscles, patients are often instructed to mimic the action of stopping the flow of urine in midstream. Some sources suggest these exercises may also improve erection in men.[5]

With extreme pelvic floor weakness or advanced prolapse, surgical intervention is recommended.

Pelvis and Hip Fractures

Fractures of the pelvis are often due to injuries involving high-velocity trauma, such as a motor vehicle accident (MVA) or a fall from a significant height. Because of their proximity, organs within the pelvic ring—the intestines, bladder, and kidneys—can also be damaged, causing life-threatening internal bleeding.

A minor pelvic fracture may be treated with bed rest, avoiding weight-bearing to keep the pelvis stable as the fracture heals. Severe fractures may require surgical fixation and a period of no weight-bearing until the fracture is sufficiently stable.

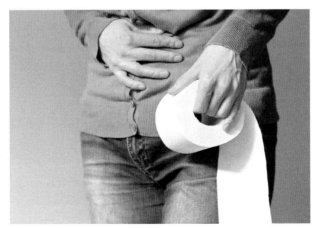

8.33 Pelvic floor dysfunction. How might occupational therapy provide a holistic approach to addressing pelvic floor dysfunction?

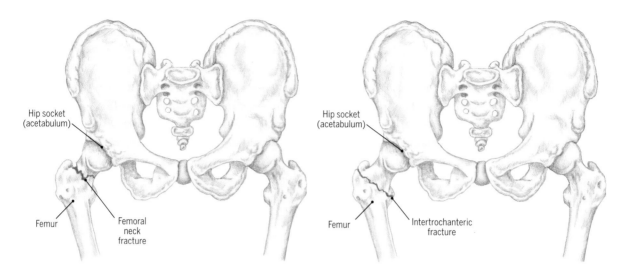

Anterior view of hip

8.34 Common fractures of the hip. How might these hip fractures have occurred?

Hip fractures are common among older adults, often from a fall on a femur weakened by age or **osteoporosis**, the loss of bone density. The majority of hip fractures involve the proximal femur, classified as either a **femoral neck fracture** or an **intertrochanteric fracture** (**8.34**). These injuries generally require internal fixation (surgery) to restore anatomical alignment and stability.

Postoperative rehabilitation begins in the acute care setting soon after the surgery and often engages both occupational and physical therapy. Occupational therapy goals may include bed mobility, functional mobility with a mobility device (walker), and tub and toilet transfers, as well as independent dressing with modified technique or adaptive equipment.

Depending on the severity of injury and surgical technique, specific hip precautions may be in place to limit certain movements of the hip or weight-bearing through the lower extremity. Most protocols encourage early weight-bearing and mobility to avoid development of secondary complications like pneumonia, deep vein thrombosis (DVT), or generalized weakness.

Occupational therapists also play a key role in giving discharge recommendations, taking into account the patient's functional level, activity tolerance, and home environment, as well as whether or not caregiver assistance is available.

Hip Arthroplasty

Like many other joints in the body, the hip is susceptible to the wear-and-tear condition of osteoarthritis due to aging or use over time. An individual's habits, roles, and routines for occupational performance place notable force demands on this essential weight-bearing joint. For example, consider an older adult who served in the military; worked in a factory, which required standing on a hard surface for many years; and played tennis as a primary leisure occupation (**8.35**).

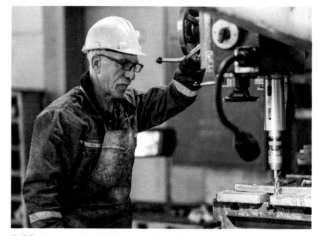

8.35 Occupational history and performance patterns affect joints. How might task demands and performance patterns affect the weight-bearing joints of the lower extremity for this worker?

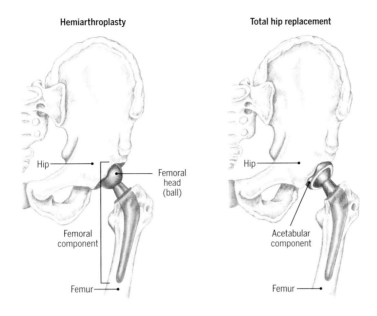

Hemiarthroplasty

Hip

Femoral
head
(ball)

Femoral
component

Femur

Total hip replacement

Hip

Acetabular
component

Femur

Anterior views of left hip

8.36 Partial and total hip arthroplasty. Can you identify the differences between these common hip replacement techniques?

Severe osteoarthritis or complex fractures of the hip may limit the benefits of surgical repair of the fracture. In these cases, an arthroplasty (replacement) may be indicated, using prosthetic implants to replicate the articular surfaces of the hip (**8.36**).

A **total hip arthroplasty (THA)** involves replacing the femoral head and acetabulum, while a **hemiarthroplasty** replaces only the femoral head. Depending on the surgical approach—anterior, lateral, or posterior—certain muscles may be damaged, requiring hip precautions for a period of time after surgery. Again, hip precautions might include avoiding hip rotation, adduction, or flexion beyond a certain point. During the acute care stay, occupational therapy could address adaptive ADLs, bed mobility, or transfers with respect to these specific precautions.

Some individuals may require inpatient rehabilitation after discharge from the hospital. These patients can receive more intensive occupational therapy services in this setting as part of a multidisciplinary rehabilitation team.

As you can see, the pelvis and hip play an essential role in positioning and aligning the entire body for occupational performance. We will continue to reference the key concepts presented in this chapter as we move forward to discuss the lower leg and examine positioning, postural alignment, and functional mobility in the remaining chapters.

APPLY AND REVIEW

Brian Kelton

After a thorough review of Brian's medical history and physician orders, you decide to talk with other health care providers involved in his care to get their perspective. The physical therapist (PT) tells you that Brian was able to get out of bed and ambulate with a walker with minimum assistance (requiring less than 25 percent assistance from the therapist) several hours ago. Brian's nurse tells you that he has been cooperative, has been eating well, and has recently had a dose of pain medication.

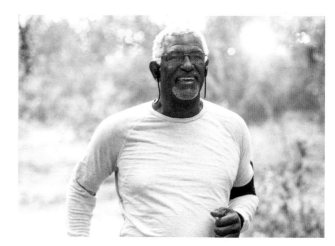

With this valuable information in mind, you proceed to Brian's room to begin his initial evaluation. You find him awake in bed, and his spouse, Brandi, is sitting nearby. You introduce yourself. How would you explain the role of occupational therapy for Brian during this acute care phase of his recovery?

You begin the subjective part of your evaluation, asking questions to determine Brian's pain level, prior level of function (PLOF), living situation, and occupational goals.

- His pain is currently 2/10 but was 4/10 when he got out of bed with physical therapy earlier.
- He and Brandi live in a single-story home with two steps to enter the front door. They have a walk-in shower and a standard toilet.
- He hopes to discharge directly home with Brandi, who will help him during his recovery.
- His main goal is to participate in the regional Senior Games qualifier events that begin in four months.

You decide to have Brian transition to sitting on the edge of the bed (EOB) to complete the rest of his evaluation. Before he moves, you remind him of the hip precautions outlined in the physician order. You instruct him to shift his pelvis and hips toward the side of the bed by pushing down on the bed with both arms.

Slowly, and with some assistance to move his surgical leg, Brian is now sitting on the side of the bed. He

demonstrates full active motion and strength (5/5 MMT) in his upper extremities. He is also able to sit without assistance and hold onto the bed rail.

- To maximize your time with Brian, what other interventions might you provide?
- Would you recommend any adaptive equipment (AE) to complete lower body dressing with respect to his hip precautions?
- What occupational therapy goals might you establish in collaboration with Brian during his acute care stay?
- Based on Brian's occupational profile, current level of function, and living situation, what are your discharge recommendations? Should he discharge to inpatient rehabilitation, home with outpatient services, home with home health, or a different type of setting? Do some research on these various options.
- What education or other training should be provided for Brian and Brandi before he leaves the acute care setting?

Review Questions

1. Which joint describes the articulation between the vertebral column and pelvis?
   a. acetabulofemoral joint
   b. sacroiliac joint
   c. pubofemoral joint
   d. lumbosacral joint

2. Tightness of which of the following muscles would be *most* likely to contribute to compression of the sciatic nerve?
   a. gluteus minimus
   b. gluteus medius
   c. superior gemellus
   d. piriformis

3. Malalignment of the ASIS in the frontal plane may indicate which of the following asymmetrical positions of the pelvis?
   a. obliquity
   b. posterior pelvic tilt
   c. anterior pelvic tilt
   d. rotation

4. Tightness of which of the following muscle groups would be associated with posterior pelvic tilt?
   a. hip flexors (iliopsoas)
   b. hip adductors
   c. hip extensors (gluteals)
   d. iliotibial tract

5. Ambulation involves which of the following motions of the pelvis?
   a. rotation
   b. elevation and depression
   c. tilt
   d. all of the above

6. Donning socks by propping one leg over the opposite knee requires which of the following motions of the hip?
   a. flexion and external rotation
   b. abduction and internal rotation
   c. flexion and internal rotation
   d. extension and external rotation

7. Anterior pelvic tilt has what impact on the lumbar spine?
   a. no impact
   b. decreases lordosis
   c. increases lordosis
   d. causes obliquity

8. Which of the following is *not* a common hip precaution after hip arthroplasty?
   a. Avoid external rotation.
   b. Avoid adduction.
   c. Avoid weight-bearing.
   d. Avoid extreme flexion.

9. You are completing a seating and mobility evaluation for an individual who requires a new wheelchair. In sitting, you measure the width of the hips as 16" and the distance from the PSIS to the back of the knee as 18". Based on these measurements, which of the following would you recommend as the ideal dimensions of the wheelchair seating surface to provide a comfortable, secure fit and allow for functional mobility?
   a. 22" wide × 24" deep
   b. 16" wide × 18" deep
   c. 18" wide × 16" deep
   d. 15" wide × 17" deep

10. Which of the following anatomical landmarks creates the highest-pressure areas when sitting and should be monitored for skin breakdown and prevention of pressure sores?
    a. pubis and iliac crest
    b. sacrum and ischial tuberosities
    c. femoral head and lesser trochanter
    d. iliac crest and lesser trochanter

See Answer Key in back of book.

Notes

1. Carol A. Oatis, *Kinesiology: The Mechanics and Pathomechanics of Human Movement*, 3rd ed. (Philadelphia: Wolters Kluwer, 2017).

2. US Census Bureau, "Americans with Disabilities: 2010," July 2012, https://www.census.gov/prod/2012pubs/p70-131.pdf.

3. Jill Sparacio et al., *The Role of Occupational Therapy in Providing Seating and Wheeled Mobility Services* (Bethesda, MD: American Occupational Therapy Association, 2017), https://www.aota.org/~/media/Corporate/Files/AboutOT/Professionals/WhatIsOT/RDP/Facts/Wheeled-Mobility-fact-sheet.pdf.

4. Pierre Lavoisier et al., "Pelvic-Floor Muscle Rehabilitation in Erectile Dysfunction and Premature Ejaculation," *Physical Therapy* 94, no. 12 (December 2014): 1731–43, https://doi.org/10.2522/ptj.20130354.

5. Lavoisier et al., "Pelvic-Floor Muscle Rehabilitation," 1731–43.

Bibliography

Biel, Andrew. *Trail Guide to Movement: Building the Body in Motion.* 2nd ed. Boulder, CO: Books of Discovery, 2019.

Biel, Andrew. *Trail Guide to the Body: A Hands-On Guide to Locating Muscles, Bones, and More.* 6th ed. Boulder, CO: Books of Discovery, 2019.

Greene, David Paul, and Susan L. Roberts. *Kinesiology: Movement in the Context of Activity.* 3rd ed. St. Louis, MO: Elsevier, 2017.

Keough, Jeremy L., Susan J. Sain, and Carolyn L. Roller. *Kinesiology for the Occupational Therapy Assistant: Essential Components of Function and Movement.* 2nd ed. Thorofare, NJ: SLACK, 2017.

Lavoisier, Pierre, Pascal Roy, Emmanuelle Dantony, Antoine Watrelot, Jean Ruggeri, and Sébastien Dumoulin. "Pelvic-Floor Muscle Rehabilitation in Erectile Dysfunction and Premature Ejaculation." *Physical Therapy* 94, no. 12 (December 2014): 1731–43. https://doi.org/10.2522/ptj.20130354.

Oatis, Carol A. *Kinesiology: The Mechanics and Pathomechanics of Human Movement.* 3rd ed. Philadelphia: Wolters Kluwer, 2017.

Pendleton, Heidi McHugh, and Winifred Schultz-Krohn. *Pedretti's Occupational Therapy: Practice Skills for Physical Dysfunction.* 8th ed. St. Louis, MO: Elsevier, 2017.

Sparacio, Jill, Chris Chovan, Cynthia Petito, Jacqueline Anne Hall, Jessica Presperin Pedersen, Leslie A. Jackson, and Theresa Lee Gregorio-Torres. *The Role of Occupational Therapy in Providing Seating and Wheeled Mobility Services.* Bethesda, MD: American Occupational Therapy Association, 2017. https://www.aota.org/~/media/Corporate/Files/AboutOT/Professionals/WhatIsOT/RDP/Facts/Wheeled-Mobility-fact-sheet.pdf.

Standring, Susan. *Gray's Anatomy: The Anatomical Basis of Clinical Practice, International Edition.* 41st ed. Cambridge, UK: Elsevier, 2016.

US Census Bureau. "Americans with Disabilities: 2010." *Current Population Reports*, July 2012. https://www.census.gov/prod/2012pubs/p70-131.pdf.

CHAPTER 9

Knee, Ankle, and Foot

Learning Objectives

- Describe the bones, joints, and muscles contributing to purposeful movement of the knee, ankle, and foot.

- Identify the primary purposeful movements of the lower extremity within the context of occupational performance.

- Develop competency in goniometry and manual muscle testing (MMT) as clinical assessment techniques for the knee, ankle, and foot.

- Use clinical reasoning to identify limitations of the knee, ankle, and foot that may affect occupational performance.

Key Concepts

above-knee amputation (AKA)	lower limb (LL) amputation
ambulation	peripheral neuropathy
arches of the foot	pes cavus
below-knee amputation (BKA)	pes planus
foot drop	plantar fasciitis
functional mobility	screw-home mechanism
genu valgum	total knee arthroplasty (TKA)
genu varum	weight-shifting

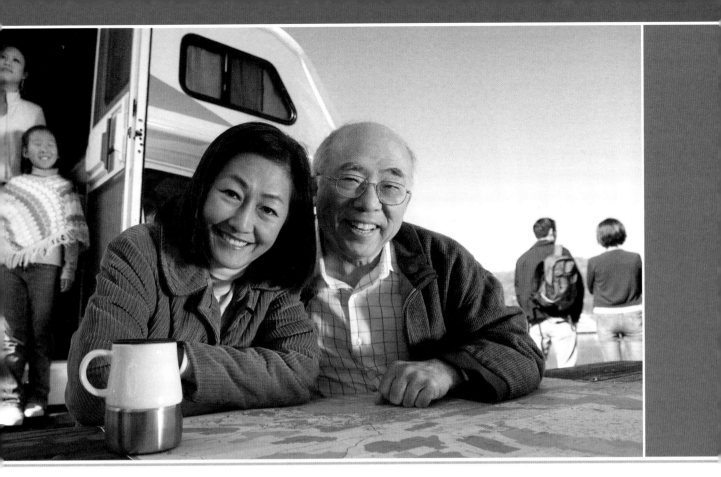

 Occupational Profile: Ruth Feng

RUTH FENG is a retired college professor who spends much of her time traveling and camping with her family in their deluxe RV. She and her spouse have a goal to visit all fifty states, and they have only ten to go. On some trips, they bring a few of their eight grandchildren along, but they also enjoy traveling on their own.

They have a consistent rhythm of life, waking up early each day to see the sunrise, eating bacon and eggs for breakfast, taking an early morning walk or hike, and spending a leisurely afternoon and evening before turning in to bed to do it all again the next day.

Over the past year, Ruth has developed pain in her dominant right knee, which makes it difficult to walk, hike, and drive—occupations she really enjoys and doesn't want to give up. She also has peripheral neuropathy with some loss of sensation in her feet as a result of chronic diabetes. She has difficulty walking at night because her feet don't feel stable beneath her. Over the past few years, she has had several falls.

As we discuss the related anatomy of the knee, think about these questions:

- Based on Ruth's occupational history and current symptoms, what do you suspect is causing her knee pain?
- What contexts, performance patterns, performance skills, or client factors should be considered in analyzing her occupational performance?

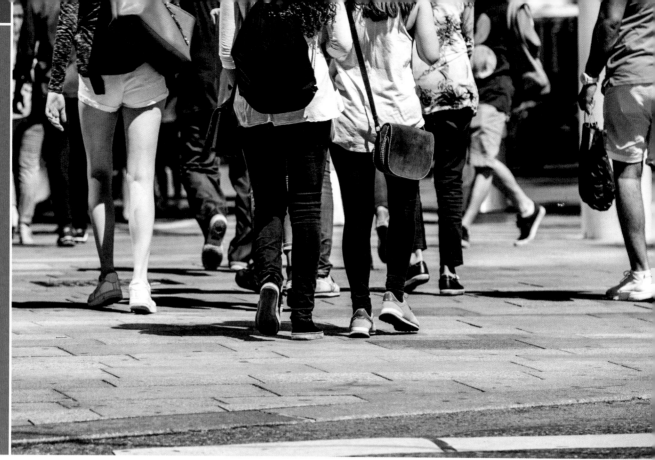

9.1 The knee, ankle, and foot are key components of functional mobility.

Knee, Ankle, and Foot: Links for Functional Mobility

Occupational performance involves the entire body, and motor performance skills are interdependent. We rely on stability and alignment of the core for effective reaching and manipulating objects, but we have to get there first. The knee, ankle, and foot cooperate as links for **functional mobility**, moving from one position or place to another (**9.1**).

Functional mobility involves much more than **ambulation**, or walking. It encompasses bed mobility, transfers, carrying objects, using stairs, and other positional changes. Positioning and moving the body require multisegment stability and mobility of the joints of the lower extremity, acting in both open- and closed-chain patterns.

RUTH FENG | Keep Ruth in mind as we discuss the bones of the leg. Consider her current and prior habits, roles, and routines. What effect might these performance patterns have had on the skeletal structures of her legs over the years?

The simple but essential functional purpose of the knee is to lengthen and shorten the lower limb. Extension of the knee raises the body out of a chair or supports standing for morning hygiene. Flexion slowly lowers the body to a commode for toileting or into a vehicle for community mobility. Repeated knee flexion, coupled with the ground contact of the foot, propels the body forward when walking or running.

During ground contact, the ankle and foot create a stable but flexible interface between the leg and variable surfaces beneath. Proprioceptive and tactile (skin) sensory input from the foot guide each step, cueing the body to accommodate surface changes. Think about walking on an icy sidewalk. The loss of surface friction is quickly communicated to the brain, with the entire body adjusting to navigate the slippery path. But what if sensation from the foot were impaired? How would this affect safe functional mobility in a bathroom at night?

Unlike the upper extremities, the legs often function in a closed-chain weight-bearing kinetic pattern with the ground beneath, supporting the weight of the body. **Weight-shifting**, or shifting the weight of the body from one leg to another, facilitates positioning and movement of the body for occupational performance. Ground reaction forces must be absorbed by the joints, similar to the shock absorbers on a vehicle, to minimize their impact on the upper body. The joints of the leg are designed to absorb these compressive forces, but they also have their limits.

This chapter presents the bones, joints, and muscles contributing to purposeful movement of the lower extremities. As you analyze their structure and function, be sure to focus on their interactions with one another to supply the purposeful movement and strength of functional mobility.

Osteology: Bones of the Lower Extremity

The bones of the lower extremity are some of the largest of the human skeleton. Their length is a primary component of a person's overall height, and they are uniquely designed to support and mobilize the body (**9.2**).

As you examine each bone, access and use the digital palpation resources provided with this text to practice identifying surface anatomy. Many of these landmarks are referenced in the *OT Guide to Goniometry & MMT* eTextbook and will serve as a guide for clinical assessment.

Femur

The **femur** provides the structural support for the superior segment of the lower extremity, or **thigh** (**9.3**).

As you know from Chapter 8, the femur angles inward from the hip, positioning the leg beneath the body and its center of gravity for stability. The downward and medial orientation of the femoral shaft creates a physiological valgus, or a lateral angulation of the tibia relative to the femur, at the knee. The distal end of the femur expands from side to side and front to back, to supply the large articular surfaces of the patella and tibia.

Bony Landmarks of the Femur

Many of the bony landmarks of the femur serve as attachment sites for the powerful muscles of the lower extremity that contribute to ambulation and functional mobility.

The two rounded projections on the inferior aspect of the distal femur are the **medial** and **lateral femoral condyles**. These convex bony prominences form the

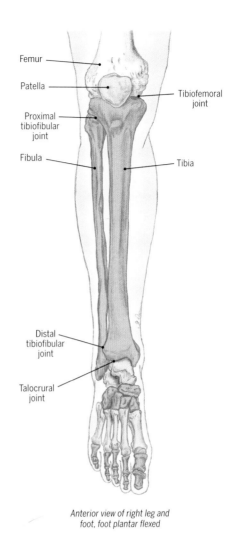

Femur
Patella
Tibiofemoral joint
Proximal tibiofibular joint
Fibula
Tibia
Distal tibiofibular joint
Talocrural joint

Anterior view of right leg and foot, foot plantar flexed

9.2 Bones of the lower extremity

superior articular surfaces of the knee joint. The medial condyle is larger and longer than the lateral condyle—a feature that helps stabilize the knee for standing, discussed later in this chapter. The gap between the condyles on the posterior aspect of the femur is the **intercondylar fossa** (**9.4**).

The **medial** and **lateral femoral epicondyles** are easily palpable on the side of the distal femur and are important attachment sites for tendons and ligaments.

Tibia

The **tibia** is the primary weight-bearing bone of the lower leg and a direct link between the knee and ankle (**9.5**).

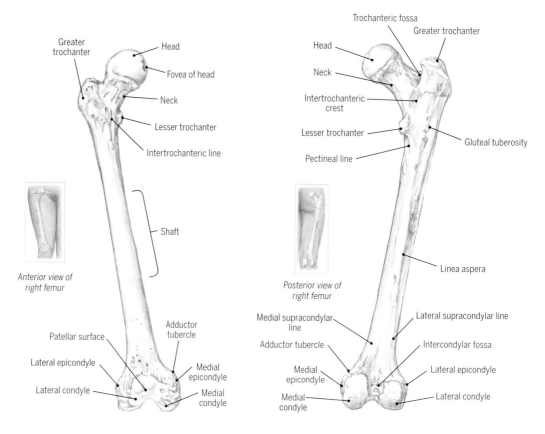

9.3 Femur

The anterior portion of the tibia is informally referred to as the shin. Its lateral surface provides attachment sites for the muscles that dorsiflex the ankle and foot.

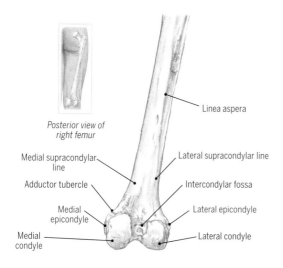

9.4 Bony landmarks of the distal femur

Bony Landmarks of the Tibia

The proximal, superior aspect of the tibia is referred to as the **tibial plateau** and features distinct medial and lateral portions designed to articulate with the femoral condyles. The medial aspect of the tibial plateau is wider and more concave—an articular counterpart to the larger femoral condyle. This design also supports function, as the medial knee bears more relative weight in standing. Projecting from both sides of the tibial plateau are the **medial** and **lateral tibial condyles** (**9.5**).

On the anterior surface of the proximal tibia is a rough bony projection called the **tibial tuberosity**. This important landmark provides the attachment site for the patellar ligament, a continuation of the quadriceps (patellar) tendon, and is the site of force application for the powerful quadriceps muscles to extend the knee.

The distal end of the tibia expands, forming the **medial malleolus** and inferior surface to articulate with the talus bone of the foot.

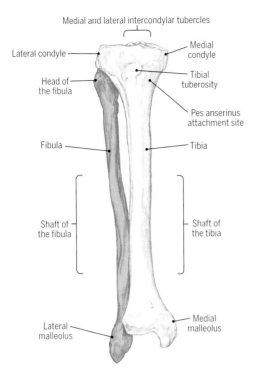
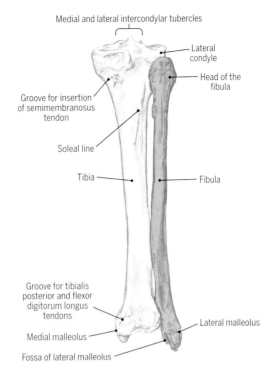

Anterior view of right tibia and fibula *Posterior view of right tibia and fibula*

9.5 Tibia and fibula

CLINICAL APPLICATION
Genu Varum and Genu Valgum

The tibia is not aligned with the femur in a straight line but has some deviation that changes over the life span.

Slight **genu varum** (bowleg), or inward angulation of the tibia relative to the femur, is present at birth and persists until around eighteen months of age. Between two and five years of age, the tibia begins to angle outward, typically up to 20°. This is called **genu valgum** (knock-knee). In adults, normal genu valgum is between 5° and 7°.

Excessive varus or valgus at the knee may create an imbalance of forces between the femur and tibia. This imbalance can eventually cause the articular surfaces of the knee to degenerate.

What specific effects might genu varum have on the knee? What about genu valgum?

Fibula

The **fibula** is a slender bone positioned parallel to the tibia between the knee and ankle (**9.5**). The proximal fibula articulates with an articular facet on the tibia (proximal tibiofibular joint) and bears little weight. The shaft of the fibula provides a rigid structure for the attachment of ligaments and tendons of the leg.

Bony Landmarks of the Fibula

The **head of the fibula** lies outside of the knee joint proper and is easily palpable just distal to the proximal end of the tibia. The **lateral malleolus** projects from the distal fibula, forming the lateral portion of the talocrural joint.

Patella

The **patella** is the largest sesamoid bone in the body, tethered against the distal femur by the quadriceps tendon (**9.6**). This small triangular bone plays a significant role in the knee. It stabilizes the anterior knee during

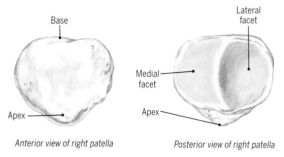

Base

Lateral facet

Medial facet

Apex

Apex

Anterior view of right patella

Posterior view of right patella

9.6 Patella

flexion and acts as a lever to increase the moment arm (leverage) of the quadriceps muscles to extend the knee.

The **quadriceps tendon** inserts into the superior border of the patella, traverses its anterior surfaces, and inserts into the tibial plateau as the **patellar ligament**. The patella has **medial** and **lateral facets** on its posterior surface that accommodate the rounded projections of the femoral condyles.

Bones of the Foot

As we examine the bones of the foot, consider their similarities to and differences from the bones of the hand. The foot is made up of seven irregularly shaped **tarsal bones**, **metatarsals**, and **phalanges** (9.8).

The **talus** projects upward, creating the rigid central portion of the talocrural (ankle) joint. Beneath the talus lies the **calcaneus**, which projects posteriorly and inferiorly to form the heel of the foot. Its superior surface features three facets that are articular surfaces with the talus, forming the subtalar joint. The rounded posterior aspect of the calcaneus is the attachment site for the powerful plantar flexor muscles of the foot and ankle via the calcaneal (Achilles) tendon. Together the calcaneus and talus are the posterior aspect of the foot, or **hindfoot**.

Similar to the carpal bones of the hand, the **navicular**, **cuboid**, and **cuneiforms (medial, intermediate, lateral)** make up the central part of the foot, or **midfoot**. The cuboid and cuneiform bones form the distal

---

CLINICAL APPLICATION
Lower Limb (LL) Amputation

Lower limb (LL) amputations are more common than upper limb amputations and are often related to peripheral vascular disease (PVD) as a complication of diabetes. Other causes include traumatic injuries due to combat or environmental hazards like land mines. Common sites of amputation include transfemoral (through the femur) **above-knee amputation (AKA)** or transtibial (through the tibia) **below-knee amputation (BKA)**.

Typically, after an amputation, a multidisciplinary rehabilitation team including occupational and physical therapists works together for optimal patient care. Postoperatively, it is essential to manage edema, prevent joint contractures, and begin to shape the residual limb in preparation for a prosthetic fitting. During this **preprosthetic phase**, adaptive and compensatory strategies facilitate functional mobility, transfers, and safe performance of ADLs and IADLs.[1]

Once a patient receives a prosthesis, **prosthetic training** is extensive and can take up to a year. It begins with learning to don and doff the prosthesis and, gradually, to bear weight. The individual must learn to distribute weight evenly into the prosthesis to restore optimal standing and ambulation (9.7).

During this phase of recovery, occupational therapy may address performance skills and performance patterns as well as environmental and personal factors to maximize occupational performance.

Think about the importance of sensation to guide motor function. How might an individual with a prosthesis compensate for the loss of sensory input from the amputated lower limb?

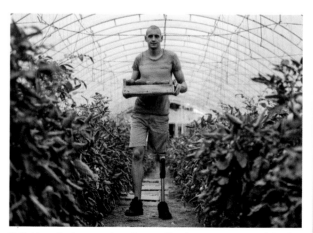

9.7 Use of a lower extremity prosthesis to support participation in occupation

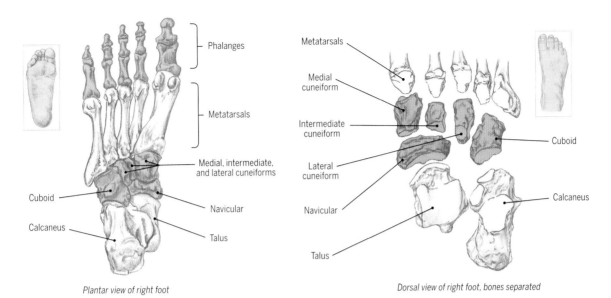

Plantar view of right foot

Dorsal view of right foot, bones separated

9.8 Bones of the foot

portion of the midfoot and articular surfaces for the five **metatarsals** (**9.9**).

The bones of the midfoot have many interconnected joints, stabilized by ligaments, that form the structure for the **arches of the foot**. The **lateral longitudinal**, **medial longitudinal**, and **transverse arches** stabilize the foot and support the weight of the body (**9.10**). The ability of the foot to absorb force is directly related to these structures, particularly the medial longitudinal arch. Dissipating ground reaction force at the level of the foot limits its impact on the structures above: the knee, hip, and spine.

The arches of the foot may be atypically higher (**pes cavus**) or flatter (**pes planus**) due to congenital differences, injuries, or occupational roles and routines. For example, a ballet dancer, consistently working to balance the weight of the body on tiptoe, can develop higher arches over time. A higher arch often contributes to instability, with less contact between the bottom of the foot and ground surface. A flatter arch is less able to absorb ground forces, transferring more of the ascending forces to the knee, hip, and spine.

The arches of the feet are stabilized by the **plantar ligaments** as well as a thick fibrous tissue called the

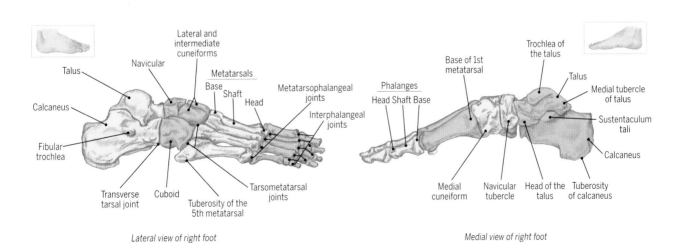

Lateral view of right foot

Medial view of right foot

9.9 Bony landmarks of the ankle and foot

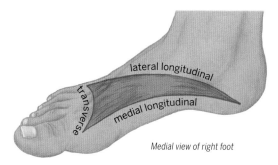

Medial view of right foot

9.10 Arches of the foot

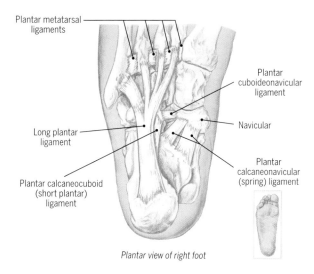

Plantar view of right foot

9.11 Ligaments of the foot

CLINICAL APPLICATION
Plantar Fasciitis

The ankle and foot are designed to support the body with repetitive weight-bearing. However, excessive or prolonged strain may lead to injury.

Inflammation of the plantar aponeurosis is called **plantar fasciitis** and may involve debilitating pain when bearing weight on the affected foot. The cause of this condition is not entirely clear, but risk factors include repetitive use (running or cycling), prolonged standing, and obesity. Similar to other inflammatory musculoskeletal pathologies, plantar fasciitis commonly features microtears, collagen breakdown, and scarring.

Conservative treatment is preferred and includes rest, orthotics, physical agent modalities, and stretching. Often the gastrocnemius and other plantar flexors are tight, resulting in increased tension on the plantar fascia. What activity modifications or compensatory strategies might decrease stress to these inflamed tissues?

plantar aponeurosis (fascia) (**9.11**). The fibers of the plantar aponeurosis arise from the calcaneus, traverse the underside of the foot, and gradually fan out into five individual bands, one for each toe.

Joints

Unlike the joints in the upper extremity, those of the lower extremity are designed to absorb and withstand the compressive forces associated with a lifetime of weight-bearing. From activities like walking, running, cycling, hiking, and gymnastics, the daily functional demands that the joints of the lower extremities endure are significant. Dysfunction of these critical joints can greatly affect functional mobility.

Knee

The knee joint consists of two distinct articulations—the tibiofemoral joint and the patellofemoral joint—contained within a single synovial-lined fibrous capsule.

Tibiofemoral Joint

Structural classification: hinge (modified)
Functional (mechanical) classification: biaxial
Movements: flexion, extension, internal (medial) and external (lateral) rotation

The **tibiofemoral joint** is a modified hinge, allowing for flexion, extension, and rotation of the tibia relative to the femur (**9.12**, **9.13**). This joint is designed to support the weight of the upper body, transferring forces between the lower and upper leg during walking and standing. As noted earlier, the tibia is not exactly linear relative to the femur but has a slight valgus, or inward angle, that increases during development into adulthood.

In part because the medial femoral condyle is larger and longer than the lateral condyle, the femur passively rotates medially as the knee extends during terminal knee extension. This arthrokinematic pattern is referred to as the **screw-home mechanism** (**9.14**).

The screw-home mechanism essentially "locks" the knee, tightening the femoral condyles within their tibial receptacles in full extension, its close-pack position, which enhances stability. "Unlocking" the joint surfaces requires activation of the popliteus muscle, which reverses the pattern, rotating the femur laterally to allow flexion of the knee. In an open-chain functional pattern, as when kicking a football, the tibia also rotates in the

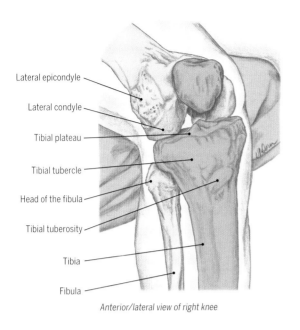

Lateral epicondyle
Lateral condyle
Tibial plateau
Tibial tubercle
Head of the fibula
Tibial tuberosity
Tibia
Fibula

Anterior/lateral view of right knee

9.12 Knee, showing tibiofemoral joint

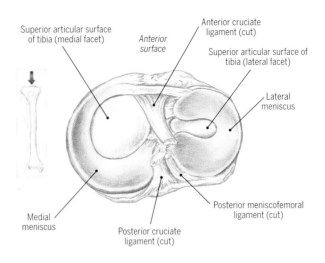

Superior articular surface of tibia (medial facet)
Anterior surface
Anterior cruciate ligament (cut)
Superior articular surface of tibia (lateral facet)
Lateral meniscus
Medial meniscus
Posterior cruciate ligament (cut)
Posterior meniscofemoral ligament (cut)

Superior view of right tibia

9.13 Tibiofemoral joint

opposite direction of the femur (laterally) with terminal extension. Additionally, there is a degree of posterior and anterior translation of the femoral condyles as the knee respectively flexes and extends.[2]

The distal femur and proximal tibia require specialized structures to withstand the considerable compressive forces imposed on them. The tibial condyles, which form the tibial plateau, are lined by specially shaped fibrocartilage discs called **menisci**. The menisci increase the depth and surface area of the tibial plateau, providing concave receptacles for the convex femoral condyles.

There is relatively little bony congruity or stability at the tibiofemoral joint, which relies heavily on surrounding ligaments and muscles for support (**9.15**).

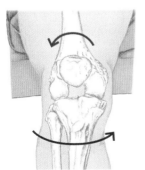
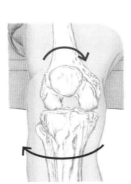

Tibia rotates medially and femur rotates laterally (unlocks) as knee flexes.

Tibia rotates laterally and femur rotates medially (locks) in full extension.

9.14 Screw-home mechanism of the knee

The **anterior cruciate ligament (ACL)** and **posterior cruciate ligament (PCL)**, named according to their cross formation, limit anterior and posterior gliding as

▶**TRY IT**

The knee functions in both open- and closed-chain positions, often alternating rapidly between the kinetic patterns as when walking, running, or playing sports. It also has the ability to support a static standing position over a prolonged period, as when completing your morning hygiene routine in front of a mirror. The screw-home mechanism increases the bony congruence and stability with full extension of the knee when standing. This mechanism decreases the muscular force required to remain standing and preserves energy.

To appreciate this phenomenon, place your hands on the powerful quadriceps muscles on the front of your thighs as you move from sitting to standing. What do you feel? Did you notice a powerful contraction? Now feel the muscles as you stand with your knees fully extended. What difference do you notice?

Maintaining full extension of the knee is essential for maintaining this stabilizing pattern. However, in the presence of swelling or pain, the knee often assumes a position of comfort—approximately 30° of flexion, its open-pack position—to decrease tension on its surrounding ligaments. Prolonged flexion may lead to a **flexion contracture**, preventing full extension and the stabilizing effect of the screw-home mechanism.

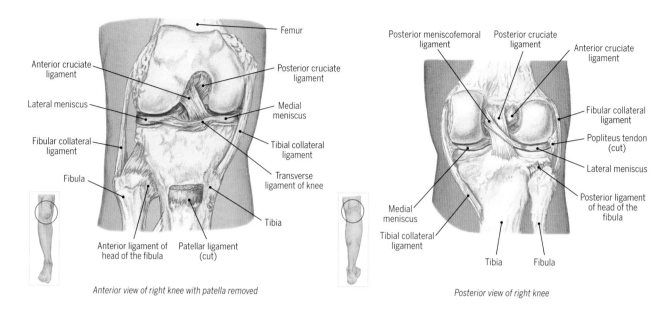

9.15 Ligaments of the knee

RUTH FENG | Ruth's pain and stiffness have increased over the past few months, and she has noticed a considerable impact on her daily life. She decides to see an orthopedic surgeon. She tells the surgeon her pain is mainly on the inside (medial aspect) of her knee and that supportive braces have not been helpful in reducing her symptoms.

The physical assessment reveals pronounced genu varum, with the tibia angled inward relative to the femur. X-rays are ordered and reveal significant osteoarthritis with joint degeneration on the articular surfaces of both the femur and tibia, predominantly on the medial aspect of the knee.

The surgeon recommends a **total knee arthroplasty (TKA)**, a complete joint replacement, as a long-term solution. Ruth is hesitant but really wants to return to doing the things she loves. She is adamant that she will not have surgery until later in the year to enjoy traveling during the warmer months.

Do some research and answer these questions about her diagnosis, its impact on her daily function, and the potential benefits of conservative or postoperative rehabilitation.

- Why does the varus deformity of her knee cause osteoarthritis of the medial aspect of the knee?
- What benefit might occupational therapy services provide prior to her seriously considering surgery? Think about adaptive or compensatory strategies regarding her occupational performance, habits, roles, and routines.

well as rotation between the femur and tibia. The PCL spans the posterior intercondylar surface of the tibia and inner surface of the medial femoral condyle. The ACL traverses the anterior intercondylar surface of the tibia to the lateral femoral condyle.

The **medial collateral ligament (MCL)** and **lateral collateral ligament (LCL)** support the hinge design of the knee, preventing varus and valgus at the knee and centralizing the tibia beneath the femur for weight-bearing. The LCL spans the lateral femoral epicondyle and fibular head, and the MCL connects the medial femoral epicondyle, tibial condyle (deep band), and medial surface of the tibia (superficial band). As discussed earlier, varus or valgus deformities of the knee can cause an imbalance in tension on the collateral ligaments, elongating one and shortening the other.

Considerable multidirectional forces are imposed on the knee when walking, running, or participating in activities like soccer or tennis. As the body moves forward, backward, or side to side, the respective anterior, posterior, and lateral/medial forces combine with compression as the foot makes contact with the ground. The cruciate and collateral ligaments counteract these complex forces and maintain the functional alignment of the femur and tibia.

Over time, malalignment can lead to an imbalance of these counterbalancing ligaments, and excessive force can cause a traumatic rupture. You have likely known someone who has had a collateral or cruciate ligament tear (or perhaps you've experienced one yourself) due to excessive medial, lateral, or rotary force at the knee.

Patellofemoral Joint
The **patellofemoral joint** is a gliding articulation between the trochlear grove of the femur and the posterior patella (**9.16**). The posterior patella has facets that accommodate the rounded surfaces of the femoral condyles.

As the knee flexes under the weight of the body, the patella glides distally and compresses against the femur and tibia, providing anterior stability to the knee. As the knee extends, the patella glides superiorly and becomes lax as the quadriceps muscles also relax. The patella also glides laterally as the knee flexes and medially as it extends.[3]

As mentioned earlier, the patella increases the moment arm and leverage of the quadriceps muscles to extend the knee. Its mobility during knee motion helps direct the force of this powerful muscle group appropriately.

Proximal and Distal Tibiofibular Joints
The **proximal** and **distal tibiofibular joints** are the two articulations between the tibia and fibula (**9.17**). The joints demonstrate slight movement and contribute to the stability of the ankle. An interosseous membrane binds the tibia and fibula together, distributes compressive loads between the two bones, and actually forms the distal joint (a fibrous and not a synovial joint).

Ankle
The ankle is made up of the talocrural joint, which provides mainly dorsiflexion and plantar flexion, and the subtalar joint, which allows for inversion, eversion, and slight rotation (**9.17**).

Talocrural Joint
Structural classification: hinge
Functional (mechanical) classification: uniaxial
Movements: dorsiflexion (extension) and plantar flexion

The **talocrural joint** is formed by the superior talus held between the lateral malleolus of the fibula and medial malleolus of the tibia (**9.18**). It is classified as a hinge joint and functions similar to a nut (talus) held on both sides by the pincers of a wrench (malleoli) (**9.19**).

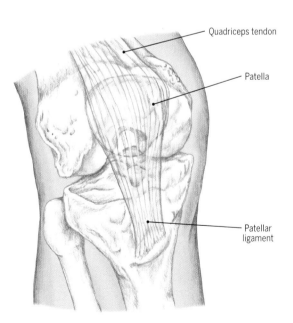

Anterior view of flexed right knee

9.16 Patellofemoral joint

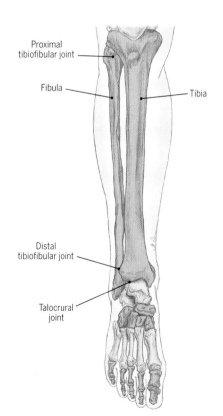

Anterior view of right leg and foot, foot plantar flexed

9.17 Joints of the lower leg

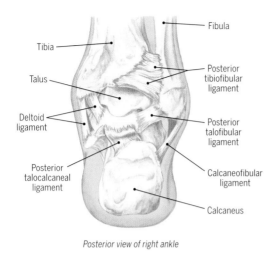

Posterior view of right ankle

9.18 Talocrural joint

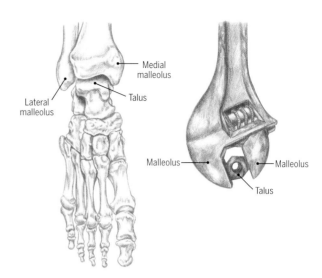

9.19 The talus is stabilized by the medial and lateral malleoli.

This design allows the talocrural joint to efficiently transition between a state of rigidity and flexibility, which accommodates the reciprocal open- and closed-chain patterns of gait. As the foot comes into contact with the ground, the malleoli stabilize the talus, supporting the weight of the body. As the weight of the body shifts forward, the ankle dorsiflexes, forcing the malleoli apart slightly and increasing stability. Once the foot comes off the ground, the talocrural joint is able to move freely in an open-chain position in preparation for the next step.

The talocrural joint's close-pack position is in maximal dorsiflexion, and the ligaments are laxer with eversion or inversion and some plantar flexion. The distal tibia and fibula are stabilized by the **posterior** and **anterior tibiofibular ligaments** (**9.20**). These ligaments are often involved in a high ankle sprain caused by forceful lateral rotation of the foot.

The lateral aspect of the talocrural joint is supported by collateral ligaments, including the **posterior** and **anterior talofibular ligaments** and the **calcaneofibular ligament**. The medial aspect of the joint is stabilized by the **deltoid ligament**, which originates from the medial malleolus and fans downward, attaching to several tarsal bones. These lateral ligament supports are commonly involved in a low ankle sprain due to excessive inversion, referred to as rolling the ankle.

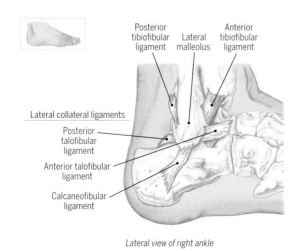

Lateral view of right ankle

Medial view of right ankle

9.20 Ligaments of the talocrural joint

Subtalar Joint

The **subtalar joint** is formed by the facets of the calcaneus and the inferior aspect of the talus (**9.21**).

This joint provides primarily inversion (supination) and eversion (pronation) of the ankle but does not contribute to dorsiflexion and plantar flexion (**9.22**). Some sources describe the joint as a hinge that rotates about an axis parallel to and at a 45° angle to the calcaneus.[4]

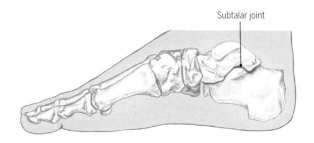

9.21 Subtalar joint

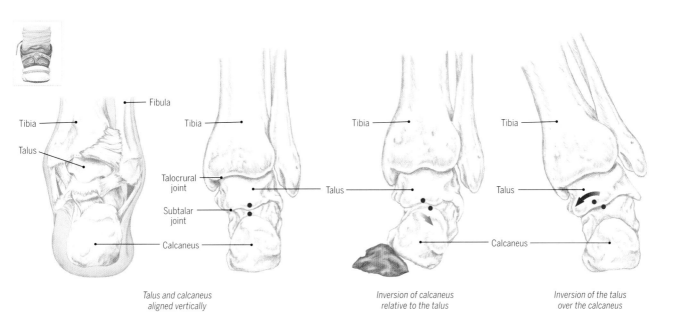

Talus and calcaneus
aligned vertically

Inversion of calcaneus
relative to the talus

Inversion of the talus
over the calcaneus

9.22 Inversion and eversion of the ankle at the subtalar joint

▶TRY IT

While we may not be as aware of sensory input from the feet as that of the hands, the feet provide an enormous amount of sensory feedback to the brain to guide the movements of the body.

To appreciate the tactile (skin) sensation provided by your feet, lightly place your bare feet on some different surfaces, such as carpet, hardwood, and grass. With your eyes closed, pay attention to the sensory details of each surface.

Now stand upright on these surfaces. Do you feel the proprioception, or joint sense, provided by the foot and ankle? This type of sensation tells the brain about the forces passing through the joint and its position relative to the ground surface.

Even without visual input, your feet communicate what type of surface you are walking on—an incline, gravel, sand, or slippery linoleum—guiding each step to accommodate the ground surface. The brain responds with motor signals to coordinate each step with the appropriate amount of muscle force to stabilize the cooperating joints of the lower extremity.

While we are able to voluntarily, or consciously, react to sensory feedback from the feet, much of this occurs involuntarily, or subconsciously, as part of the sensorimotor loop of the lower extremities.

RUTH FENG | Ruth's past medical history includes **peripheral neuropathy**, and she complains of consistent numbness and tingling in her lower legs and feet. Do some research on this diagnosis and answer the following questions:

- What effect might peripheral neuropathy have on the sensorimotor loop of her lower extremities?
- How would this impact her functional mobility, such as walking across the bathroom floor at night, hiking, or driving?
- What adaptive or compensatory strategies might improve her functional mobility and safety related to these symptoms?

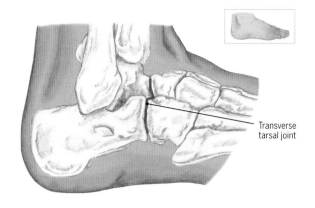

Lateral view of right ankle

9.23 Transverse tarsal joint

Transverse Tarsal Joint

The calcaneus and talus articulate, respectively, with the cuboid and navicular to form the **transverse tarsal joint (Chopart's joint)** (**9.23**). This joint permits some rotation and gliding between the midfoot and hindfoot, primarily for eversion and inversion of the ankle and foot.

Intertarsal Joints

Distal to the transverse tarsal joint are several **intertarsal joints**: the **naviculocuneiform**, **intercuneiform**, **cuboidocuneiform**, **cuneiometatarsal**, **cuboidometatarsal**, and **intermetatarsal** articulations (**9.24**).

These joints, similar to the carpal bones of the hand, permit varying degrees of gliding to facilitate global motions of the foot and ankle. Many ligaments, named according to the bones to which they attach, bind the tarsal bones together, providing rigidity for weight-bearing on the foot.

Metatarsophalangeal and Interphalangeal Joints

The **metatarsophalangeal (MTP)** and **interphalangeal (IP) joints** of the toes are similar to their counterparts in the hand (**9.25**).

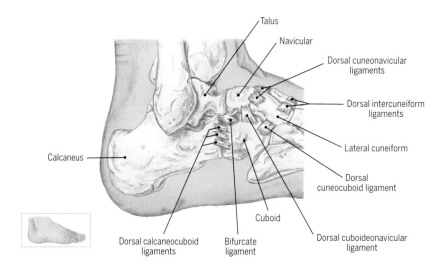

Lateral view of right ankle

9.24 Intertarsal joints

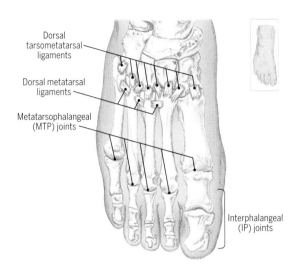

Dorsal tarsometatarsal ligaments

Dorsal metatarsal ligaments

Metatarsophalangeal (MTP) joints

Interphalangeal (IP) joints

Dorsal view of right foot

9.25 Metatarsophalangeal and interphalangeal joints

The MTPs allow flexion and extension and some abduction and adduction, while the IPs are simple hinge joints that flex and extend. The great toe is the most mobile, and the toes become successively less mobile moving toward the small toe.

Functional mobility is fluid and rapidly changes the demands on the lower extremities. Think about the demands placed on the legs from your morning ADL routine, including getting out of bed, standing on a slippery shower or tub surface, and lower extremity dressing. As you continue to develop your activity analysis and clinical reasoning skills, consider the specific joints involved and their unique contribution to occupational performance.

RUTH FENG | Before we leave joints and move on to muscles, think about Ruth. How might her symptoms and loss of knee mobility impact her performance of IADLs and ADLs involving weight-bearing and weight-shifting? How might other joints of her body compensate for loss of knee motion?

▶TRY IT

When completing an activity analysis involving the lower extremities, you must consider several unique factors. You might find it helpful to think about the big picture, or broad perspective, first, and then analyze more specifically. For example, let's think about loading a dishwasher as an IADL (**9.26**).

When placing a dish in the lower rack of a dishwasher, the legs function in a closed-chain pattern with the feet planted in a stagger stance. What is required of the knees, hips, and trunk to lower the body to place the dish? How do a stagger stance (see Chapter 3) and weight-shifting facilitate performance of this IADL and limit stress to other parts of the body?

Now imagine putting the clean dish away in an overhead cabinet on the right side of your body that you can barely reach. As you try to place the dish, you move your ankle into plantar flexion, standing on tiptoe, and shift your weight onto the right leg with the left toe barely touching the ground. How does this posture change the position and load-bearing on the joints of your legs? How do the specific joints contribute to mobility or stability? What is required of the trunk? How are your center of gravity and base of support (see Chapter 10) affected by these positional changes?

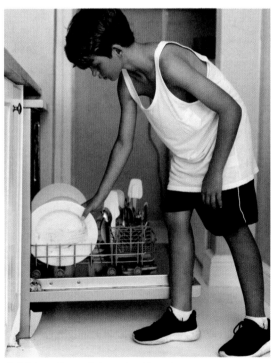

9.26 Loading a dishwasher. How does a stagger stance facilitate weight-shifting for occupational performance?

Musculature and Movement

The force demands on the powerful muscles of the lower extremity are often significantly more than solely the weight of the body. Standing from a sitting position, climbing stairs, or jumping exponentially increases the forces required of these muscles to stabilize and mobilize the body. As you examine the muscles acting on the lower extremity, try to conceptualize them in a functional context. Some examples are provided as a starting point.

Flexors of the Knee

Hamstrings

Popliteus

These muscles supply forces that flex the knee as a component of functional mobility and serve as a counterbalance to the powerful quadriceps muscles, which extend the knee (**9.27**).

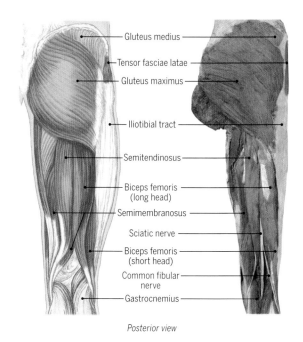

Posterior view

9.27 Flexors of the knee

Hamstrings

Semimembranosus

Semitendinosus

Biceps femoris

The muscles of the posterior thigh are the **hamstrings**, which cross and act upon both the hip and knee (**9.28**). This muscle group shares a common origin at the ischial tuberosity of the pelvis and splits distally, inserting into the medial and lateral aspects of the knee. The medial hamstrings are the **semimembranosus** and **semitendinosus**. The lateral hamstring is the **biceps femoris**, which features long and short heads.

The hamstrings collectively extend the hip, flex the knee, and tilt the pelvis posteriorly. Some force for medial and lateral rotation of the hip and knee is also available.

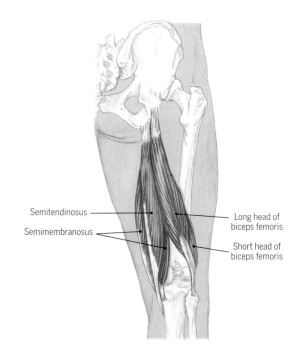

Posterior view of right thigh, showing superficial hamstrings

9.28 Hamstrings

SEMIMEMBRANOSUS	SEMITENDINOSUS	BICEPS FEMORIS
Purposeful Activity	**Purposeful Activity**	**Purposeful Activity**
P Functional mobility (acceleration when walking)	P Functional mobility (acceleration when walking)	P Functional mobility (acceleration when walking)
A Flex the knee (tibiofemoral joint) **Internally (medially) rotate** the flexed knee (tibiofemoral joint) **Extend** the hip (coxal joint) Assist to **internally (medially) rotate** the hip (coxal joint) **Tilt** the pelvis posteriorly	A Flex the knee (tibiofemoral joint) **Internally (medially) rotate** the flexed knee (tibiofemoral joint) **Extend** the hip (coxal joint) Assist to **internally (medially) rotate** the hip (coxal joint) **Tilt** the pelvis posteriorly	A Flex the knee (tibiofemoral joint) **Externally (laterally) rotate** the flexed knee (tibiofemoral joint) Long head: **Extend** the hip (coxal joint) Assist to **externally (laterally) rotate** the hip (coxal joint) **Tilt** the pelvis posteriorly
O Ischial tuberosity	O Ischial tuberosity	O Long head: Ischial tuberosity Short head: Lateral lip of linea aspera
I Posterior aspect of medial condyle of tibia	I Proximal, medial shaft of the tibia at pes anserinus tendon	I Head of the fibula
N Sciatic (tibial branch) L4 and L5, S1 and S2	N Sciatic (tibial branch) L4 and L5, S1 and S2	N Long head: Sciatic (tibial branch) L5, S1 to S3 Short head: Sciatic (fibular branch) L5, S1 and S2

Popliteus

The **popliteus** is a small but important muscle of the posterior knee (**9.29**). While it can generate weak force for knee flexion, more importantly it medially rotates the tibia to unlock the knee prior to flexion. Recall that the screw-home mechanism involves lateral rotation of the tibia and medial rotation of the femur. The popliteus contracts before knee flexion, rotating the tibia medially to unlock these same bony surfaces. This ability has earned the popliteus its nickname, "the key that unlocks the knee."

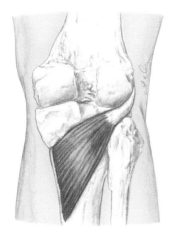

Posterior view of right knee

9.29 Popliteus

POPLITEUS
Purposeful Activity
P Facilitates knee flexion for sitting and ambulation
A **Internally (medially) rotate** the flexed knee (tibiofemoral joint) **Flex** the knee (tibiofemoral joint)
O Lateral condyle of the femur
I Proximal, posterior aspect of tibia
N Tibial L4 and L5, S1

Extensors of the Knee (Quadriceps)

Rectus femoris
Vastus lateralis
Vastus medialis
Vastus intermedius

This powerful muscle group extends the knee while often supporting the weight of the body, as when moving into a sitting or standing position. The muscles of the anterior thigh are the **quadriceps**, which are typically divided into four separate muscles: **rectus femoris**, **vastus lateralis**, **vastus medialis**, and **vastus intermedius** (9.30).

This muscle group is the powerful and only extensor of the knee. The rectus femoris arises from the anterior inferior iliac spine (AIIS) of the pelvis and crosses both the hip and knee. As a result, it can also flex the hip. The other muscles of the quadriceps group arise from various aspects of the proximal femur and share a common terminal pathway.

The muscles converge to form the patellar tendon, span the top and sides of the patella, and insert at the tibial tuberosity via the patellar ligament, sometimes referred to as the patellar tendon. The knee is positioned medial relative to the hip, creating a somewhat oblique pathway for the quadriceps. As a result, this muscle group as a whole exerts an upward and lateral force on the patella. The vastus medialis, on the medial aspect of the thigh, supplies a counterbalance to limit excessive lateral movement of the patella.

EXTENSORS OF THE KNEE (QUADRICEPS)	
Purposeful Activity	
P	**Transfers (standing from a chair, toilet, or other seating surface)**
A	**Extend** the knee (tibiofemoral joint) Rectus femoris: **Flex** the hip (coxal joint)
O	Rectus femoris: Anterior inferior iliac spine (AIIS) Vastus lateralis: Lateral lip of linea aspera, gluteal tuberosity, and greater trochanter Vastus medialis: Medial lip of linea aspera Vastus intermedius: Anterior and lateral shaft of the femur
I	Tibial tuberosity (via the patella and patellar ligament)
N	Femoral L2 to L4

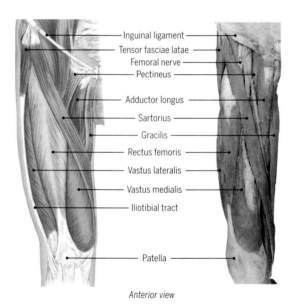

Inguinal ligament
Tensor fasciae latae
Femoral nerve
Pectineus
Adductor longus
Sartorius
Gracilis
Rectus femoris
Vastus lateralis
Vastus medialis
Iliotibial tract
Patella

Anterior view

9.30 Extensors of the knee

Dorsiflexors of the Ankle and Foot

Tibialis anterior

Extensor hallucis longus (EHL)

Extensor digitorum longus (EDL)

By dorsiflexing (extending) the ankle and foot, this muscle group allows the foot to clear the ground as it swings from the back to the front of the body when ambulating. These muscles are considerably smaller than the plantar flexors on the posterior aspect of the lower leg, which must support the weight of the body.

The three muscles that dorsiflex (extend) the ankle and foot lie on the anterior aspect of the lower leg: **tibialis anterior**, **extensor hallucis longus (EHL)**, and **extensor digitorum longus (EDL)** (9.31).

From the medial side, the tibialis anterior crosses the ankle only and as a result can both dorsiflex and invert the ankle but has no direct action on the toes. The other muscles span the ankle, foot, and toes. Similar to the extrinsic muscles of the hand, these muscles exert force on each joint crossed, including the ankle and the MTPs and IPs of the toes.

An injury to the fibular nerve or hemiparesis as a result of a stroke may weaken or paralyze this muscle group, resulting in foot drop (discussed later in this chapter).

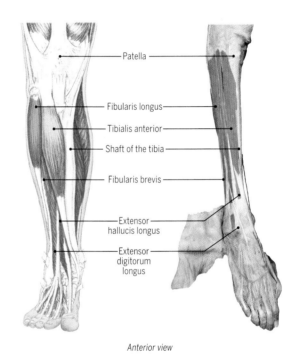

Anterior view

9.31 Dorsiflexors of the ankle and foot

TIBIALIS ANTERIOR

Purposeful Activity

P Functional mobility (ground clearance of foot during swing phase)

A Invert the foot
   Dorsiflex the ankle (talocrural joint)

O Lateral condyle of tibia; proximal, lateral surface of tibia; and interosseous membrane

I Medial cuneiform and base of the 1st metatarsal

N Deep fibular L4 and L5, S1

EXTENSOR HALLUCIS LONGUS

Purposeful Activity

P Functional mobility (ground clearance of foot during swing phase)

A Extend the 1st toe (metatarsophalangeal and interphalangeal joints)
   Dorsiflex the ankle (talocrural joint)
   Invert the foot

O Middle, anterior surface of fibula and interosseous membrane

I Distal phalanx of 1st toe

N Deep fibular L4 and L5, S1

EXTENSOR DIGITORUM LONGUS

Purposeful Activity

P Functional mobility (ground clearance of foot during swing phase)

A Extend the 2nd through 5th toes (metatarsophalangeal and interphalangeal joints)
   Dorsiflex the ankle (talocrural joint)
   Evert the foot

O Lateral condyle of tibia; proximal, anterior shaft of fibula; and interosseous membrane

I Middle and distal phalanges of 2nd through 5th toes

N Deep fibular L4 and L5, S1

Plantar Flexors of the Ankle and Foot

Superficial

Gastrocnemius

Soleus

Plantaris

Deep

Tibialis posterior

Flexor digitorum longus (FDL)

Flexor hallucis longus (FHL)

Lateral compartment

Fibularis longus

Fibularis brevis

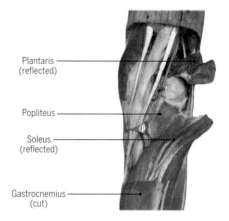

Plantar flexion of the ankle and foot in a closed-chain pattern involves elevating the entire body, as when ambulating, ascending stairs, or jumping.

The muscles on the posterior aspect of the lower leg are categorized as superficial or deep. The superficial muscles are the **gastrocnemius** and **soleus**—together referred to as the triceps surae—and the **plantaris** (**9.32**).

Collectively, these muscles plantar flex the ankle, often against the weight of the entire body. For this reason, the muscle bellies of this group are much larger than the anterior dorsiflexor muscles of the foot and ankle.

The gastrocnemius and plantaris originate above the knee and, as a result, contribute some force for knee flexion. The soleus originates below the knee and plantar flexes the ankle only. The muscles of this group share a common insertion at the calcaneus via the **calcaneal (Achilles) tendon**.

The plantaris is a thin strand of muscle fiber that is absent in some individuals, similar to the palmaris longus.

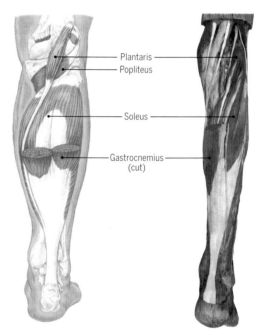

Posterior views

9.32 Superficial plantar flexors of the ankle and foot

GASTROCNEMIUS	
Purposeful Activity	
P	Cycling, running (acceleration)
A	**Flex** the knee (tibiofemoral joint) **Plantar flex** the ankle (talocrural joint)
O	Condyles of the femur, posterior surfaces
I	Calcaneus via calcaneal tendon
N	Tibial S1 and S2

SOLEUS
Purposeful Activity

P Cycling, running (acceleration)

A **Plantar flex** the ankle (talocrural joint)

O Soleal line; proximal, posterior surface of tibia; and posterior aspect of head of fibula

I Calcaneus via calcaneal tendon

N Tibial L5, S1 and S2

PLANTARIS
Purposeful Activity

P Cycling, running (acceleration)

A Weak **plantar flexion** of the ankle (talocrural joint)
Weak **flexion** of the knee (tibiofemoral joint)

O Lateral supracondylar line of femur

I Calcaneus via calcaneal tendon

N Tibial L4 and L5, S1 and S2

The **tibialis posterior, flexor digitorum longus (FDL)**, and **flexor hallucis longus (FHL)** lie deep to the gastrocnemius and soleus (**9.33**). These muscles pass behind the medial malleolus of the tibia, which acts as a lever, and insert in their respective tarsal or phalangeal bones. As a result, the muscles plantar flex each joint they cross and collectively invert the ankle. An easy way to remember these muscles and their order relative to the medial malleolus is the mnemonic Tom, Dick, and Harry (tibialis, digitorum, hallucis).

TIBIALIS POSTERIOR
Purposeful Activity

P **Reaching for an object in an overhead cabinet (standing on tiptoe)**

A **Invert** the foot
Plantar flex the ankle (talocrural joint)

O Proximal, posterior shafts of tibia and fibula; and interosseous membrane

I All five tarsal bones and bases of 2nd through 4th metatarsals

N Tibial L4 and L5, S1

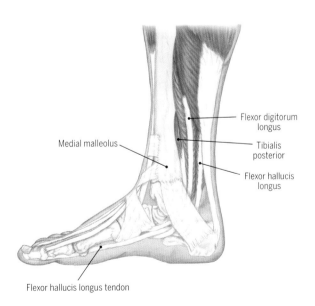

Medial view of right ankle and foot

9.33 Deep plantar flexors of the ankle and foot

FLEXOR DIGITORUM LONGUS
Purposeful Activity

P Ballet dancing

A **Flex** the 2nd through 5th toes (metatarsophalangeal and interphalangeal joints)
Weak **plantar flexion** of ankle (talocrural joint)
Invert the foot

O Middle, posterior surface of tibia

I Distal phalanges of 2nd through 5th toes

N Tibial L5, S1 and S2

FLEXOR HALLUCIS LONGUS
Purposeful Activity

P Ballet dancing

A **Flex** the 1st toe (metatarsophalangeal and interphalangeal joints)
Weak **plantar flexion** of ankle (talocrural joint)
Invert the foot

O Middle half of posterior fibula

I Distal phalanx of 1st toe

N Tibial L5, S1 and S2

The **fibularis longus** and **fibularis brevis** are on the lateral aspect of the lower leg and lend some force to plantar flex the ankle (**9.34**). As a result of their lateral orientation and pathway behind the lateral malleolus, which acts as a lever, their primary action is eversion of the ankle.

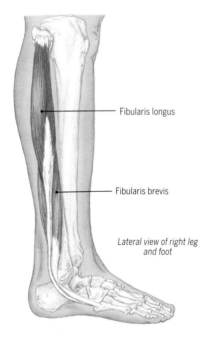

Lateral view of right leg and foot

— Fibularis longus

— Fibularis brevis

9.34 Fibularis longus and brevis

FIBULARIS LONGUS
Purposeful Activity

P Walking on sand or a nature trail (uneven surface)

A **Evert** the foot
Assist to **plantar flex** the ankle (talocrural joint)

O Head of fibula and proximal two-thirds of lateral fibula

I Base of the 1st metatarsal and medial cuneiform

N Superficial fibular L4 and L5, S1

FIBULARIS BREVIS
Purposeful Activity

P Walking on sand or a nature trail (uneven surface)

A **Evert** the foot
Assist to **plantar flex** the ankle (talocrural joint)

O Distal two-thirds of lateral fibula

I Tuberosity of 5th metatarsal

N Superficial fibular L4 and L5, S1

Intrinsic Muscles of the Foot

Similar in many ways to their counterparts in the hand, the intrinsic muscles of the foot are entirely contained within the foot (**9.35**, **9.36**). They are arranged in layers with attachments throughout the bones of the foot. While they are able to exert force on individual bones, collectively their primary function is to stabilize and move the toes.

Now that we have examined the functional anatomy of this region in detail, let's link this foundational knowledge to motion and function.

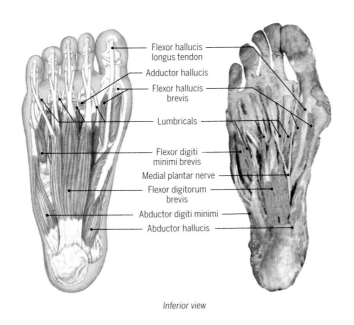

Inferior view

9.35 Intrinsic muscles of the foot, superficial layer

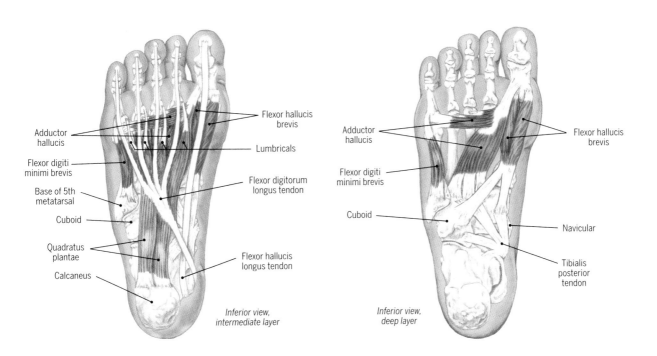

9.36 Intrinsic muscles of the foot, intermediate and deep layers

Purposeful Movement of the Knee, Ankle, and Foot

Many of the muscles of the lower extremities cross multiple joints. The respective joint positions will have an impact on the length-tension relationship and function of these muscles. As an example, consider the impact of hip position on knee flexion and extension. End-range hip flexion with knee extension requires passive elongation of the hamstrings. The opposite position requires elongation of the rectus femoris. As we examine specific movements, think about the relative position of the joints involved and their impact on muscle function.

Figures **9.37–9.46** feature muscles of the knee, ankle, and foot in the context of functional mobility, with prime movers listed first. Asterisks indicate muscles not shown.

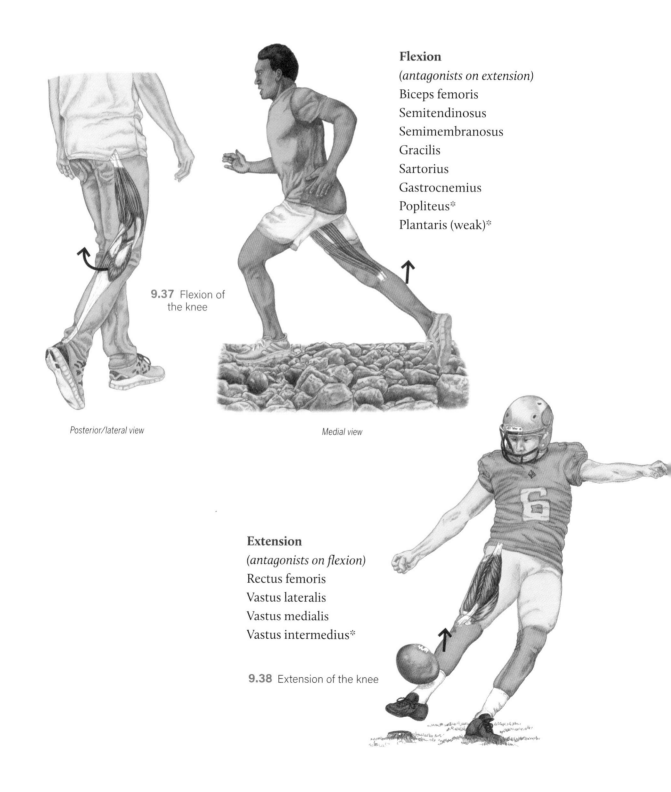

9.37 Flexion of the knee

Posterior/lateral view

Medial view

Flexion

(*antagonists on extension*)

Biceps femoris

Semitendinosus

Semimembranosus

Gracilis

Sartorius

Gastrocnemius

Popliteus*

Plantaris (weak)*

Extension

(*antagonists on flexion*)

Rectus femoris

Vastus lateralis

Vastus medialis

Vastus intermedius*

9.38 Extension of the knee

Internal (medial) Rotation of Flexed Knee

(antagonists on external rotation)

Semitendinosus

Semimembranosus

Gracilis

Sartorius

Popliteus*

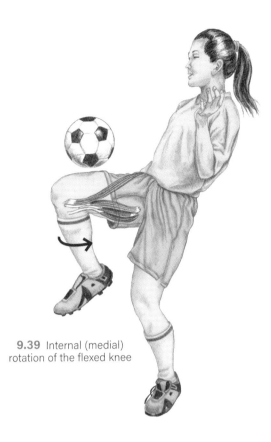

9.39 Internal (medial) rotation of the flexed knee

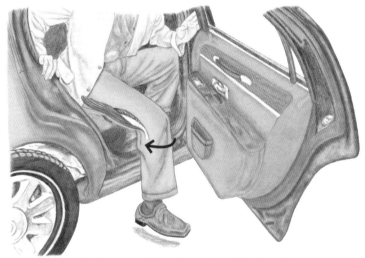

9.40 External (lateral) rotation of the flexed knee

External (lateral) Rotation of Flexed Knee

(antagonist on internal rotation)

Biceps femoris

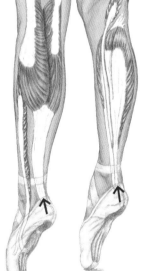

Posterior/lateral view

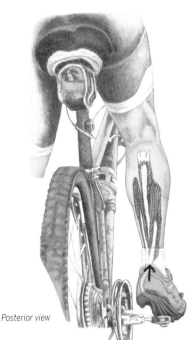

Posterior view

Plantar Flexion

(antagonists on dorsiflexion)

Gastrocnemius

Soleus

Tibialis posterior

Fibularis longus (assists)

Fibularis brevis (assists)

Flexor digitorum longus (weak)

Flexor hallucis longus (weak)

Plantaris (weak)

9.41 Plantar flexion of the ankle

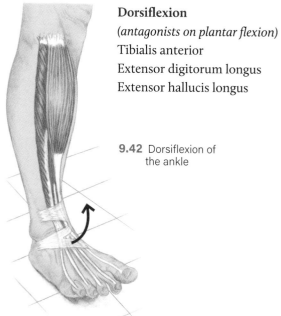

Dorsiflexion
(*antagonists on plantar flexion*)
Tibialis anterior
Extensor digitorum longus
Extensor hallucis longus

9.42 Dorsiflexion of the ankle

Anterior/lateral view

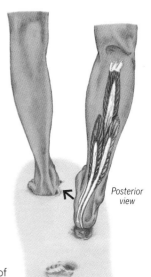

Posterior view

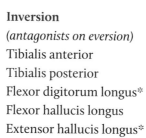

Anterior view

9.43 Inversion of the foot

Inversion
(*antagonists on eversion*)
Tibialis anterior
Tibialis posterior
Flexor digitorum longus*
Flexor hallucis longus
Extensor hallucis longus*

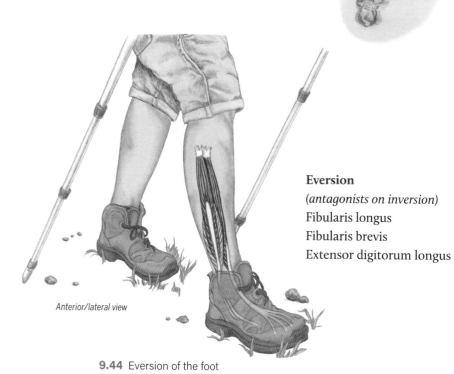

Eversion
(*antagonists on inversion*)
Fibularis longus
Fibularis brevis
Extensor digitorum longus

Anterior/lateral view

9.44 Eversion of the foot

Flexion of 2nd through 5th Toes

(antagonists on extension of toes)

Flexor digitorum longus

Flexor digitorum brevis

Lumbricals*

Quadratus plantae (assists)*

Dorsal interossei (2nd–4th)*

Plantar interossei (3rd–5th)

Abductor digiti minimi (5th)

Flexor digiti minimi brevis (5th)*

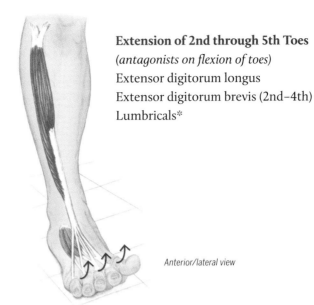

Extension of 2nd through 5th Toes

(antagonists on flexion of toes)

Extensor digitorum longus

Extensor digitorum brevis (2nd–4th)

Lumbricals*

Anterior/lateral view

9.46 Extension of the toes

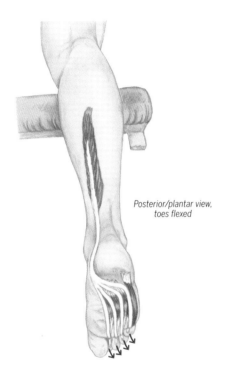

Posterior/plantar view, toes flexed

9.45 Flexion of the toes

Think about the muscles of the legs in a functional context, such as when sitting down on a toilet. Which muscles act concentrically or eccentrically? What is the effect of gravity? Do any muscles demonstrate isometric contraction to stabilize specific joints? How do these patterns change when standing from the toilet? What impact does the height of the toilet have on the forces required of the muscles? Thinking through these personal and environmental factors, or the context, will promote safe and effective occupational performance for your future patients.

OT Guide to Goniometry & MMT: Knee, Ankle, and Foot

Now that you are familiar with the bones, joints, and muscles that contribute to purposeful movement of the knee, ankle, and foot, let's practice goniometry and MMT using the *OT Guide to Goniometry & MMT* eTextbook. Remember that these joints often frequently alternate between open- and closed-chain kinematic patterns. How might a limitation in one joint impact the motion of another? How should an adjacent joint be positioned to allow maximal motion of the joint being measured?

As you practice the techniques, describe the bony landmarks and underlying anatomy associated with each motion and its measurement. Also think about lower extremity motion in the context of functional mobility. How much motion of each joint is required for toilet transfers, getting in and out of a vehicle, walking, or running? How might one joint compensate for loss of motion in another?

Occupational and Clinical Perspectives

While the upper extremities provide the motor performance skills required for reaching, gripping, and manipulating, the lower extremities facilitate walking, aligning, and positioning the body for occupational performance. These functions should not be thought of as separate or independent of one another; they must be integrated and coordinated. The occupation-based practitioner analyzes the motor performance skills of the entire body to facilitate engagement in occupation.

Functional Mobility

Each joint of the lower extremity serves a unique purpose in positioning and moving the body. The simple functional purpose of the knee is to shorten and lengthen the lower extremity for ambulation, standing, and sitting. Repetitive knee flexion propels the body forward and controls the speed of walking or running.

The quadriceps are essential for safe transfers: eccentric contraction lowers the body to a seated position while concentric contraction enables standing. This muscle group is vital to maintaining functional mobility in older adults, ensuring safe transfers from the commode or other functional surfaces (**9.47**).

The lower the seating surface, the more force demands are placed on the quadriceps to extend the knee and raise the body. Elevating or increasing firmness of seating surfaces decreases demand on the quadriceps to facilitate safer transfers.

As noted earlier, the screw-home mechanism stabilizes the articular surfaces of the knee, limiting the amount of muscle force needed to maintain a static standing position. In other words, the tibia and fibula are aligned vertically and locked in place. However, the screw-home mechanism depends on full active extension of the knee.

Lack of full knee extension places significantly more demand on the quadriceps to remain standing. Postoperative edema or contracture of the knee joint often limits full active extension. Preserving and/or restoring full knee extension after surgery or injury is critical to maintain this stabilizing mechanism for standing.

The foot and ankle represent the first line of defense against the ground reaction forces ascending through the lower extremity. Much of this ground reaction force is absorbed directly by the noncontractile arches of the foot, which act as passive shock absorbers.

Additional shock absorption comes from the subtalar and talocrural joints of the ankle. These joints allow positional changes to accommodate to the changing ground surfaces beneath. When walking on an incline, for example, ankle inversion or dorsiflexion may be required to keep the body upright on an uneven surface.

Neurological Impairment of the Lower Extremity

The joints and skin of the foot are highly innervated, sending valuable proprioceptive and tactile (skin) sensory input to the brain. For example, when walking on sand, the surface instability is quickly perceived, and the muscles work harder to stabilize and propel the body forward. These sensations also allow for safe mobility without visual input, as when walking across a cold bathroom floor at night.

Damage to the joint capsule during surgery may affect joint proprioception. Tactile sensation can be impaired by vascular disorders like peripheral neuropathy, with

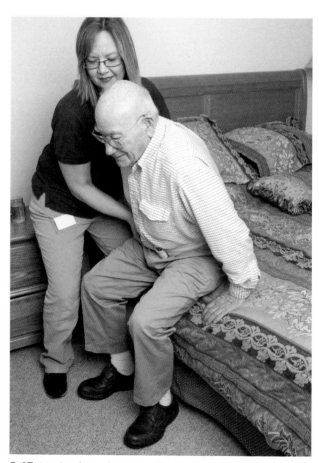

9.47 Moving from sit to stand from a bed with assistance. What modifications could be made to improve safety and efficiency?

damage to nerve endings in the distal extremities due to lack of blood flow.

Central nervous system disorders, such as a stroke or traumatic brain injury (TBI), may also cause significant sensorimotor impairments of the lower extremity. Damage to the sensory cortex or motor cortex of the brain can cause partial or total loss of sensation and motor control.

Often an individual with hemiparesis (partial paralysis) of the leg will develop **foot drop**, or inability to actively dorsiflex the ankle and foot. Attempts to propel the leg forward may cause the foot to drag against the ground, creating a fall risk. An ankle-foot orthosis (AFO) holds the foot in a passive, neutral position, to help restore a modified gait pattern and functional mobility (**9.48**).

Global weakness of the leg may also lead to a **circumduction gait** pattern. If the hip flexors and knee extensors are too weak to advance the leg, the pelvis and trunk rotate to swing the leg forward. This and other abnormal gait patterns are presented in Chapter 10.

Fall Prevention

More than one in four adults age sixty-five or older experience a fall each year, and many of these falls go unreported to health care providers. Falls often cause significant debilitating injuries like a hip fracture or TBI. Health care costs associated with falls and resulting injuries amount to more than $50 billion annually.[5]

Falls are caused by a variety of contributing factors. Loss of sensation, lower body weakness, or visual impairment may contribute to a lack of confidence, fear, or impaired balance.

Physical barriers in walking paths, poor lighting, or unstable ground surface are environmental risk factors. Certain medications may also cause dizziness with walking or standing (**9.49**).

Occupational therapy practitioners, applying holistic evaluation of the person, their environment, and their occupations, have an important role to play in the prevention of falls. Environmental modifications like removing rugs or other obstacles in the home, use of stable footwear with rubber soles to increase surface friction, and improving visibility with lighting or reflective surfaces reduces fall risk for older adults. Installing handrails in the shower or around the commode provides additional support in these high-risk areas. Mobility devices, when properly fitted and used, increase an individual's base of support and, as a result, stability.

Musculoskeletal Injuries of the Lower Extremity

The demands placed on the lower extremities related to performance patterns—habits, routines, roles, and rituals—may contribute to musculoskeletal disorders like osteoarthritis, which often develop gradually over time. High-impact forces, such as with motor vehicle accidents (MVAs) or athletic injuries, are more likely to result in traumatic injuries.

As the knee has limited bony congruity, multidirectional support is provided by the collateral (medial and

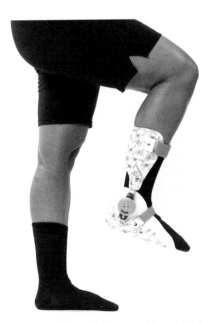

9.48 Ankle-foot orthosis (AFO). How would an AFO improve functional mobility for an individual with foot drop?

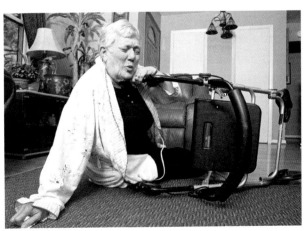

9.49 A fall in the home environment. What factors may have contributed to this fall? How could fall risk be minimized for this older adult?

lateral) and cruciate (anterior and posterior) ligaments. Load imbalance may increase tensile force through one collateral ligament while creating laxity on the opposing ligament. For example, genu varum effectively creates a bend at the medial knee, shortening the MCL and elongating the LCL.

Over time, these noncontractile supportive tissues will adapt to the load placed upon them and contribute to long-term imbalance of the joint. Additionally, high-impact injuries involving inward or outward force with the knee in a closed-chain position—for example, due to being tackled from the outside of the leg while the foot is planted—may result in traumatic rupture of individual or multiple ligaments of the knee.

The collateral ligaments are susceptible to injury with lateral or medial force, while the cruciate ligaments are susceptible to anterior, posterior, or torsional forces. Also, the menisci may be injured with excessive rotation at the knee during weight-bearing activity, grinding the supportive tissue between the compressed femur and tibia. These injuries often require surgical repair, including debridement (removal) of damaged tissue, direct repair, or grafting.

If soccer, basketball, running, or tennis are currently, or have ever been, among your leisure occupations, you likely have rolled your ankle (9.50). Typically, this involves inversion of the ankle, elongating or rupturing the lateral collateral (talofibular or calcaneofibular) ligaments. Mild injuries, or sprains, may heal with immobilization in an orthopedic walking boot, which maintains the foot and ankle in a neutral position to allow tissue healing. More severe injuries often require surgical repair.

Bones of the lower leg can fracture through high-impact injuries from falling, MVAs, or crush injuries. Nondisplaced injuries may be treated nonoperatively with immobilization, while more complex fractures require surgical repair with a period of non-weight-bearing depending on the severity. ADL modifications, mobility devices, and adaptive equipment are common interventions used by occupational therapy practitioners after lower extremity injuries.

How many steps per day does the average person take? It depends on your geographical location, surrounding environment, and performance patterns. Americans on average take approximately 5,000 steps per day, while in

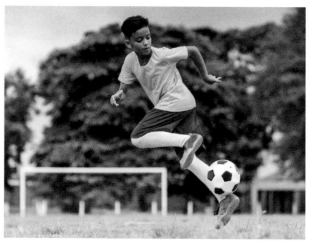

9.50 Force demands on the lower extremity. How do leisure occupations like soccer impact the ligaments of the knee and ankle?

Switzerland the average is nearly double that, at 9,650 daily steps.[6] Among Amish communities, children and adults may average between 14,000 to 18,000 steps per day, which may contribute to low rates of obesity.[7] The lower extremity is designed to absorb compressive forces sustained over a lifetime of functional mobility.

Excessive loading related to injury, work tasks, or the strain of obesity may result in premature breakdown of the protective structures, leading to **osteoarthritis**, or degeneration of joint surfaces due to wear and tear (9.51).

Joint bracing, ADL modifications, mobility devices (cane or walker), and pain management are conservative interventions that often provide some symptom relief and functional benefit. Severe osteoarthritis can necessitate joint replacement, or knee joint arthroplasty. Knee arthroplasties are very common. Depending on the severity of joint degeneration, they may involve a partial (medial or lateral femoral condyle and tibial plateau) or total (both femoral condyles and the tibial plateau) replacement. These surgical procedures may be completed on an outpatient basis or involve a short hospital stay, with the individual returning to normal ADLs and driving within three to six weeks.

This chapter concludes our look at regional functional anatomy. The next chapter provides a broader perspective of movement of the entire body for occupational performance. Many of the concepts from this chapter will be applied further as we examine functional mobility in greater detail.

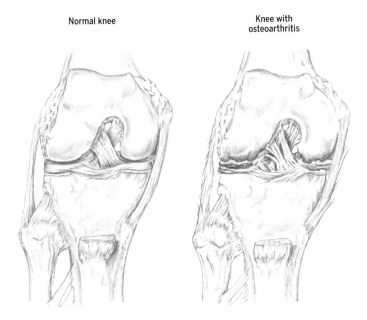

Normal knee

Knee with
osteoarthritis

Anterior view of right knee with patella removed

9.51 Comparison of normal and arthritic knees. What changes do you notice?

APPLY AND REVIEW

Ruth Feng

Before Ruth considers a TKA (replacement), the physician has referred her to both occupational and physical therapy for conservative (nonoperative) therapy services. The orders are broad and general: "Maximize mobility/function and decrease pain."

Review Ruth's occupational profile and the other case information in the chapter. Then answer the following questions:

- An interdisciplinary team approach to rehabilitation utilizes various disciplines for optimal patient outcomes. How do you see occupational therapy and physical therapy working together before surgery to optimize Ruth's functional outcome?
- Think about compensatory or adaptive strategies. What specific modifications to Ruth's occupational performance might be beneficial?

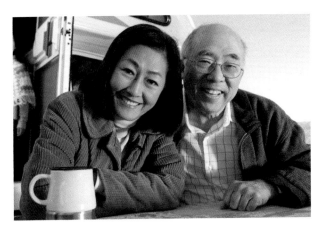

- Do some research on the role of occupational therapy for individuals with a knee arthroplasty. If she decides to proceed with the knee arthroplasty later on, how would your approach change postoperatively?

Review Questions

1. The functional purpose of the patella includes all of the following *except*
   a. increasing the moment arm (leverage) of the quadriceps for knee extension.
   b. providing anterior stability to the knee during flexion.
   c. remaining static with motion of the knee.
   d. providing a protective covering.

2. To decrease the force demands of the quadriceps and improve safety with bathroom transfers, which of the following would be the *most* beneficial modification?
   a. Provide a raised toilet seat.
   b. Install a tub shower.
   c. Install hardwood or linoleum flooring.
   d. Lower the toilet seat.

3. The screw-home mechanism involves which of the following to stabilize the joint surfaces of the knee in standing?
   a. medial rotation of the fibula relative to the tibia
   b. lateral rotation of the tibia relative to the femur
   c. lateral rotation of the femur relative to the tibia
   d. medial rotation of the tibia relative to the femur

4. Genu varum, or excessive inward (medial) angulation of the tibia relative to the femur, would most likely contribute to osteoarthritis on which aspect of the tibial plateau?
   a. posterior
   b. lateral
   c. medial
   d. anterior

5. What is the essential functional purpose of the intrinsic muscles of the foot?
   a. Provide individual motion of toes.
   b. Generate force for dorsiflexion and plantar flexion of the foot and ankle.
   c. Generate force for eversion and inversion of the ankle and foot.
   d. Stabilize the arches of the foot during weight-bearing.

6. Which of the following joints separates the hindfoot and midfoot?
   a. transverse tarsal joint
   b. intertarsal joint
   c. talocrural joint
   d. subtalar joint

7. What joint provides eversion and inversion of the ankle, accommodating functional mobility on uneven surfaces?
   a. talocrural
   b. subtalar
   c. intertarsal
   d. transverse tarsal

8. The arches of the foot provide all of the following benefits to the lower extremity *except*
   a. providing shock absorption at the most inferior aspect of the lower extremity.
   b. reducing the impact of ascending forces on the knee, hip, and spine.
   c. stabilizing the bones of the foot.
   d. providing active force for plantar flexion of the foot and ankle.

9. An injury to the fibular nerve would most likely result in which of the following?
   a. plantar fasciitis
   b. circumduction gait pattern
   c. foot drop
   d. Trendelenburg gait pattern

10. Leisure occupations that involve repetitive weight-bearing through the foot may contribute to which of the following?
    a. foot drop
    b. circumduction gait
    c. plantar fasciitis
    d. hemiparesis

See Answer Key in back of book.

Notes

1. Heidi McHugh Pendleton and Winifred Schultz-Krohn, *Pedretti's Occupational Therapy: Practice Skills for Physical Dysfunction*, 8th ed. (St. Louis, MO: Elsevier, 2017), 1107–13.

2. Carol A. Oatis, *Kinesiology: The Mechanics and Pathomechanics of Human Movement*, 3rd ed. (Philadelphia: Wolters Kluwer, 2017), 786.

3. Oatis, *Kinesiology*, 803–4.

4. Oatis, *Kinesiology*, 872–73.

5. Centers for Disease Control and Prevention, National Center for Injury Prevention and Control, "Important Facts about Falls," Home and Recreational Safety, last reviewed February 10, 2017, https://www.cdc.gov/homeandrecreationalsafety/falls/adultfalls.html.

6. David R. Bassett Jr. et al., "Pedometer-Measured Physical Activity and Health Behaviors in U.S. Adults," *Medicine and Science in Sports and Exercise* 42, no. 10 (October 2010): 1819–25, https://doi.org/10.1249/MSS.0b013e3181dc2e54.

7. David R. Bassett Jr., Patrick L. Schneider, and Gertrude E. Huntington, "Physical Activity in an Old Order Amish Community," *Medicine and Science in Sports and Exercise* 36, no. 1 (January 2004): 79–85, https://doi.org/10.1249/01.MSS.0000106184.71258.32; David R. Bassett Jr. et al., "Physical Activity and Body Mass Index of Children in an Old Order Amish Community," *Medicine and Science in Sports and Exercise* 39, no. 3 (March 2007): 410–15, https://doi.org/10.1249/mss.0b013e31802d3aa7.

Bibliography

American Occupational Therapy Association. *Occupational Therapy Practice Framework: Domain and Process.* 4th ed. Bethesda, MD: AOTA Press, 2020.

Avers, Dale, and Marybeth Brown. *Daniels and Worthingham's Muscle Testing: Techniques of Manual Examination and Performance Testing.* 10th ed. St. Louis, MO: Saunders, 2019.

Biel, Andrew. *Trail Guide to Movement: Building the Body in Motion.* 2nd ed. Boulder, CO: Books of Discovery, 2019.

Biel, Andrew. *Trail Guide to the Body: A Hands-On Guide to Locating Muscles, Bones, and More.* 6th ed. Boulder, CO: Books of Discovery, 2019.

Bassett, David R., Jr., Patrick L. Schneider, and Gertrude E. Huntington. "Physical Activity in an Old Order Amish Community." *Medicine and Science in Sports and Exercise* 36, no. 1 (January 2004): 79–85. https://doi.org/10.1249/01.MSS.0000106184.71258.32.

Bassett, David R., Jr., Mark S. Tremblay, Dale W. Esliger, Jennifer L. Copeland, Joel D. Barnes, and Gertrude E. Huntington. "Physical Activity and Body Mass Index of Children in an Old Order Amish Community." *Medicine and Science in Sports and Exercise* 39, no. 3 (March 2007): 410–15. https://doi.org/10.1249/mss.0b013e31802d3aa7.

Bassett, David R., Jr., Holly R. Wyatt, Helen Thompson, John C. Peters, and James O. Hill. "Pedometer-Measured Physical Activity and Health Behaviors in U.S. Adults." *Medicine and Science in Sports and Exercise* 42, no. 10 (October 2010): 1819–25. https://doi.org/10.1249/MSS.0b013e3181dc2e54.

Centers for Disease Control and Prevention, National Center for Injury Prevention and Control. "Important Facts about Falls." Home and Recreational Safety. Last reviewed February 10, 2017. https://www.cdc.gov/homeandrecreationalsafety/falls/adultfalls.html.

Clarkson, Hazel M. *Joint Motion, Muscle Length, and Function Assessment: A Research-Based Practical Guide.* 2nd ed. Philadelphia: Wolters Kluwer, 2020.

Keough, Jeremy L., Susan J. Sain, and Carolyn L. Roller. *Kinesiology for the Occupational Therapy Assistant: Essential Components of Function and Movement.* 2nd ed. Thorofare, NJ: SLACK, 2017.

Lundy-Ekman, Laurie. *Neuroscience: Fundamentals for Rehabilitation.* 5th ed. St. Louis, MO: Elsevier, 2018.

Oatis, Carol A. *Kinesiology: The Mechanics and Pathomechanics of Human Movement.* 3rd ed. Philadelphia: Wolters Kluwer, 2017.

Pendleton, Heidi McHugh, and Winifred Schultz-Krohn. *Pedretti's Occupational Therapy: Practice Skills for Physical Dysfunction.* 8th ed. St. Louis, MO: Elsevier, 2017.

Standring, Susan. *Gray's Anatomy: The Anatomical Basis of Clinical Practice, International Edition.* 41st ed. Cambridge, UK: Elsevier, 2016.

CHAPTER 10

Positioning, Postural Alignment, and Functional Mobility

Learning Objectives

- Describe positioning, postural alignment, and functional mobility as they relate to occupational performance.

- Understand the typical human gait pattern as a component of functional mobility.

- Analyze atypical posture and gait patterns and their impact on occupational performance.

- Apply knowledge related to anatomy, biomechanics, and functional mobility to safe patient transfers.

Key Concepts

ambulation

anatomical stability

antalgic gait

ataxic gait

base of support (BOS)

bridging

center of gravity (COG)

circumduction gait

dependent transfer

dowager's hump

forward head posture (FHP)

functional (dynamic) stability

functional mobility

gait

gait cycle

hemiplegic gait

joint contracture

leg length discrepancy

line of gravity (LOG)

logroll

mobility device

Parkinsonian gait

pelvic tilt

postural alignment

postural control

posture

pressure sore

quiet standing

scissor gait

scoliosis

sliding board transfer

squat-pivot transfer

stability

stand-pivot transfer

step

stride

Trendelenburg gait

two-person squat-pivot transfer

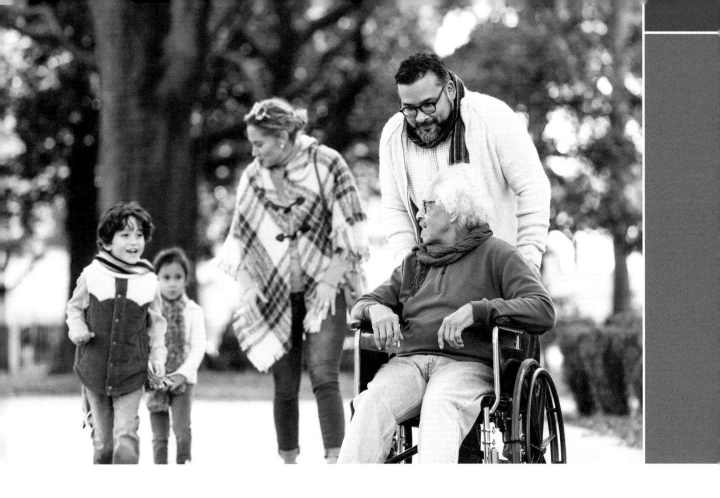

Movement through the Lens of Occupation

Think about your daily occupations—bathing, dressing, studying, or leisure pursuits like reading, running, or yoga. All of these purposeful activities involve a unique position or pattern of movement engaging the entire body. They take place within specific environmental contexts, each of which either supports or inhibits occupational performance (**10.1**). Purposeful movement of the entire body is also linked to client factors such as values, beliefs, spirituality, body structures, and body functions.

In previous chapters, you have learned the functional anatomy of separate regions of the body. Of course, the segments of the human body do not operate independently. Like interconnected links in a chain, the position and function of one segment of the body impacts the others (**10.2**).

As a future practitioner, you should develop the ability to zoom in on individual body regions or structures and zoom out to analyze motor performance of the body as a whole. Understanding how these body segments align and move together prepares you to analyze and promote the motor performance skills of occupational performance.

In this chapter, we put the pieces of purposeful movement together, analyzing movement and position of the entire body in relation to occupational performance. We will look at stability, positioning, postural alignment, and functional mobility with an emphasis on context, performance patterns, performance skills, and client factors.

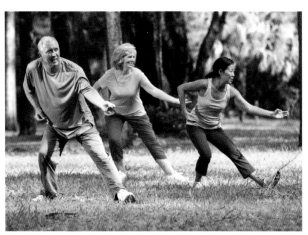

10.1 Occupational performance is influenced by context (environmental and personal) and client factors.

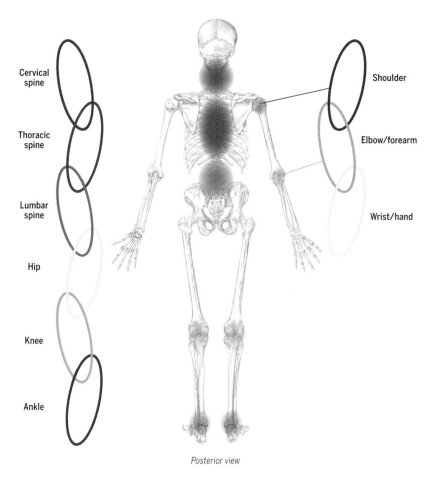

Posterior view

10.2 Interconnected segments of the body

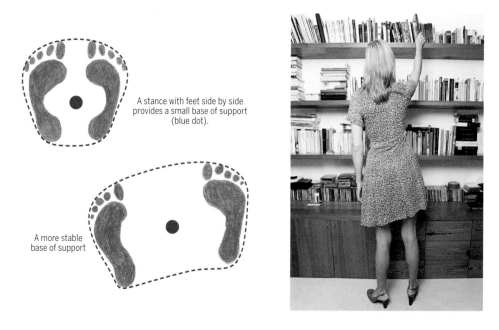

10.3 A wider base of support increases functional stability.

Stability

As it relates to functional anatomy, **stability** refers to the ability to maintain control over the position or movement of your body. Whether you are maintaining a complex yoga pose or simply sitting upright to enjoy a meal, the segments of your body cooperate to provide complimentary stability and mobility for purposeful activity.

The sensorimotor system integrates sensory input—visual, vestibular, and somatosensory (proprioceptive, tactile)—sending appropriate motor responses to maintain equilibrium to position and move the body. When analyzing the positional stability of the human body, specific biomechanical concepts to consider are base of support, center of gravity, and line of gravity.

Base of support (BOS) refers to the parts of the body, or a mobility device like a walker or cane, that come into contact with the ground surface and the distance between those points of contact. The more points of contact and the larger the distance between them, the better the base of support and stability. For example, standing with the feet shoulder-width apart gives greater stability than a narrow stance (**10.3**).

In a seated position, the base of support may be the legs of a chair or the wheels of a wheelchair, as well as the feet if they are in contact with the ground. When walking or running, our base of support constantly changes according to the varying contact between the feet and the ground surface beneath (**10.4**).

Mobility devices such as canes, crutches, and walkers add points of contact, increasing stability. A walker, for example, adds four points of contact for greater stability while standing and walking (**10.5**). What effect would a cane or crutches have on an individual's base of support?

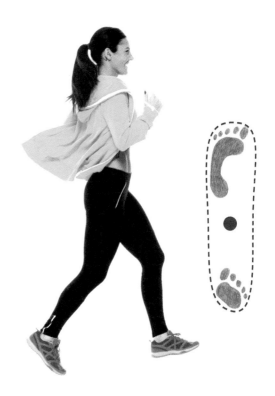

10.4 Walking or running changes the base of support.

The position of the body at any given moment significantly affects functional balance. The **center of gravity (COG)** is the focal point at which gravity acts and around which the weight of an object is evenly distributed. Lowering a person's COG increases stability: a football player crouching before the snap is much more stable than a ballerina standing on tiptoe.

In the anatomical position, the human body's COG is around the second sacral level. However, as weight distribution through the body shifts with movement, the COG migrates in proportion to the direction and

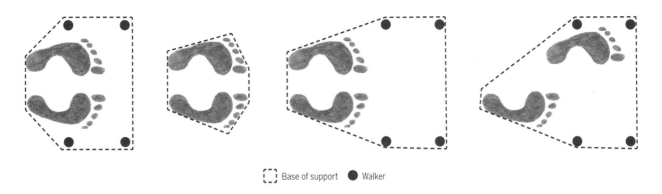

☐ Base of support   ● Walker

10.5 Base of support while using a walker. The left foot is the affected foot.

magnitude of movement. For example, bending forward to touch your toes shifts your COG anteriorly and inferiorly (**10.6**).

COG can also change based on the weight of an object or the way it is carried. When someone carries an object, its weight and distribution become part of the body with respect to gravity. In order to maintain balance, the body's position and weight distribution shift to accommodate the object's weight (**10.7**). The farther an object is held from the body, the greater its effect on an individual's COG.

In Chapter 1 we explained that the muscles generate internal force to lift objects, but objects also exert external forces on the body. An object applies greater leverage and force the farther it is held from the body. Keeping the object close to the body decreases its external moment arm and the joint reaction force (JRF) necessary to hold the object up against the force of gravity. Holding objects closer to the body relies more upon the larger proximal muscle groups and joints, which are better suited for carrying and lifting.

Holding objects close to the body, a key principle of safe lifting and joint protection techniques, is often beneficial for ADL/IADL training, workers who handle materials, and individuals with musculoskeletal conditions like osteoarthritis. The specific ways people lift or carry objects may be ingrained in their habits and routines, and it may take time to implement helpful modifications (**10.8**).

The **line of gravity (LOG)** is a vertical line extending downward from the COG of an individual or object to the ground beneath. This line represents the downward force of gravity acting on the body.

Identifying the LOG and base of support helps to identify and promote **anatomical stability**. When the LOG falls *within* the base of support, the body is anatomically stable. When the LOG falls *outside* the base of support, the body is anatomically unstable.

Think of an older adult with postural compromise leaning forward due to kyphosis of the spine (**10.9**).

▶TRY IT

To appreciate the benefits of carrying objects closer to the body, hold your backpack or a similar object by its straps with your arms extended away from your body. What do you notice? Do you feel the strain on the joints of your fingers and wrist? Do you feel the muscles of your back and shoulder contract to counteract this anterior shift in your COG?

Now hold the same object close against your body using only your shoulders, elbows, and forearms. Did you notice the difference? How does this change your COG and the joint reaction forces required to hold the object?

What does this exercise tell you about educating individuals on safe lifting and joint protection techniques? What other environmental or personal factors affect lifting and carrying objects?

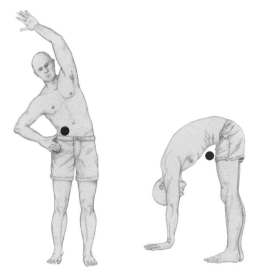

10.6 Changing the position of your body causes a proportional change to the center of gravity (*red dots*).

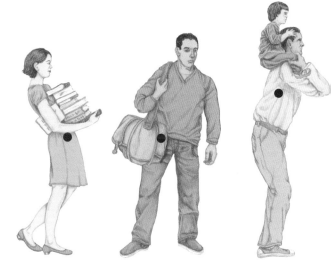

10.7 Describe the way each person's body position changes in order to maintain balance when carrying an object or child. (*Red dots* represent the center of gravity.)

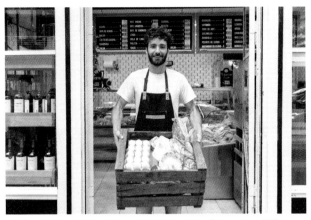

10.8 Lifting and transporting as motor performance skills. How might this worker modify his lifting technique to decrease joint reaction forces and improve his balance?

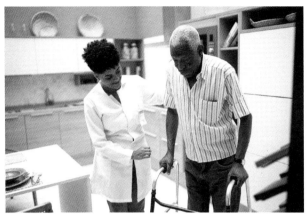

10.9 Mobility devices may be used to increase anatomical stability to promote safe functional mobility. How does using a walker impact this individual's base of support and overall stability?

Flexion of the trunk positions the upper body anterior in relation to the feet beneath. As a result, the LOG moves outside the base of support. This pattern creates instability and increases fall risk and related injuries. What might you recommend for an individual with this clinical presentation to bring their LOG within the base of support?

Clinically, addressing stability as a component of occupational performance is vital. Enhancing stability not only improves mobility and function but also decreases

▶TRY IT

As a future practitioner, you should remember that anatomical stability does not necessarily indicate **functional (dynamic) stability**, the stability required for an individual to perform a particular task in a specific environmental context. Functional stability is much more complex and depends on body structure and function (client factors) as well as environmental and personal factors (context).[1] It involves the ability to maintain balance while the body is in motion, changing positions, or navigating the surrounding environment.

Refer to the client and personal factors sections in the *Occupational Therapy Practice Framework*, fourth edition (OTPF-4) to analyze anatomical and functional stability for the individuals and specific activities shown in Figure **10.10**. Analyze the position of the body, LOG, and base of support relative to anatomical stability. Also consider environmental factors that affect functional stability like ground surface, lighting, and footwear, as well as client and personal factors like age, emotional state, motivation, and cognition.

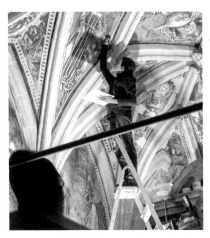
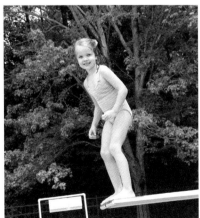
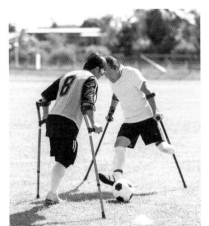

10.10 Analyze the anatomical and functional stability of these individuals performing specific occupations.

the risk of falls and other injuries. Here are some practical recommendations using base of support, COG, and LOG to enhance stability:

- Increase the base of support and maintain the LOG within its boundaries.
  ◦ Widen the stance.
  ◦ Add a mobility device, such as a walker, cane, or crutches (depending on the diagnosis and functional level of the individual).
  ◦ Encourage upright walking with optimal posture (discussed in the next section).
- Increase the surface area and friction of points of contact with the ground.
  ◦ Wear stable, well-fitted footwear that supports the arches of the foot and the neutral position of the ankle.
  ◦ Use shoes with durable rubber-like soles to increase friction with ground surface.
  ◦ Add nonslip tips to the ends of canes, walkers, or crutches.
- Carry objects close to the body and distribute weight as evenly as possible.
  ◦ When wearing a backpack, use both shoulder straps at an equal length.
  ◦ Carry objects on forearms with elbows bent at sides when possible.
  ◦ Bend at the knees and maintain an upright trunk when lifting.

Positioning and Postural Alignment

Occupational performance also relies on effective positioning and alignment of the segments of the body within the surrounding environment.

Position

Position refers to the general static location of an object or individual in space. An individual's position includes their body's general position, angles, dimensions, and location within the environment.

Occupational therapists and occupational therapy assistants often analyze and make recommendations regarding positioning. Here are a few examples:

- In an acute care setting, changing positions frequently is often recommended for individuals with limited mobility in order to vary and distribute pressure to prevent skin breakdown while lying in bed.

- After a neurological injury with hemiparesis (weakness on one side of the body), such as a stroke or traumatic brain injury (TBI), positioning might focus on maintaining optimal alignment of the weakened trunk or limbs.
- In a burn unit, specific joint positions may be recommended to prevent **joint contractures** (see Chapter 1) from scar tissue that develops during the healing process.
- When working with a child, the OT/OTA might suggest playing in the prone position to encourage development of head and neck control.

CLINICAL APPLICATION
Position and Respiratory Function

Occupational therapy practitioners often serve on interdisciplinary teams, providing positioning and mobility recommendations for patients in acute care or an **intensive care unit (ICU)**. Optimal positioning and movement are essential for cardiovascular, respiratory, and musculoskeletal function. Specific recommendations are often made based on an individual's diagnosis and level of activity tolerance.

For example, early in the COVID-19 crisis, researchers discovered that for some individuals, the prone position improved respiratory function.[2] Many occupational therapists on the frontlines of the crisis gave guidance on positioning and mobility as well as rehabilitation for individuals diagnosed with COVID-19 (**10.11**).

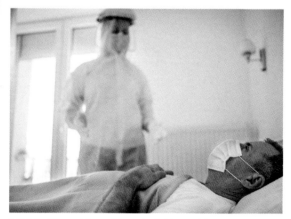

10.11 OT working with an individual with COVID-19 and limited mobility. What recommendations might an occupational therapist make regarding positioning for this individual?

For individuals who spend a lot of time in bed or in a wheelchair, occupational therapy addresses areas of high pressure that can lead to **pressure sores**. These areas often involve a **bony prominence**, or an area where a bone protrudes beneath the skin. There are specific areas associated with high pressure in the seated, supine, side lying, and prone positions (**10.12**).

Pillows or other soft external supports may be used to limit pressure in these areas, and the individual's position should be changed often. The skin in these areas should be checked frequently for redness, inflammation, or breakdown as indicators of pressure sores. In some cases, a specialized mattress or seat cushion is necessary to ensure pressure distribution.

Posture

Posture is more complex and dynamic than position. It refers to the relative position of the segments of the body—trunk, extremities, and head—that changes in response to the demands of an activity. **Postural alignment** is the collective position of these body segments at any given moment and affects occupational performance.

Postural control is the ability to achieve or maintain a balanced body position for a given activity. It depends on sensory input and motor output to accommodate task and environmental demands. Postural control involves both voluntary and involuntary adjustments as the body responds to these changing demands.

As you read this book, whether you are sitting up or lying down, your entire body is working to position your head and neck in front of a book or screen (**10.13**). Maybe you are seated with the book on a desktop, your trunk and neck flexing to keep the words within your visual field. Or perhaps you are lying on your stomach, propped on your elbows, with your trunk and neck extended. Regardless, each of these functional positions requires an integrated response and reaction from the entire body. As your muscles fatigue, or pressure on certain joints becomes uncomfortable, the position of your body and the posture necessary to support your functional position will change.

How does your surrounding environment support or inhibit this activity? How is the lighting? Does your workstation support your body position, or could it be improved?

Daily occupations rely on a variety of postures that are continually changing to meet the demands of the particular activity. Consider your daily ADLs and IADLs as well as your performance patterns—habits, roles, routines, or rituals. Think about the unique posture involved with each of these activities as well as the alignment and demands placed on the musculoskeletal system.

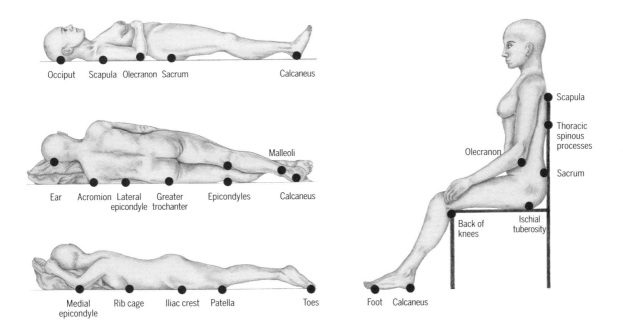

10.12 Areas associated with high pressure in various body positions

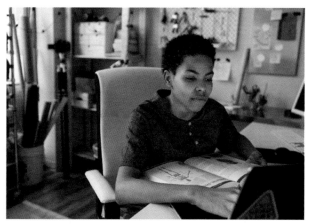

10.13 Consider the body position, environmental factors, and personal factors associated with the study habits of a student.

While there is no "perfect" posture that eliminates all imbalance within the tissues of the body, certain positions are more conducive to function with less impact on the musculoskeletal system. Ideal posture features anatomical symmetry of the core and extremities for equal force distribution and balance.

Standing Posture

Optimal standing posture features neutral alignment of the joints of the body, requiring minimal effort to remain standing and minimizing strain. The alignment of the segments of the body when standing is directly linked to balance and function. When you analyze posture, begin centrally at the pelvis and spine, as the position of these proximal structures will affect the position of the distal arms and legs.

The position of the pelvis, or **pelvic tilt**, can be assessed by examining the relative position of the **anterior superior iliac spine (ASIS)** and **posterior superior iliac spine (PSIS)**. When the pelvis is level, the ASIS and PSIS should be relatively aligned in the transverse plane (across the top of the pelvis) (**10.14**). This neutral position supports the natural lordosis of the lumbar spine as well as symmetry of the arms and legs.

An asymmetrical pelvis affects the position of the spine and extremities, contributing to suboptimal postures. We will look at several of these later in this chapter.

A level pelvis supporting the natural curvature of the spine is the foundation of optimal standing posture (**10.15**). In this position, the weight-bearing joints of the lower extremities (ankles, knees, and hips) align vertically, limiting the amount of muscle contraction needed to maintain standing.

The upper body is vertically balanced above the pelvis, supporting the head, neck, and upper extremities. This position is also referred to as **quiet standing**. While the body appears static, it actually makes small movements from side to side and front to back, called **postural sway**.

Notice the large muscle groups on either side of the LOG: the ankle plantar flexors, quadriceps, gluteals, and muscles of the core. These muscle groups counterbalance one another with small contractions to maintain joint alignment and balance during quiet standing.

Also think about the opposing muscles of the core on either side of the LOG, predominantly the abdominals and erector spinae. In standing, the slow-twitch fibers of these muscles supply low-intensity contraction to resist the downward pull of gravity and maintain an upright position.

Begin to examine the alignment of these landmarks when you observe individuals standing upright. This is basic clinical reasoning for assessing posture.

Seated Posture

Many occupations involve prolonged sitting, such as office work, driving, gaming, or having a meal. The same principles apply for optimal upper body posture when seated: neutral pelvic tilt, upright trunk with balanced curvature of the spine, and neutral head and neck, with the ears aligned with the shoulders. However, sitting involves hip and knee flexion, which will naturally shorten the hamstrings and hip flexors over time. Stretching these muscle groups, along with intermittent

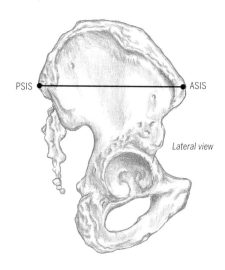

10.14 Neutral pelvic tilt

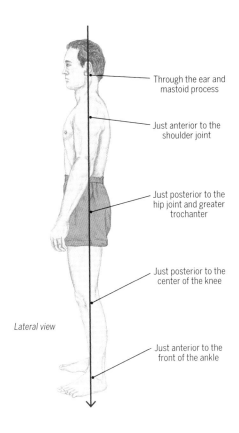

10.15 Optimal standing posture, showing the line of gravity passing through key anatomical landmarks

Through the ear and mastoid process

Just anterior to the shoulder joint

Just posterior to the hip joint and greater trochanter

Just posterior to the center of the knee

Lateral view

Just anterior to the front of the ankle

may require adjustments to their workstation to promote slight anterior pelvic tilt and trunk extension to avoid propping their elbows and forearms on the work surface.

The use of a computer workstation presents unique considerations regarding seated or standing posture. Typing generally requires flexion of the elbows as well as positioning the wrists and hands to interface with the keyboard. The position of the head and neck must also place the monitor(s) within the visual field.

Ergonomics is the study of human interaction and efficiency within the work environment, a unique area of practice for occupational therapy practitioners. In order to optimize posture, minimize musculoskeletal strain, and prevent injury, a common ergonomic principle is to fit the workstation to the worker. This means allowing for adjustability in workstation dimensions and seating to accommodate a wide variety of individual body types.

Although ergonomics is a broad topic and beyond the scope of this text, here are a few common principles for workstation setup to promote musculoskeletal balance and prevent strain (**10.16**):

- The lumbar spine should be supported against the back of the chair with the feet flat on the floor.
- The hips, knees, and elbows should be positioned at roughly 90° angles.
- The wrist should be in neutral, not flexed, extended, or deviated.
- The monitor should be 18–24 inches from the face (within arm's reach) with the top of the monitor at eye level.
- The head and neck should be neutral, not flexed, extended, or rotated.

standing and walking, may limit the musculoskeletal impact of prolonged sitting.

Environmental and personal factors also affect seated posture and function. Remember, a stable proximal core is necessary for distal function of the extremities. Individuals with poor core strength might need a more supportive chair. A person seated at a desk or tabletop

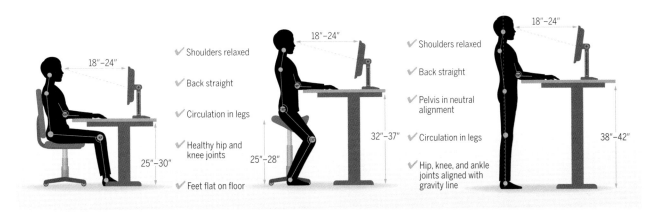

10.16 Ideal ergonomic workstation design

Common Postural Abnormalities

Postural analysis, as it relates to occupational performance, is used to examine the individual, their environment, and the purposeful activity involved. Think about the artist shown in Figure **10.17**. How will environmental factors like the height of his easel, footwear, or ground surface impact his posture? How does his body type or the way he paints contribute to his overall body position?

When addressing the physical aspect of posture, it is helpful to think about **ascending** or **descending forces** relative to the pelvis that can create imbalance throughout the body. As an example, consider a child born with one leg longer than the other, known as a congenital **leg length discrepancy**. The longer leg will generate an ascending force that contributes to pelvic and upper body asymmetry as a result.

In contrast, **scoliosis**, or abnormal curvature of the spine, can contribute to pelvic obliquity (see Chapter 8) and an imbalance in the lower extremities through descending forces from the spine (**10.18**).

Determining the primary cause of postural imbalance is essential because your approach to intervention will largely depend on the source of the issue. Remember, postural control requires sensory input—visual, vestibular, and somatosensory—to guide motor output for both voluntary and involuntary postural control. An individual

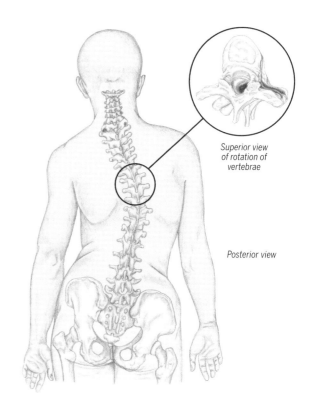

Superior view of rotation of vertebrae

Posterior view

10.18 Scoliosis. How does abnormal curvature of the spine impact the position of superior and inferior body segments as well as overall posture?

with sensory impairment, such as peripheral neuropathy, often has difficulty with postural control due to lack of sensory input regarding placement of the feet.

For some individuals, issues are related to musculoskeletal imbalance. For example, someone with a leg length discrepancy may benefit from a compensatory lift in their shoe to restore symmetry of the lower extremities.

The environment can support or inhibit postural control and, as a result, occupational performance. Workstation adjustments, for instance, can promote healthier posture by accommodating an individual's height or body type.

Postural reeducation could take the form of activities or occupations that promote balanced, neutral posture. If reeducation is limited due to a specific pathology, compensatory or adaptive approaches might be more appropriate.

Note that asymmetry of the extremities is often a result of an issue more proximally located in the pelvis or spine. Identifying the source of the imbalance is important in order to properly intervene.

Bear in mind that the body will do everything it can to maintain its midline (centered) position based on visual and vestibular input unless there is an underlying neu-

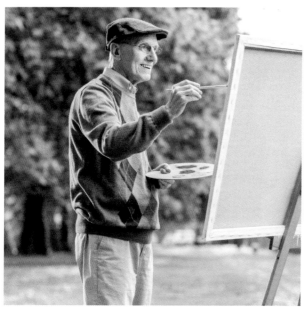

10.17 Functional standing posture while painting

rological impairment. With imbalance in the proximal pelvis or trunk, the rest of the body will compensate to keep the body upright. Optimal seated or standing posture serves as a reference point to analyze suboptimal postures that impede occupational performance.

Posterior Pelvic Tilt

A level, balanced pelvis is essential to the overall posture and function of the upper body. Pelvic asymmetry has a chain reaction through the spine and extremities, affecting the position and function of the entire body.

Posterior pelvic tilt is backward rotation of the pelvis out of the neutral position. In this tilted position, the ASIS is higher than the PSIS (**10.19**).

Posterior pelvic tilt can occur after prolonged sitting, due to fatigue of the postural muscles. You may be experiencing it as you read this text. Individuals who use wheelchairs for mobility and others who spend much of their day in a seated position are at particular risk for this postural pattern.

Over time, posterior pelvic tilt contributes to muscle imbalance, with tightness of the hip extensors, abdominals, and pectoral muscles and elongation of the hip

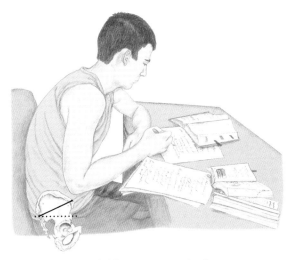

10.19 Posterior pelvic tilt

flexors, erector spinae, and scapular stabilizers. With the pelvis out of neutral position, the spine and lower extremities compensate to keep the body upright.

Several common postural abnormalities are associated with posterior pelvic tilt. Posterior pelvic tilt increases thoracic kyphosis and a generally **rounded back** and shoulders (protraction of the scapula) (**10.20**).

CLINICAL APPLICATION
Fixed or Mobile Postural Abnormalities

Postural abnormalities can lead to joint contractures (see Chapter 1). Fixed contractures cannot be adjusted; the skeleton is permanently in that position and motion cannot be improved with conservative treatment. Mobile contractures demonstrate some flexibility, which suggests the position can be improved.

In clinical practice, determining whether the position is fixed or mobile is important for choosing your approach to treatment. Individuals with mobile abnormalities may benefit from a rehabilitative approach to restore musculoskeletal balance through postural reeducation and occupation-based interventions that promote healthy posture. Individuals with fixed postural compromise or contractures often require a more adaptive or compensatory approach, such as environmental modifications or adaptive equipment to support occupation in the fixed position.

In future clinical practice, how could you safely determine if a contracture is fixed or flexible?

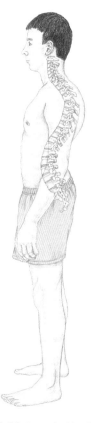

10.20 Rounded back

The extensor muscles of the upper back are elongated and weakened, while the anterior pectoral muscles become short and tight. Thoracic kyphosis also orients the scapula downward and weakens its stabilizing muscles. This position limits the ability of the scapula to upwardly rotate, impairing overhead motion and the function of the humerus.

Think about how a rounded back position might affect vision, safety awareness, breathing, and social interaction. Practitioners should educate patients and caregivers on how to identify and safely prevent this pattern of postural compromise. How might you promote a posture that is more conducive to occupational performance?

Posterior pelvic tilt often leads to abnormalities in standing posture. **Swayback** refers to posterior tilt and shifting of the pelvis relative to the feet (**10.21**).

The hips compensate by extending, ultimately shortening the hamstrings. Lumbar lordosis and thoracic kyphosis also increase.

Eventually, excessive thoracic kyphosis can become a fixed postural abnormality called **dowager's hump**, a permanent flexion of the thoracic spine and orientation of the upper body downward (**10.22**).

How would this fixed posture impact occupational performance? Think about specific ADLs, IADLs, and social interactions. How might the posture impact movement of the shoulders? What compensatory or adaptive strategies might support occupational performance?

Excessive lumbar lordosis contributes to rounding of the thoracic spine, but a significant loss of lordosis is undesirable as well. **Flat back** refers to a decrease in lumbar lordosis and general flattening of the thoracolumbar spine (**10.23**). This leads to tightness of the hamstrings as well as overstretching of the hip flexors.

Anterior Pelvic Tilt

In many ways, **anterior pelvic tilt** is anatomically the opposite of posterior pelvic tilt. The top of the pelvis tilts forward, with the PSIS elevated relative to the ASIS. This results in increased lumbar lordosis and extension of the upper trunk as well as retraction of the scapulae.

When standing, this posture resembles a soldier at attention, with the chest puffed out and the head and neck vertical. For sitting, slight anterior pelvic tilt is often preferred to prevent slouching and encourage the core muscles to contract to maintain an upright position (**10.24**).

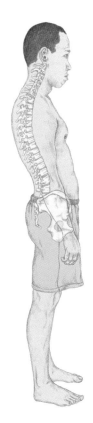

10.21 Swayback

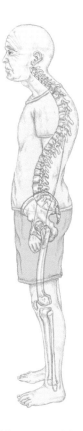

10.22 Dowager's hump

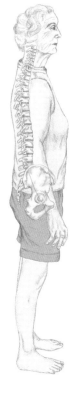

10.23 Flat back

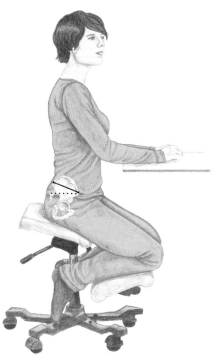

10.24 Anterior pelvic tilt

10.25 Right pelvic obliquity

Excessive anterior pelvic tilt, however, can increase strain on the lumbar spine and fatigue the postural muscles. Anterior pelvic tilt may be present in pathologies that involve abnormal muscle tone, like cerebral palsy.

Pelvic Obliquity

Pelvic obliquity is asymmetry of the pelvis in the frontal plane with one side elevated relative to the other. This position causes a compensatory chain reaction in the rest of the body to maintain the midline position of the trunk.

Can you identify the compensatory patterns occurring in the spine and shoulders in Figure **10.25**? On the right side of the body, the pelvis is elevated, the spine is slightly laterally flexed, and the shoulder is depressed. On the left side, the pelvis is depressed with opposite compensatory reactions of the spine and shoulder.

Think about how this pelvic position would impact the lower extremities in terms of ground force through the foot and pressure distribution in the joints. Over time, pelvic obliquity contributes to an imbalance of forces when sitting, standing, or walking.

If the person is a wheelchair user, pelvic obliquity may also increase the risk of skin breakdown with increased pressure over the ischial tuberosity of the lower side

of the pelvis. Figure **10.26** is a pressure map (a digital visual representation of pressure distribution) of someone sitting in a wheelchair. Can you see the imbalance in pressure distribution? How might you decrease and distribute pressure when developing a seating system for an individual with pelvic obliquity?

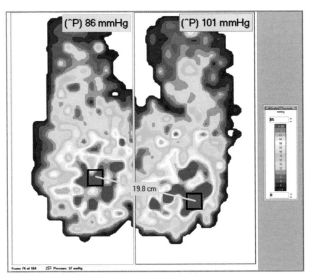

10.26 Pressure map of the pelvis and hips while sitting. What does this pressure map suggest about the position of the pelvis?

Forward Head Posture

Forward head posture (FHP), or protraction of the head and neck anterior to the trunk, may be a result of postural issues in the pelvis or trunk or can be present despite otherwise optimal posture (**10.27**).

FHP can result from prolonged suboptimal positioning in a wheelchair or at a workstation with the head and neck protruding forward and flexed. Over time, the cervical vertebrae lose their natural lordosis and musculoskeletal imbalance occurs, with shortening of the neck extensors and lengthening of the flexors. This posture can cause general neck pain and tension as well as functional impairment of the temporomandibular joint (TMJ).

Posture and Occupation

Performance of specific occupations, driven by roles, habits, routines, and rituals, also affects overall posture. Your role as a student likely includes spending hours poring over notes, working on a laptop computer, and sitting through lectures. How does this impact the postural tendency of your body?

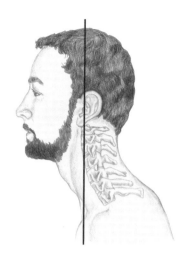

10.27 Forward head posture

Consider the individuals, environments, and occupations shown in Figure **10.28**. How are these elements reflected in each individual's posture? How does posture facilitate or inhibit occupation?

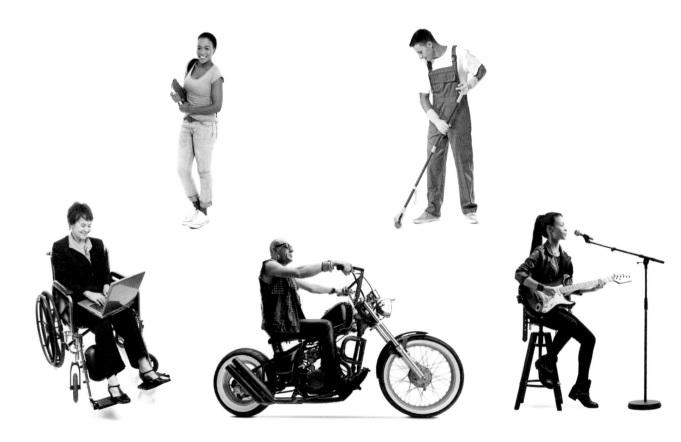

10.28 Posture affects and is affected by occupational performance, performance patterns, and context (environmental and personal factors).

Functional Mobility

To align the body within the surrounding environment for occupational performance, we must first move ourselves into the right position.

Functional mobility is described in the OTPF-4 as

> *moving from one position or place to another (during performance of everyday activities), such as in-bed mobility, wheelchair mobility, and transfers (e.g., wheelchair, bed, car, shower, tub, toilet, chair, floor). Includes functional ambulation and transportation of objects.*[3]

Functional mobility includes **ambulation** (walking) through a particular environment, such as navigating to the bathroom at night across a cold tile floor or walking a dog on a wet, sandy beach. It encompasses bed mobility, wheelchair mobility, and transfers from various functional surfaces like a toilet or shower chair, as well as transporting functional objects, such as carrying a bag of groceries up the stairs to a third-floor apartment (**10.29**).

Functional mobility has many components: environmental factors like wheelchair accessibility, ground surface, and lighting; personal factors including age or underlying health conditions; and client factors like body structure and function. As a future practitioner, you should understand the impact of these factors on safety. Recommending or modifying mobility devices, appropriate use of a gait belt, or the addition of grab bars in a shower are examples of ways practitioners can promote safe functional mobility.

Safe ambulation is guided by somatosensory input from the foot and lower extremity. Cutaneous (skin) sensation informs the brain as to the quality of ground surface, whether hard asphalt, sand, or gravel. Proprioceptive input from the joint capsule and surrounding ligaments guides pressure and placement of the foot and ankle, such as when walking on an incline or hiking on a mountain trail. Without guiding somatosensation, the ankle and foot are limited in their ability to accommodate changes in ground surface, increasing the risk of fall and injury.

A holistic approach to functional mobility addresses the sensorimotor system, psychosocial factors, and cognition, as well as the surrounding environment, to promote safety and occupational engagement.

Bed Mobility

Bed mobility describes the ability to move and change positions while in bed—something many of us take for granted as an automatic part of our morning and evening routines.

Postoperative pain, paralysis, and general weakness considerably affect an individual's ability to mobilize against the weight of gravity while in bed. A lack of bed mobility can lead to skin breakdown from prolonged pressure over bony prominences like the sacrum, ischial tuberosities, or heels, as well as general deconditioning.

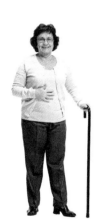 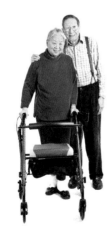 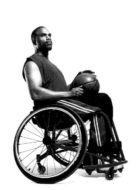 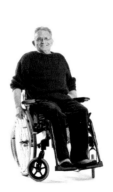 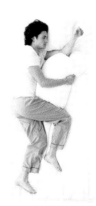

10.29 Identify the environmental and personal contexts and client factors affecting functional mobility for these individuals.

OT practitioners should educate patients who must spend a large amount of time in bed and their health care teams on the importance of changing positions frequently and positioning to avoid pressure around bony prominences. Several common modified techniques and adaptive aids may facilitate bed mobility.

For example, after some hip or spinal surgeries, certain precautions limit movement to protect the surgical repair—specifically, rotation of the back and hips. One modified technique to transition from lying on the back (supine) to sitting on the edge of the bed, or moving from sitting to supine, without rotating the back or hips is called a **logroll** (**10.30**). A modified version of logrolling may also be beneficial for an individual with hemiplegia as a result of a stroke, with or without assistance, depending on the person's functional level.

An individual with general fatigue or weak upper body strength may have difficulty changing positions in bed. **Bridging** involves flexing the hips and knees and pushing with the feet against the bed to elevate and shift the pelvis

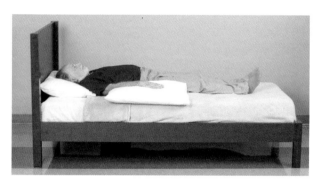

1. The patient is lying in the supine position.

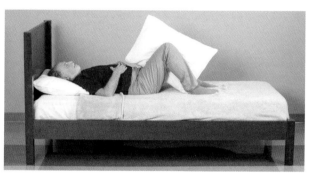

2. The knees are flexed and a pillow is placed between them.

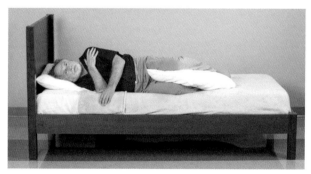

3. The patient rolls onto the side of the body toward the edge of the bed.

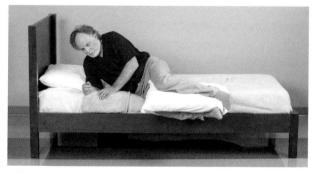

4. The legs are moved off the edge of the bed toward the floor as the patient pushes through the arm to sit upright.

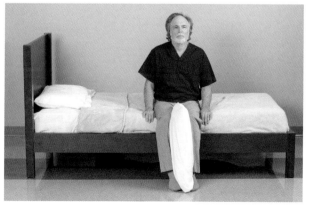

5. To move from sitting upright to supine, the steps are reversed.

10.30 A logroll is a modified bed mobility technique to move from supine to sit or sit to supine without rotating the back or hips.

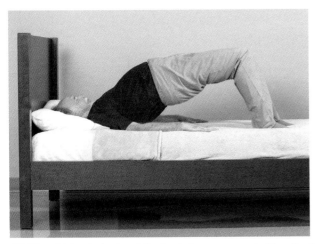

10.31 Bridging for bed mobility (technique exaggerated for effect)

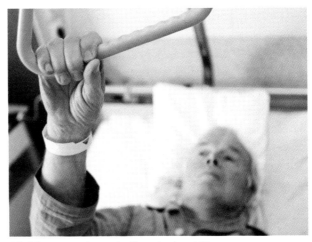

10.32 Trapeze bar to facilitate bed mobility

and upper body in bed (**10.31**). This technique is used to move higher in the bed or toward the edge of the bed in preparation for sitting.

For an individual with significant weakness or paralysis of the lower body, such as someone with a spinal cord injury (SCI), a **trapeze bar** helps maximize the use of the upper extremities for bed mobility. The trapeze bar is arranged over the top of the bed on a stable frame, providing overhead support for bed mobility using the strength of the arms (**10.32**).

Wheelchair Mobility

People who use wheelchairs should have the ability to mobilize through their homes and communities as seamlessly as non–wheelchair users. Fortunately, in many countries, laws require accessible infrastructure design for sidewalks, buildings, bathrooms, and other public areas.

If someone who uses a wheelchair cannot access an area, it is the environment, not the individual's limitation, that restricts access and function (**10.33**).

Occupational therapy practitioners routinely address environmental restrictions and advocate for access for individuals with disabilities. While addressing seating and mobility in detail is beyond the scope of this text, **wheelchair mobility** is important to include as a common type of mobility for many individuals.

Wheelchair mobility, whether manual or powered, requires a supportive seating surface to promote postural alignment and stability for occupational performance. The chair and its components should be customized to meet the unique needs of the individual, supporting safe functional mobility as unobtrusively as possible.

▶**TRY IT**

Building empathy—understanding and relating to the feelings and experience of others—is key for effective practice and developing compassion in general. One way to intentionally practice empathy with your future patients is to put yourself in their place.

You might try completing your daily routine using only one arm to troubleshoot functional modifications, such as for a patient experiencing hemiplegia as a result of a stroke. Or you might begin with logrolling or bridging for bed mobility, limiting yourself to the use of one side of your body.

Then try other ADLs or IADLs. What specific strategies or modifications do you find yourself using? If you find a unique solution, write it down. You might identify a better method or even a piece of adaptive equipment that could improve occupational performance or safety for an individual, group, or entire population.

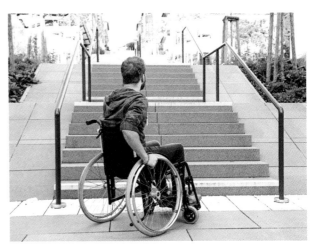

10.33 Environmental barriers to mobility and occupation

There are several general anatomical and mechanical considerations. The chair should encourage a neutral pelvic tilt with a neutral or slightly extended trunk to facilitate an upright posture. The footrests should support the legs in approximately 90° of hip and knee flexion, similar to an ergonomic workstation position (**10.34**). The hands must be able to reach the rim of a manual chair or the controller of a power chair to mobilize. Arm and leg rests may be removable to facilitate transfers.

For individuals with lower muscle tone, a customized seat or backrest may improve trunk support. If patients have loss of sensation or paralysis in the lower body, the seat cushion should be optimized to decrease pressure. There are many different pressure-relieving cushions available commercially. Specialty cushions, like the ROHO®, decrease pressure by contouring air-filled domes to the body to increase surface contact and distribute force (**10.35**).

Practitioners also encourage wheelchair users to weight-shift, changing the position of their body while in the wheelchair, or change the position of a power chair frequently, essential techniques for preventing skin breakdown and pressure sores.

Wheelchair design and various components should facilitate the occupational performance of the individual (**10.36**). Someone who plans to participate in adaptive sports likely needs a wheelchair that moves and turns more quickly with additional stability. A student might benefit from a removable tray table. Individuals who plan to return to driving will need additional components to integrate their seating system into an adapted vehicle.

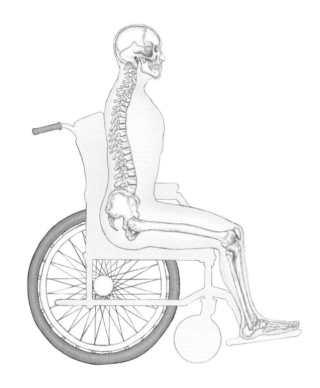

10.34 Wheelchair positioning

Simple modifications or additions, like extensions to better access wheel locks or a wheelchair bag for carrying items, have a positive impact on safety and function.

Keep the broader occupational perspective in mind as we explore human gait as a component of functional mobility.

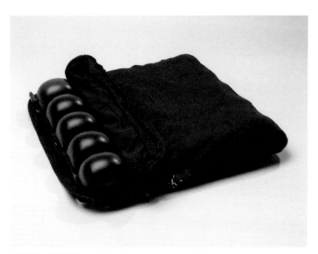

10.35 ROHO® cushion for pressure relief

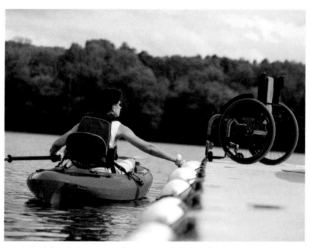

10.36 Wheelchairs can be customized to facilitate desired occupations. How have this wheelchair and kayak been adapted for this active individual?

Typical Human Gait

The way human beings are designed supports a certain pattern of typical movement. Are you a people watcher? If so, you will notice both variation and key similarities in the ways people walk. Humans are bipedal, walking on two legs, whereas many animals are quadrupedal, moving on four legs.

Typical **gait** (ambulation) features a repeating, reciprocal pattern of lower extremity movement, called the **gait cycle**, to propel the body forward. Throughout the gait cycle, the weight of the body shifts as the feet alternately contact the ground and advance to take the next step.[4]

Gait is generally described in reference to foot contact with the ground with an alternating **stance phase** and **swing phase** of each lower extremity. During this cyclical pattern, each leg alternates the tasks of **weight acceptance**, **single leg support**, and **double leg support** (10.37).

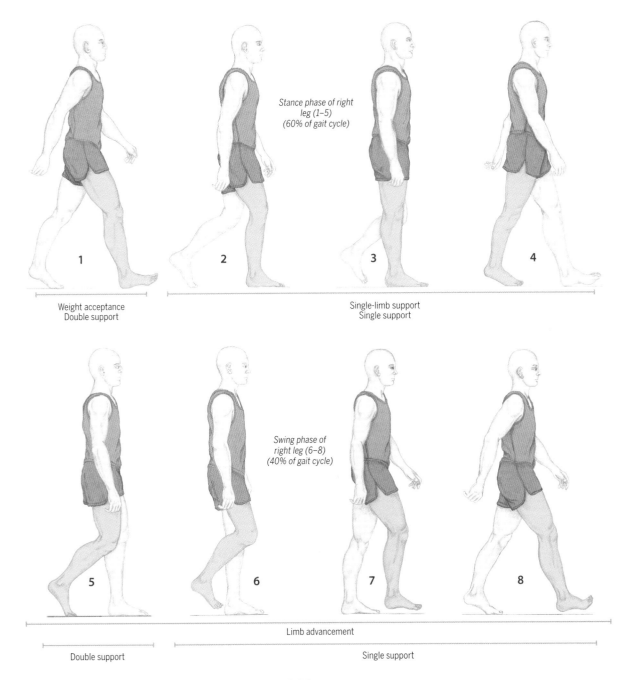

Stance phase of right leg (1–5) (60% of gait cycle)

1   2   3   4

Weight acceptance
Double support

Single-limb support
Single support

Swing phase of right leg (6–8) (40% of gait cycle)

5   6   7   8

Limb advancement

Double support   Single support

10.37 Gait cycle

The stance phase of gait has five parts: heel strike, foot flat, midstance, heel-off, and toe-off (**10.38**). The swing phase of gait has three parts: acceleration, midswing, and deceleration (**10.39**).

The gait cycle features cyclical concentric, eccentric, and isometric contractions of the muscles of the lower extremities. Propulsion occurs through the shear force (friction) created between the bottom of the foot (or shoe) and the ground beneath.

Acceleration involves an anterior shear force applied to the foot from the ground. This force is achieved through ankle plantar flexion, knee flexion, and hip extension. The muscles primarily involved with acceleration are the

gluteals (hip extension), hamstrings (knee flexion), and gastrocnemius/soleus (ankle plantar flexion) (**10.40**). The more rapidly and forcefully these muscles contract, the faster the speed of walking or running.

Deceleration involves posterior shear force applied to the foot from the ground to slow the propulsion of the lower extremity. This is achieved through slowing the overall motion of the legs when ambulating as well as increasing knee extension during the heel strike phase. Concentric contraction of the quadriceps and eccentric contraction of the hamstrings extend and stabilize the knee, firmly planting the heel in the ground, which acts as a brake to slow forward progression (**10.41**).

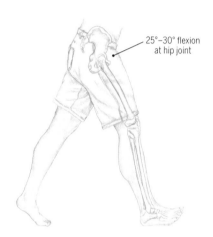

25°–30° flexion at hip joint

Heel strike. Heel of the foot strikes the ground; anterior rotation of the trunk toward the stance leg; 25° flexion of the hip; slight knee flexion.

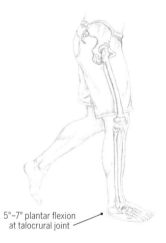

5°–7° plantar flexion at talocrural joint

Foot flat. Entire foot in contact with the ground; hip begins to extend with 20° of knee flexion; slight plantar flexion of the foot.

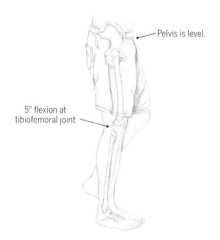

Pelvis is level.

5° flexion at tibiofemoral joint

Midstance. Body passes over stance leg; neutral pelvis and trunk; knee and hip extended; ankle begins to plantar flex to accelerate.

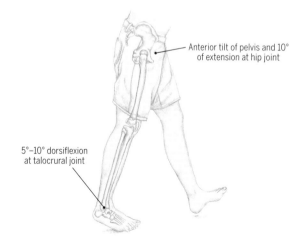

Anterior tilt of pelvis and 10° of extension at hip joint

5°–10° dorsiflexion at talocrural joint

Heel-off. Heel rises from ground surface; pelvis and trunk rotate away from stance leg (advancing the opposite leg); knee and hip are extended; rapid ankle plantar flexion (propulsion).

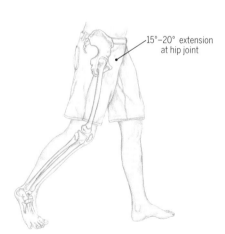

15°–20° extension at hip joint

Toe-off. End of propulsion and stance phase; hip and knee begin to flex; slight ankle plantar flexion.

10.38 Stance phase

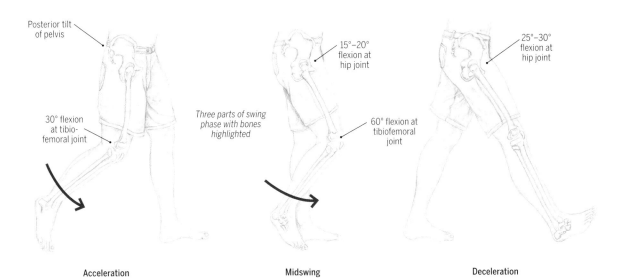

Acceleration

The pelvis rotates forward with hip and knee flexion to rapidly move the swing leg anteriorly, "catching up with" the stance leg.

Midswing

The hip and knee flex farther to ensure the foot clears the ground surface as it passes the stance leg.

Deceleration

The pelvis rotates forward with continued hip flexion to advance the leg; the knee is extended with the ankle neutral in preparation for heel strike.

10.39 Swing phase

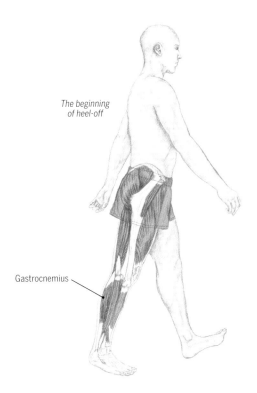

10.40 Acceleration during heel-off

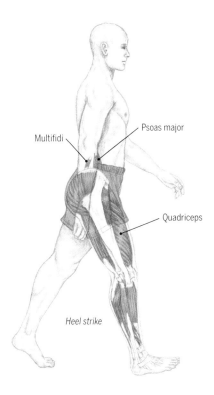

10.41 Deceleration during heel strike

The pelvis plays an essential role in the gait cycle, with cyclical motions to facilitate movement of the legs. As you know from Chapter 8, the pelvis is formed by two separate bones (coxae) that move in opposite directions: as one side elevates or rotates anteriorly, the other side depresses or rotates posteriorly. The pelvis demonstrates movement in three different planes throughout the gait cycle:

- anterior/posterior (forward and back)—rotates anteriorly to advance the swing leg and rotates posteriorly with the stance leg through the toe-off position (**10.42**)
- superior/inferior (up and down)—elevates with the stance leg during weight acceptance and depresses with the swing leg as it advances (**10.43**)
- lateral (side to side)—shifts laterally toward the stance leg in midstance, ensuring the swing leg clears the stance leg (**10.44**)

A gait cycle involves a single stance and swing phase for each extremity, or a **stride**. Stride can be measured

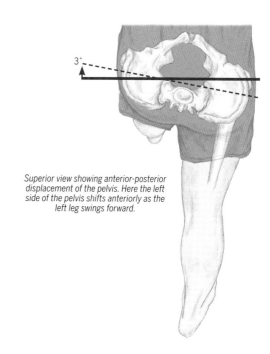

Superior view showing anterior-posterior displacement of the pelvis. Here the left side of the pelvis shifts anteriorly as the left leg swings forward.

10.42 Anterior/posterior movement of the pelvis during ambulation

▶ TRY IT

To visualize and better understand the movement of the pelvis and hip during ambulation, hold the bottom of a dry-erase marker against your hip with the tip against a whiteboard. Holding the marker steady against the whiteboard, walk forward, allowing the marker to draw along with the movement (see **10.43**).

Now step back and take a look at the line on the board. Did you notice the wave pattern? This illustrates the reciprocal elevation and depression of the pelvis and hip during typical ambulation.[5]

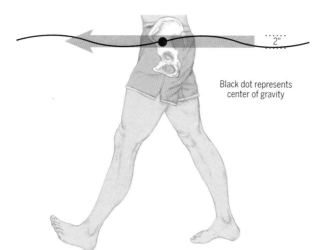

Black dot represents center of gravity

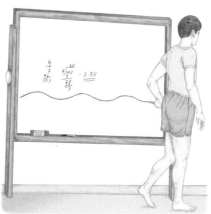

Drawing a line on a whiteboard with a marker at the hip

10.43 Superior/inferior movement of the pelvis during ambulation

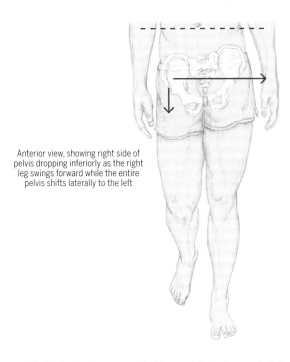

Anterior view, showing right side of pelvis dropping inferiorly as the right leg swings forward while the entire pelvis shifts laterally to the left

10.44 Lateral movement of the pelvis during ambulation

from the point at which the foot comes into contact with the ground to the next point of contact from the same foot—for example, heel strike to heel strike.

A **step** is the distance the foot advances in relation to the other and is measured as the distance from the same point on opposite feet (right heel strike to left heel strike). The distance between heels is **step width**, which determines an individual's base of support while ambulating (**10.45**).

Additionally, the foot is angled outward approximately 5°–8°, and this angle decreases as the pace increases. **Cadence** refers to the number of steps taken per minute.

While human gait follows the patterns described above, real-world functional mobility is much more complicated as it relates to occupational performance. A gait pattern is often a component of occupational performance. However, there are many other factors to consider: the specific occupation, ground surface, footwear, and the surrounding environment, to name a few.

For example, an older adult may have sufficient motion and strength to ambulate to the bathroom, but without adequate lighting, a safe ground surface, and appropriate footwear, they could still have a high risk of falling.

Home and community mobility require us to adapt our normal gait cycle to meet environmental and task demands. When walking on a stable, even surface, we are likely to use a typical balanced gait pattern.

This changes, however, when we walk on uneven or slippery surfaces like grass, sand, or a recently washed floor. Our sensory input informs the body as to the quality of the ground surface beneath, and the body responds accordingly.

Walking safely on a slippery surface usually means spreading the feet and lowering the body to increase the base of support and lower the COG. When we feel unstable, we often hold our arms out, away from the body, as an additional counterbalance. Walking on a soft surface like sand requires more effort from the muscles of the legs to advance the body as the feet sink into the surface beneath.

Because carrying an object shifts the COG, more of the body's weight may be focused on the opposite leg as a counterbalance when we transport objects as part of occupational performance.

Consider the occupations shown in Figure **10.46**. How does each purposeful activity and surrounding environment affect the individual's gait pattern?

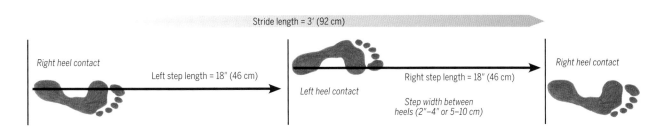

Stride length = 3′ (92 cm)

Right heel contact

Left step length = 18″ (46 cm)

Left heel contact

Right step length = 18″ (46 cm)

Step width between heels (2″–4″ or 5–10 cm)

Right heel contact

10.45 Measuring gait

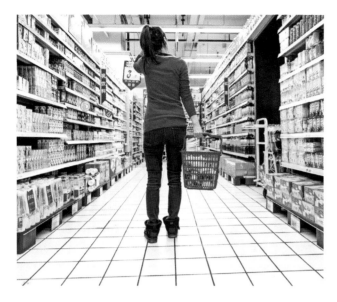

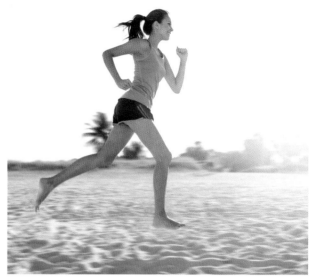

10.46 Ambulating with an uneven load or on an uneven surface

Abnormal or Pathological Gait Patterns

The skilled occupational therapy practitioner begins the process of assessment at first sight, analyzing the subtleties of a patient's position, posture, and gait pattern. While each person has a somewhat unique gait pattern, several atypical patterns of ambulation correlate to specific impairments in strength, range of motion, or underlying neurological impairment. Because each of the links of the human body affects the others, impaired motion of the upper extremities can also create imbalances in gait.[6]

As the following abnormal gait patterns are discussed, try them. This might feel awkward, but it will help you understand how a pattern of weakness or paralysis affects movement. This may help you relate to your future patients and collaborate on functional solutions.

Trendelenburg Gait

The gluteus medius muscle plays an important role in stabilizing the pelvis during ambulation. As the swing leg advances, the gluteus medius of the opposite (stance) leg contracts to prevent the contralateral pelvis from dropping inferiorly.

If the gluteus medius is weak, the pelvis will drop excessively on the swing leg side with each step, called **Trendelenburg gait**. The trunk will also lean toward the stance leg to maximize the force of the weakened gluteus medius (**10.47**).

Circumduction Gait

Normal gait raises the leg during the swing phase to clear the ground and advance forward. This requires simultaneous flexion of the hip and knee as well as dorsiflexion of the ankle.

With limited range of motion, or with weakness of the muscles contributing to typical movements of the legs for ambulation, the trunk and pelvis often compensate by rotating anteriorly, circumducting (swinging) the leg

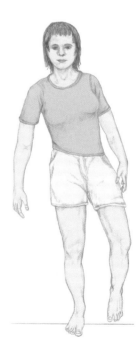

10.47 Trendelenburg gait

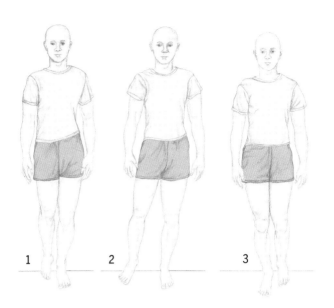

10.48 Circumduction gait

out to the side of the body to propel it forward. Called **circumduction gait**, this compensatory pattern occurs in patients with general muscle weakness, hemiplegia, or osteoarthritis of the knee (**10.48**).

Foot Drop

Ankle dorsiflexion is a key component of functional gait, allowing ground clearance with each step. The ankle dorsiflexors also eccentrically contract to transition from heel strike to foot flat, counterbalancing plantar flexion to bring the foot gently to the ground.

Weakness or paralysis of the ankle dorsiflexors can impair heel strike, with the toes coming into contact with the ground prior to the heel. This pattern is called **equinus gait**. During the swing phase, the toes often drag against the ground due to **foot drop**, the formal term for the loss of ankle dorsiflexion, and it is common after a stroke or TBI (**10.49**).

Isolated weakness of the dorsiflexors can result from injury to the deep fibular nerve, with the strength of the hip and knee preserved. In this case, the hip compensates through excessive flexion to allow the foot to clear the ground, termed high-stepping or **steppage gait**.

An **ankle-foot orthosis (AFO)** is used to keep the ankle in a neutral position, preventing the foot from dragging, in conjunction with a mobility device to improve stability depending on the clinical presentation (**10.50**).

Hemiplegic Gait

A **hemiplegic gait** pattern involves paralysis or weakness of an entire side of the body resulting from a neurological pathology like a stroke, TBI, or cerebral palsy. This gait pattern may include circumduction of the leg with foot drop, but it also includes common positions of the upper and lower extremities. The hip is often internally rotated and adducted, with an unstable knee extended against the weight of gravity. Distally,

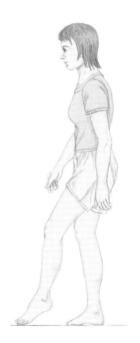

10.49 Foot drop

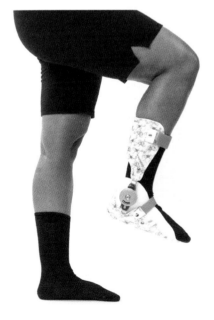

10.50 Ankle-foot orthosis to prevent foot drop

the ankle is usually inverted in plantar flexion. The arm is often flexed at the elbow and wrist, held against the body, limiting arm swing and balance (**10.51**).

After a neurological injury, some individuals recover a certain degree of muscle strength, relearning the ambulatory patterns they used prior to the injury. In other cases, permanent paralysis or weakness requires an adaptive approach to ambulation. While circumduction gait is not ideal, it serves as a modified approach to functional mobility when coupled with an AFO and a mobility device.

Antalgic Gait

Antalgic gait literally means ambulating against (*anti*), or to avoid, pain (*algos*). For example, suppose you experience an ankle sprain and limp for several days afterward due to the pain of weight-bearing through the affected leg. This pattern shortens the stance phase through the painful leg and shifts the weight onto the noninjured opposite side.

You might see an antalgic gait in patients for a short duration after they have had a minor soft tissue strain. Or it can be a subtle, chronic pattern with prolonged pain, associated with osteoarthritis of the hip or knee. Additionally, patients with postoperative pain after surgery of the hip, knee, or ankle often demonstrate this antalgic pattern. For these patients, you could focus their rehabilitation on accepting weight on the surgical limb to restore symmetrical, balanced ambulation.

Ataxic Gait

An **ataxic gait** is unique in that range of motion and strength are not compromised; rather, a lack of coordination causes the impairment. Generally, due to neurological impairment of the cerebellum, the individual strives for a wider base of support with jerky, staggering movements in attempts to ambulate. The loss of global coordination and impaired proximal stability have a considerable effect on upper extremity function.

Scissor Gait

As noted earlier, the width between the heels is usually two to four inches for a stable base of support during ambulation. Individuals with a **scissor gait** pattern demonstrate a narrowing, or even crossing-over, of the legs as they walk (**10.52**). This is often due to abnormal muscle tone with tightness of the hip adductors and is associated with cerebral palsy or other neurological pathologies that cause muscle spasticity.

Parkinsonian Gait

For individuals with Parkinson's disease, gait is affected by impaired perception and modulation of motor movements. **Parkinsonian gait** includes shuffling the feet—small forward motions with limited elevation of the legs—with flexion of the trunk, placing the weight of the body on the balls of the feet (**10.53**). This gait pattern increases the risk of falls and injury.

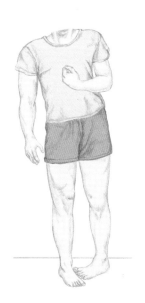

10.51 Hemiplegic gait

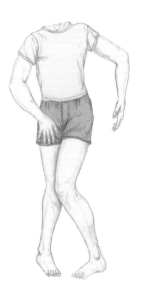

10.52 Scissor gait

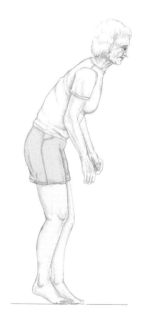

10.53 Parkinsonian gait

Mobility Devices

Patients with gait impairments due to weakness, loss of stability, pain, or recent surgery may benefit from a temporary or long-term **mobility device** to enhance their safe functional mobility. A mobility device adds points of contact with the ground surface, increasing the base of support and, as a result, stability.

Occupational therapists and physical therapists, individually or collaboratively, recommend mobility devices or their modification to ensure a person's safe mobility. These recommendations are based on an individual's medical history, functional level, physical strength, cognition, vision, and surrounding environment. Occupational therapists also consider adaptations to facilitate occupational performance, such as the addition of a walker bag or modified grip.

The following sections give general information about common mobility devices—canes, walkers, and crutches—used as adaptive techniques for functional mobility.

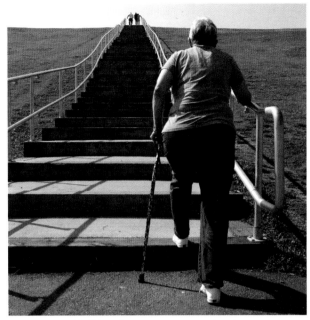

10.54 Using a cane to ascend stairs

Cane

A **cane** is usually prescribed to an individual with minor weakness, impairment in balance, or pain. Single-point canes have one projection to the ground, and a quad cane has four projections at its base. The quad cane can support more weight and may be better on flat, slippery floors, whereas a single-point cane is lighter and easier to use in tight spaces.

To be the proper height, the top of the cane should be around the level of the patient's wrist crease when they are standing upright with arms at the sides. This ensures slight flexion of the elbow for leverage when using the cane.

The cane is held in the hand opposite the weaker or painful leg and is advanced first with the weaker leg when possible. For example, if the patient's left leg is weak, the cane is held with the right hand, and their left leg and the cane initiate ambulation by taking the first step together. This allows the individual to shift their weight onto the stronger leg and cane, reducing compressive forces through the joints of the weaker or painful leg.

When ascending stairs, individuals should use the cane and handrail and step up with the stronger leg first (**10.54**). When descending stairs, individuals should step with the cane and weaker leg first. To help you—and the patient—remember, the good leg goes to heaven (first when going upstairs) and the bad leg goes to hell (first when going downstairs).

Walker

An individual with more severe instability, postural compromise, or recent surgery may benefit from the use of a **walker** (**10.55**). A static or rolling (with wheels) walker provides additional stability, with four additional points of contact with the ground, expanding an individual's base of support. Additional types of walkers include a forearm platform for individuals with hemiparesis or limited grip and upright walkers to promote a more neutral posture. A person's cognitive status must also be considered for safe and effective use of a walker. For example, a rolling walker is simpler, as it does not require lifting to advance.

The arms are used to support the upper body and can reduce or eliminate weight-bearing through a weak or

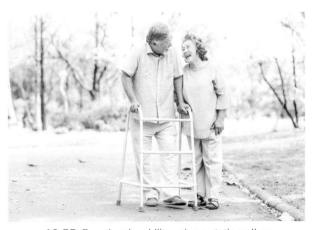

10.55 Functional mobility using a static walker

painful leg if necessary. The walker is advanced *with* the weaker or painful leg first, allowing the stronger leg to absorb the weight of the body. As with a properly fitted cane, the handles of the walker should be level with the wrist crease when the arms are by the side while providing some elbow flexion for leverage to advance the walker.

Crutches

Crutches are not a long-term compensatory solution for functional mobility but rather a temporary method of keeping weight off an injured limb (**10.56**). Crutches provide two additional points of contact with the ground, supporting the body bilaterally. The ambulatory pattern requires advancing the crutches, bringing the weaker leg and weight of your body forward, and finishing the step with the noninjured leg.

When fitting crutches, ensure the top of the crutch is one to two inches below the patient's armpit to avoid compression of axillary neurovasculature structures. The handgrips should align with the person's hips to allow the hands to push downward through the crutches and support the weight of the body.

Transfers

In occupational therapy practice, a **transfer** refers to moving from one functional surface to another, such as from the toilet to a wheelchair. The type of transfer technique used depends on the diagnosis, medical status, and functional level of the individual. Overall strength, ability to follow instructions, pain level, and weight-bearing status are primary considerations.

Often patients are functionally classified based on the level of assistance they require to complete specific ADLs, including functional mobility. While specifics vary and clinical guidelines are constantly evolving, general functional categories specify the level of need for assistance as minimum (1–25 percent assistance), moderate (26–50 percent), maximum (51–75 percent), or dependent (greater than 75 percent).

The transfer technique must give enough support to ensure safety and minimize risk for both the patient and the therapist. General transfer safety recommendations include the following:

- Review the patient's medical history for pertinent information, such as diagnosis, level of assistance required, cognitive status, weight-bearing precautions, medications, or pain.

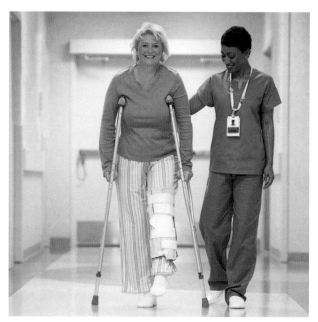

10.56 Temporary use of crutches after injury

- Ensure a safe environment. Transfer surfaces should be placed close together with a clear path between.
- Make sure any lines, such as oxygen, catheter, IV, or telemetry, have sufficient length and will not be in the way.
- Use a gait belt around the abdomen (between the pelvis and rib cage) to ensure stable contact with the patient (**10.57**).
- Always check to make sure there is no colostomy bag, feeding tube, or abdominal pain prior to securing the gait belt.
- Use clear, concise verbal instructions or visually demonstrate prior to implementing the transfer.

The next sections describe several common transfer techniques, applying biomechanical principles and optimal body mechanics.

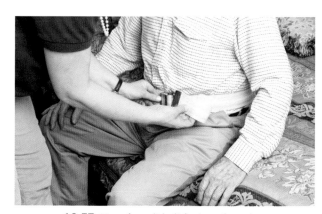

10.57 Use of a gait belt for transfer safety

Stand- or Squat-Pivot Transfer

A **stand-pivot transfer** is often appropriate for an individual requiring minimum or moderate assistance, depending on the relative size of the patient and clinician. This type of transfer includes an assisted stand, pivoting on a stance leg, and sitting on a surface placed next to (or as close as possible to) the original surface (**10.58**). It is frequently used to transfer from a toilet or bed and requires the individual to demonstrate the ability to safely bear weight through the legs and come to a full stand.[7]

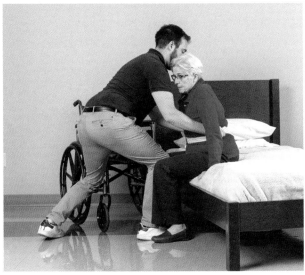

1. Transfer surfaces are positioned adjacent to one another with minimal space between. The patient is seated near the edge of the seating surface with feet shoulder-width apart. The therapist places one foot between the feet of the patient, with the other foot free to move toward the transfer surface.

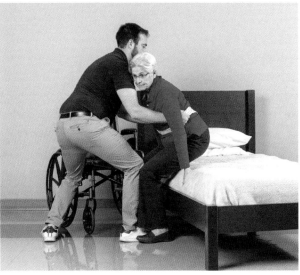

2. Flexing the hips and knees with the spine neutral, the clinician holds the gait belt, providing an appropriate amount of assistance to stand, while the patient pushes up from the seating surface or armrests.

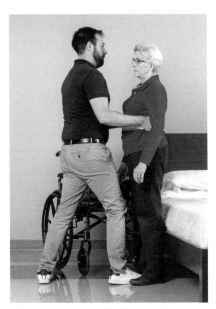

3. Once the patient is standing, the therapist ensures stability prior to turning.

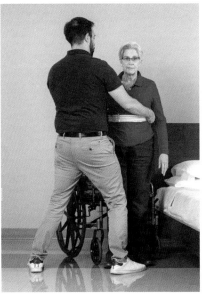

4. The patient and therapist then pivot together toward the transfer surface. The patient steps back until they feel the transfer surface on the back of their legs, reaches for the armrests, and lowers themselves to the seating surface with support from the therapist.

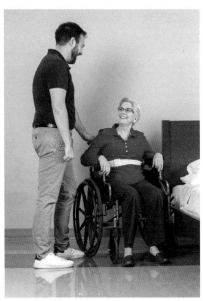

5. The therapist ensures stability and removes the gait belt.

10.58 Steps for a stand-pivot transfer

A **squat-pivot transfer** follows similar steps but is used when the patient does not have the strength to come to a complete stand. Rather, the patient comes to a squat, or half-standing position, with assistance from the clinician to pivot toward the transfer surface. Because the patient does not come to a full stand, bed rails or wheelchair armrests may need to be adjusted to ensure a clear path to the transfer surface. Leg rests should also be moved out of the way to avoid a trip hazard.

Sliding Board Transfer

A **sliding board transfer** may be the most appropriate option for an individual with lower extremity paralysis or someone who cannot safely complete a standing transfer. It is most frequently used for individuals with SCI, bariatric patients, or those with lower extremity amputations.

The sliding board is placed between the two functional surfaces, serving as a bridge for the individual to slide over, with or without assistance (**10.59**).[8] With practice, some patients who have good upper body strength and stability may be able to safely complete a sliding board transfer independently. This type of transfer may be used to transfer from many different functional surfaces including a wheelchair, commode, bed, or the seat of a vehicle, to name a few.

A sliding board transfer is completed as follows:

1. Transfer surfaces are positioned adjacent to one another, such as a wheelchair positioned next to a bed.
2. The individual shifts their weight onto the opposite hip, and the sliding board is placed under the hip closest to the intended transfer surface.
3. The opposite end of the sliding board is placed on the transfer surface, such as the seat of a wheelchair (it may be necessary to remove the armrest).
4. While leaning the trunk forward, the patient uses their arms to advance along the sliding board to the new surface.
5. The therapist provides assistance as needed in front of the individual, blocking the knees and assisting with weight-shifting.
6. Once the transfer is complete and the individual is stable, the sliding board is removed.

Dependent Transfer

A **dependent transfer** technique is used for individuals who can contribute minimal to no assistance to move from one surface to another. A sliding board technique may be used with additional support to the trunk and lower extremities from the therapist in front of the indi-

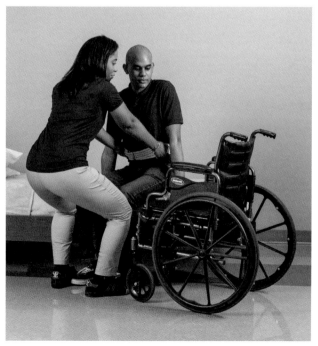
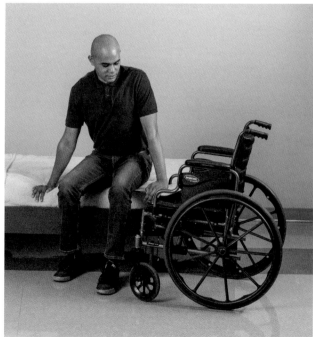

10.59 A sliding board transfer can be employed with or without assistance.

vidual. Another option is the **two-person squat-pivot transfer**, with an additional therapist standing behind the individual to help support and shift the hips and weight of the body to the intended surface.

These techniques are advanced, and you should develop competency before implementing them clinically. Know your own physical limitations: do not attempt a dependent transfer without sufficient strength, assistance, or proper technique. An improper transfer could injure you or the patient.

In certain situations, body size, functional status, or comfort level indicate the need for a **mechanical lift transfer**. Some mechanical lifts are mobile and able to transfer an individual throughout their environment (**10.60**).

Other mechanical lift systems are installed in the ceiling, with tracks to important areas of the home like the toilet or shower. Either type of system involves a harness placed securely around the individual, with multiple points of contact between the patient and lift to ensure safety.

Positioning, postural alignment and control, and functional mobility are essential considerations for occupational performance regardless of the practice setting or population. Continue to build on these foundational concepts as you learn more about assessment and intervention to help your patients maximize their participation in the occupations that are meaningful to them.

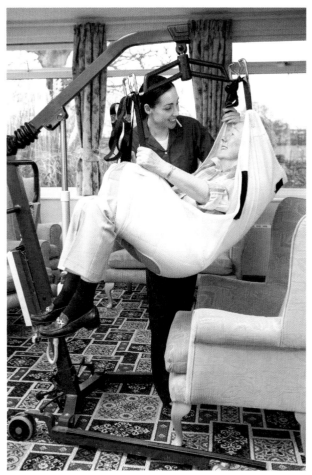

10.60 Mechanical lift for a dependent transfer

APPLY AND REVIEW

Review Questions

1. Which of the following motions of the lower extremity does not contribute to acceleration of gait?
   a. ankle plantar flexion
   b. knee flexion
   c. hip flexion
   d. pelvic rotation

2. All of the following would enhance an individual's functional stability *except*
   a. narrowing the stance.
   b. carrying objects closer to the body.
   c. using a mobility device like a cane or walker.
   d. using footwear that fits well with rubber-like soles.

3. What type of transfer would an individual with complete paralysis of the lower extremities but good upper body strength and core stability be able to complete independently?
   a. stand-pivot
   b. squat-pivot
   c. sliding board
   d. dependent

4. An individual with hemiplegia demonstrating weakness of one side of the body would be most likely to demonstrate which of the following gait patterns?
   a. antalgic gait
   b. scissor gait
   c. Trendelenburg gait
   d. circumduction gait

5. Trendelenburg gait involves dropping of the pelvis on the ipsilateral leg during the swing phase of gait. Weakness of which muscle may contribute to this pattern of ambulation?
   a. psoas major
   b. gluteus maximus
   c. gluteus medius
   d. hamstrings

6. Posterior pelvic tilt may contribute to all *but* which of the following?
   a. decreased chest expansion for respiration
   b. downward orientation of the upper body and head
   c. elongation of the abdominals
   d. decreased lumbar lordosis

7. Anterior pelvic tilt is *most* likely to result in which of the following?
   a. tightness of the hip flexors
   b. tightness of the hamstrings
   c. downward orientation of the upper body, head, and neck
   d. rounding of the upper back

8. All of the following are general recommendations for optimal seated workstation positioning *except*
   a. maintaining a 90° bend at the hips, knees, and elbows.
   b. keeping the wrists extended when typing.
   c. setting the top of the monitor at eye level.
   d. using lumbar support.

9. The line of gravity (LOG) in optimal standing posture traverses all of the following anatomical landmarks *except*
   a. the ear.
   b. slightly anterior to shoulder.
   c. slightly posterior to the greater trochanter.
   d. anterior to the patella.

10. Which of the following would contribute to *deceleration* of the body while ambulating?
    a. concentric contraction of the gastrocnemius
    b. concentric contraction of the hamstrings
    c. eccentric contraction of the hamstrings
    d. concentric contraction of the gluteals

See Answer Key in back of book.

Notes

1. American Occupational Therapy Association, *Occupational Therapy Practice Framework: Domain and Process*, 4th ed. (Bethesda, MD: AOTA Press, 2020).

2. Parisa Ghelichkhani and Maryam Esmaeili, "Prone Position in Management of COVID-19 Patients: A Commentary," *Archives of Academic Emergency Medicine* 8, no. 1 (April 11, 2020): e48, https://www.ncbi.nlm.nih.gov/pmc/articles/PMC7158870/.

3. American Occupational Therapy Association, *Occupational Therapy Practice Framework*.

4. Discussion of gait cycle is based on Andrew Biel, *Trail Guide to Movement: Building the Body in Motion*, 2nd ed. (Boulder, CO: Books of Discovery, 2019), 227–33.

5. Biel, *Trail Guide to Movement*, 230.

6. Discussion of abnormal gaits is based on Biel, *Trail Guide to Movement*, 238–41.

7. Heidi McHugh Pendleton and Winifred Schultz-Krohn, *Pedretti's Occupational Therapy: Practice Skills for Physical Dysfunction*, 8th ed. (St. Louis, MO: Elsevier, 2017), 249–50.

8. Pendleton and Schultz-Krohn, *Pedretti's Occupational Therapy*, 252–53.

Bibliography

American Occupational Therapy Association. *Occupational Therapy Practice Framework: Domain and Process*. 4th ed. Bethesda, MD: AOTA Press, 2020.

Biel, Andrew. *Trail Guide to Movement: Building the Body in Motion*. 2nd ed. Boulder, CO: Books of Discovery, 2019.

Biel, Andrew. *Trail Guide to the Body: A Hands-On Guide to Locating Muscles, Bones, and More*. 6th ed. Boulder, CO: Books of Discovery, 2019.

Ghelichkhani, Parisa, and Maryam Esmaeili. "Prone Position in Management of COVID-19 Patients: A Commentary." *Archives of Academic Emergency Medicine* 8, no. 1 (April 11, 2020): e48. https://www.ncbi.nlm.nih.gov/pmc/articles/PMC7158870/.

Greene, David Paul, and Susan L. Roberts. *Kinesiology: Movement in the Context of Activity*. 3rd ed. St. Louis, MO: Elsevier, 2017.

Keough, Jeremy L., Susan J. Sain, and Carolyn L. Roller. *Kinesiology for the Occupational Therapy Assistant: Essential Components of Function and Movement*. 2nd ed. Thorofare, NJ: SLACK, 2017.

Oatis, Carol A. *Kinesiology: The Mechanics and Pathomechanics of Human Movement*. 3rd ed. Philadelphia: Wolters Kluwer, 2017.

Pendleton, Heidi McHugh, and Winifred Schultz-Krohn. *Pedretti's Occupational Therapy: Practice Skills for Physical Dysfunction*. 8th ed. St. Louis, MO: Elsevier, 2017.

Appendix

Cardiovascular and Lymphatic Systems

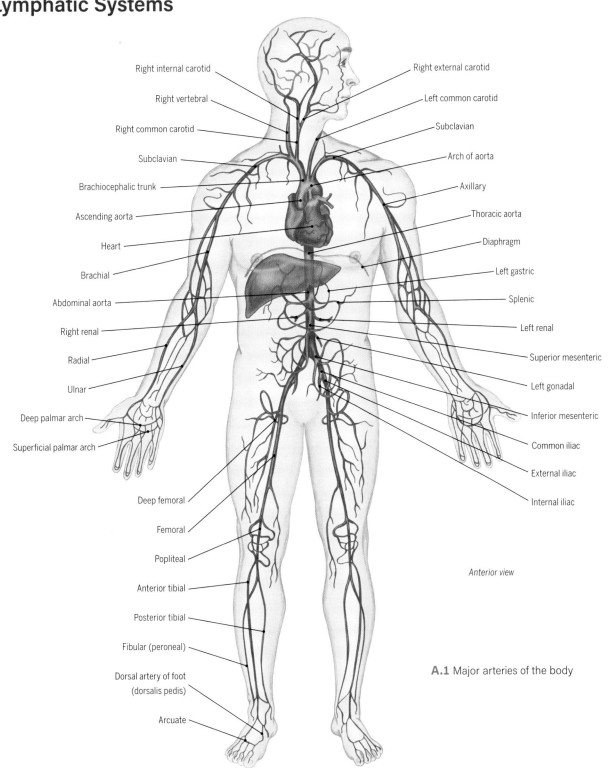

Right internal carotid

Right vertebral

Right common carotid

Subclavian

Brachiocephalic trunk

Ascending aorta

Heart

Brachial

Abdominal aorta

Right renal

Radial

Ulnar

Deep palmar arch

Superficial palmar arch

Deep femoral

Femoral

Popliteal

Anterior tibial

Posterior tibial

Fibular (peroneal)

Dorsal artery of foot (dorsalis pedis)

Arcuate

Right external carotid

Left common carotid

Subclavian

Arch of aorta

Axillary

Thoracic aorta

Diaphragm

Left gastric

Splenic

Left renal

Superior mesenteric

Left gonadal

Inferior mesenteric

Common iliac

External iliac

Internal iliac

Anterior view

A.1 Major arteries of the body

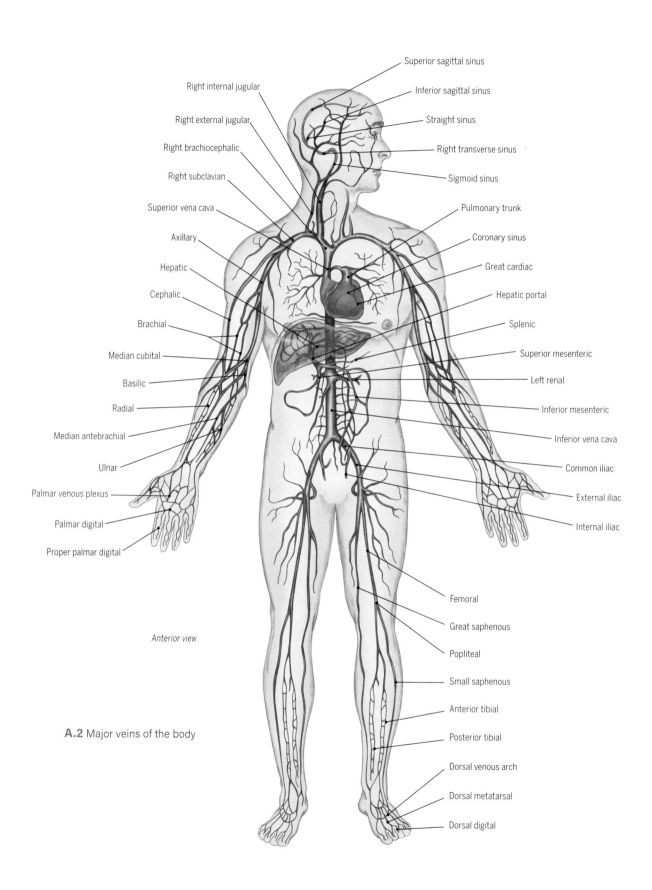

Right internal jugular

Right external jugular

Right brachiocephalic

Right subclavian

Superior vena cava

Axillary

Hepatic

Cephalic

Brachial

Median cubital

Basilic

Radial

Median antebrachial

Ulnar

Palmar venous plexus

Palmar digital

Proper palmar digital

Superior sagittal sinus

Inferior sagittal sinus

Straight sinus

Right transverse sinus

Sigmoid sinus

Pulmonary trunk

Coronary sinus

Great cardiac

Hepatic portal

Splenic

Superior mesenteric

Left renal

Inferior mesenteric

Inferior vena cava

Common iliac

External iliac

Internal iliac

Femoral

Great saphenous

Popliteal

Small saphenous

Anterior tibial

Posterior tibial

Dorsal venous arch

Dorsal metatarsal

Dorsal digital

Anterior view

A.2 Major veins of the body

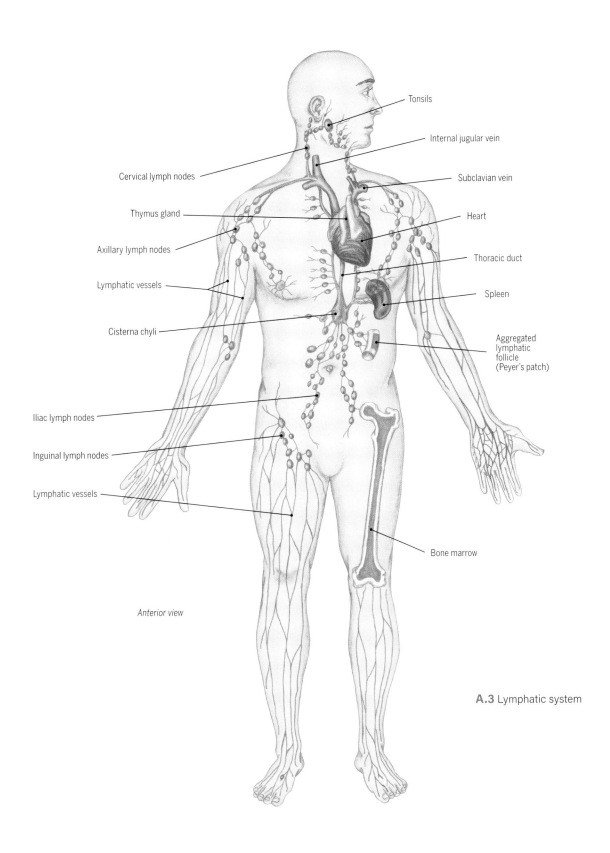

Tonsils

Internal jugular vein

Cervical lymph nodes

Subclavian vein

Thymus gland

Heart

Axillary lymph nodes

Thoracic duct

Lymphatic vessels

Spleen

Cisterna chyli

Aggregated
lymphatic
follicle
(Peyer's patch)

Iliac lymph nodes

Inguinal lymph nodes

Lymphatic vessels

Bone marrow

Anterior view

A.3 Lymphatic system

Answer Key

CHAPTER 1	CHAPTER 2	CHAPTER 3	CHAPTER 4
1. a	1. c	1. a	1. a
2. c	2. d	2. c	2. c
3. d	3. b	3. d	3. d
4. b	4. a	4. b	4. b
5. a	5. b	5. c	5. b
6. d	6. c	6. d	6. d
7. c	7. a	7. a	7. b
8. a	8. b	8. c	8. d
9. b	9. d	9. b	9. c
10. c	10. b	10. d	10. b

CHAPTER 5	CHAPTER 6	CHAPTER 7
1. d	1. a	1. c
2. b	2. d	2. b
3. c	3. c	3. a
4. d	4. a	4. b
5. a	5. b	5. d
6. c	6. b	6. b
7. d	7. d	7. d
8. d	8. a	8. b
9. d	9. c	9. d
10. c	10. c	10. c

CHAPTER 8	CHAPTER 9	CHAPTER 10
1. b	1. c	1. c
2. d	2. a	2. a
3. d	3. b	3. c
4. c	4. c	4. d
5. d	5. d	5. c
6. a	6. a	6. c
7. c	7. b	7. a
8. c	8. d	8. b
9. c	9. c	9. d
10. b	10. c	10. c

Glossary

above-knee amputation (AKA): lower limb amputation proximal to the knee

acquired amputation: the surgical amputation of a limb

active insufficiency: the inability of a joint to move further due to maximal shortening of the muscle acting upon it

adaptive equipment (AE): devices that may be used to facilitate compensatory methods for performing occupations

adaptive shortening: a decrease in the length of soft tissue due to remaining in a shortened position without sufficient elongation over time; may contribute to loss of joint mobility and function

adhesive capsulitis: a painful condition of the shoulder that involves inflammation, thickening, and adherence of the glenohumeral joint capsule with restriction of motion

afferent: in the context of the nervous system, conducting sensory information toward the central nervous system

agonist: a muscle producing a desired movement

ambulation: walking or moving from place to place

anatomical position: in the human body, standing upright with the legs straight, head facing forward, arms at the sides, and palms facing forward

anatomical stability: a body position in which the line of gravity falls within the base of support

angle of inclination: the angle of the femoral neck that positions the femur medial relative to the pelvis, positioning the feet beneath the body

ankylosing spondylitis: an inflammatory condition in the spine that can lead to fusion of its skeletal structures

antagonist: a muscle that resists a desired movement

antalgic gait: a gait pattern used to avoid pain, typically limiting weight-bearing on the affected side

anterior pelvic tilt: the position of the pelvis in which its posterior portion is elevated relative to its anterior portion

aphasia: any loss of the ability to understand or express speech

arches of the foot: anatomical features that help to support the weight of the body and absorb ground reaction forces

arthrokinematics: the specific pattern of relative bone surface movement within a joint

aspiration: the entry of food, liquid, or other foreign object into the airway

ataxic gait: a gait pattern involving lack of coordination; associated with cerebellar dysfunction

autonomic nervous system (ANS): the part of the nervous system that directs and regulates primarily subconscious, involuntary processes

axial skeleton: bones along the vertical axis of the skeleton including the vertebral column, ribs, sternum, and skull

axis of motion: a straight line around which an object rotates; typically lying within the joint

axon: the portion of a neuron that transmits information away from the cell body to other neurons

axonotmesis: a peripheral nerve injury in which the axon remains continuous while the surrounding epineurium, perineurium, and endoneurium are damaged

base of support (BOS): the parts of the body or mobility device that come into contact with the ground to stabilize the body

Bell's palsy: paralysis of the muscles on one side of the face due to facial nerve dysfunction

below-knee amputation (BKA): lower limb amputation distal to the knee

bicipital tendinitis: a painful inflammation of the long head of the biceps related to strain or overuse

biomechanics: the study of movement of living organisms

bony congruity: the degree of conformity of bone surfaces at a joint

boutonniere deformity: a dysfunctional position of the finger with flexion of the proximal interphalangeal joint and hyperextension of the distal interphalangeal joint; related to central slip injury

brachial plexus: an interconnected network of nerves from which primary nerves emanate to innervate the upper extremity

bridging: pushing through the legs to elevate the pelvis and hips while lying supine; may facilitate bed mobility

carpal tunnel syndrome (CTS): a cumulative trauma disorder involving compression of the median nerve at the level of the wrist

carrying angle: the natural valgus angulation of the elbows that allows the arms to swing wide of the hips

center of gravity (COG): the focal point at which gravity acts, around which the weight of an object is evenly distributed

central nervous system (CNS): the brain and spinal cord, which process and control the activity of the entire nervous system

cerebral palsy (CP): a congenital disorder related to abnormal brain development or damage that commonly affects movement, balance, and muscle tone

cervical plexus: an interconnected network of nerves that innervates structures primarily of the head and neck

cervical spine: the uppermost portion of the vertebral column, formed by seven cervical vertebrae

circumduction gait: a gait pattern featuring circumduction of the hip to advance the leg

claw hand: a deficit in the hand with hyperextension of the metacarpophalangeal joint and flexion of the interphalangeal joints associated with an ulnar or combined median/ulnar nerve injury

cleft palate: an opening in the hard or soft palate (in the roof of the oral cavity), which often significantly affects speech and swallowing

close-pack position: a joint position in which there is maximal contact between articular surfaces and maximal tension on the surrounding ligaments; the joint's most stable position

closed-chain movement: functional movement involving a fixed (nonmoving) distal segment such that the proximal joint(s) move together in relation to this fixed point

co-contraction: the simultaneous contraction of antagonist and agonist muscles to provide joint stability

composite grasp: the simultaneous flexion of all the joints of all the fingers in order to grip

concentric contraction: muscle contraction in which the muscle shortens

core: the central region of the body, including the back, abdomen, thorax, and pelvis; sometimes used synonymously with trunk

cranial nerves: the nerves that arise from the brainstem and innervate structures within the head and neck, glands, and some viscera

cubital tunnel syndrome: a condition of chronic compression or tension on the ulnar nerve within the cubital tunnel of the elbow

cubitus valgus: angulation of the elbow positioning the forearm farther (laterally) from the body than normal

cubitus varus: angulation of the elbow positioning the forearm closer to the body (medially) than normal

cumulative trauma disorder (CTD): a musculoskeletal pathology that involves repetitive trauma to soft tissues leading to painful inflammation and fatigue

cylindrical grasp: a pattern of grasp involving midrange flexion of the digits around a tube-shaped object

dart thrower's motion: a diagonal pattern of wrist motion involving combined flexion or extension with ulnar or radial deviation

de Quervain's tenosynovitis: a cumulative trauma disorder involving the abductor pollicis longus and extensor pollicis brevis tendons in the 1st dorsal compartment of the wrist

deglutition: the movement of food from the mouth to the stomach; swallowing

dendrite: the portion of a neuron that receives information and conducts it toward the cell body

dependent transfer: a transfer technique for individuals who can contribute minimal to no assistance

dermatome: an area of skin supplied by nerve fibers that arise from an individual spinal nerve root

differential diagnosis: the process of differentiating between multiple possible conditions based on patient history, symptoms, and clinical presentation

diplopia: double vision

dorsal nerve root: the portion of a spinal nerve that connects directly to the spinal cord via nerve rootlets and transmits sensory information

dowager's hump: excessive flexion of the thoracic spine that is fixed and permanent

Dupuytren's contracture: a pathological thickening of the palmar aponeurosis that may eventually lead to joint contractures of the fingers

dynamic stability: stability of a joint in motion; active stability

dysarthria: any disorder of speech caused by muscle weakness of the face, tongue, or throat

dysphagia: any impairment in swallowing

eccentric contraction: muscle contraction in which the muscle elongates

efferent: in the context of the nervous system, conducting motor signal information away from the central nervous system to the tissues of the body

elasticity: the ability to stretch and return to the original shape after tensile force is removed

end-feel: the feel of a joint at the end of its passive range; can indicate a general source of restriction

esophageal phase: the phase of swallowing that involves peristalsis to advance the bolus through the esophagus and into the stomach

extensor tendon injury: a rupture of an extensor tendon (or tendons) of the wrist, fingers, or thumb; classified by anatomical zone of injury

extrinsic muscle: a muscle that acts on and originates outside of the foot or hand

fall on outstretched hands (FOOSH): a fall that is broken on the hand(s) with the elbow and wrist extended; a common mechanism of injury to the upper extremity

first-class lever: a lever arranged with the exerted and resistive forces on opposite sides of an axis

fixator: a muscle that stabilizes one part of the body to facilitate movement of another part

flexion contracture: a type of joint contracture in which the joint is positioned in some degree of flexion due to restrictions of surrounding soft tissues and the passive and active extension of the joint are limited

flexor tendon injury: a rupture of a flexor tendon (or tendons) of the wrist, fingers, or thumb; classified by anatomical zone of injury

foot drop: a loss of the ability to dorsiflex the ankle and foot; often related to hemiparesis or fibular nerve dysfunction

force: push or pull

force couple: a system of muscles working together, though often in different directions, to produce the same movement or to stabilize a joint

forward head posture (FHP): a posture that involves protraction of the head and neck anterior relative to the trunk

functional anatomy: the underlying body structures and movements involved in daily function

functional (dynamic) stability: the stability required to safely and effectively complete a specific functional activity

functional mobility: moving the body from one position or place to another

fusion: surgical fixation of a joint

gait: manner of walking

gait cycle: a reciprocal pattern of lower extremity movement

genu valgum: increased inward (medial) angulation of the knee, bringing the knees closer together

genu varum: increased outward (lateral) angulation of the knee, bringing the knees farther apart

glenohumeral subluxation: a partial dislocation, typically inferiorly, of the humeral head relative to the glenoid fossa; often a result of weakness of surrounding muscles due to hemiparesis

hand of benediction: a deficit in the hand involving loss of thumb, index, and middle finger flexion as well as atrophy of the thenar muscles and web space; associated with a high median nerve injury

hard palate: the bony roof of the mouth

head, arms, and trunk (HAT): the upper portion of the body that is stabilized and supported by the pelvis

hemiarthroplasty: the partial replacement of a joint with a surgical implant

hemiparesis: unilateral weakness often related to a stroke or brain injury

hemiplegic gait: a gait pattern associated with weakness of one side of the body related to a brain injury; may include circumduction of the leg as well as common contractures of the upper and lower extremities

hip fracture: a fracture of the proximal femur

hip precautions: specific restrictions to movement or weight-bearing that may be in place after a hip fracture or surgery

homeostasis: equilibrium within the systems of the body

homonymous hemianopsia: a loss of vision on the same side of each visual field

hook grasp: a pattern of grasp involving simultaneous flexion of the proximal interphalangeal and distal interphalangeal joints with the metacarpophalangeal joints extended

iliotibial (IT) band syndrome: an overuse condition from repetitive strain of the IT band; common in athletes such as long-distance runners and cyclists

incontinence: the loss of bowel or bladder control

intra-abdominal pressure: pressure generated in the abdominal area from contraction of the abdominals, diaphragm, and pelvic floor that stabilizes the lumbar spine

intrinsic minus: hyperextension of the metacarpophalangeal joints and flexion of the interphalangeal joints of the fingers; may be present with intrinsic muscle weakness or paralysis

intrinsic muscle: a muscle that is contained entirely within the foot or hand

intrinsic plus: flexion of the metacarpophalangeal joints of the fingers with extension of the interphalangeal joints; elongates the interossei and lumbricals and keeps tension on the collateral ligaments of the fingers

isometric contraction: muscle contraction that does not change muscle length or produce joint motion

isotonic contraction: muscle contraction that changes muscle length and produces joint motion

joint contracture: the loss of passive mobility of a joint

joint dislocation: the displacement of a joint with complete loss of contact between articular surfaces

joint reaction force: the force generated within the joint in response to external forces acting upon it

kinesiology: the study of anatomy and mechanics in relation to human movement

kinetic chain: cooperative, interdependent movement of the segments and joints of the body

laminectomy: the removal of the lamina of a vertebra or vertebrae

lateral (key) pinch: a pinch pattern involving the pad of the thumb pressed against the radial side of the index finger

lateral epicondylosis: degenerative tendinopathy involving the extensor muscles of the wrist and hand

leg length discrepancy: a lower extremity abnormality in which one leg is longer than the other

length-tension relationship: the concept that a muscle's strength is relative to its length at time of contraction

lever: a pulley system that increases the mechanical advantage of a force to move an object

line of gravity (LOG): a vertical line extending downward from the center of gravity of an individual or object to the ground beneath

logroll: a technique to transition from lying on the back (supine) to sitting on the edge of the bed without rotating the trunk or hips

low back pain (LBP): a common location of pain in the vertebral column due to the load-bearing nature of the lumbar spine

lower limb (LL) amputation: the loss of a portion of or the entire lower extremity due to disease process, trauma, or surgical removal

lumbar plexus: an interconnected network of nerves from which primary nerves emanate to innervate muscles of the pelvis and thigh

lumbar spine: the lowermost portion of the vertebral column formed by five lumbar vertebrae

mechanical advantage: leverage affected by the type of lever and length of moment arm

medial epicondylosis: degenerative tendinopathy involving the flexor muscles of the wrist and hand

mobility device: a device used to enhance safe functional mobility by increasing points of contact with the ground and expanding the base of support

modified barium swallow study: radiologic imaging technique to examine the physiology of the swallow and identify aspiration or other dysfunction

moment: the turning effect of a force or its tendency to cause rotation

moment arm: the distance from an axis to the force acting upon it; in functional anatomy, the perpendicular distance from a joint's center of rotation to the muscle moving it

motor cortex: the part of the brain that sends motor commands

motor nerve: a peripheral nerve that transmits efferent motor signals

motor planning area: the part of the brain responsible for planning purposeful movements

motor skills: performance skills that include physical movement of the body

muscle memory: the tendency for motor commands and coordinated muscle actions for repeated activities to become seemingly subconscious and automatic

myotome: a group of muscles innervated by a particular spinal nerve

neuron: a nerve cell

neurotmesis: a peripheral nerve injury that disrupts the continuity of the entire nerve

occupational performance: the act of completing meaningful activities by a person, group, or population

occupations: everyday activities that people do to bring meaning and purpose to life

open-chain movement: free movement of the joints and segments of the body in space; joints move together or independently of the others

open-pack position: a joint position with the least articular surface contact and laxity of the surrounding ligaments; the joint's most mobile position

optokinetic reflex: reflexive activity of the eyes that stabilizes the visual field as the head moves through the surrounding environment

oral preparatory phase: the phase of swallowing in which food is mixed with saliva and undergoes mastication to form a manageable bolus

oral transit phase: the phase of swallowing in which the tongue propels the bolus posteriorly through the oral cavity toward the pharynx

osteoarthritis (OA): the degeneration of joint cartilage and underlying bone within a joint

osteokinematics: the gross movement of bones in relation to one another; often an externally visible pattern of movement

palmar arch: an anatomical arch within the palm that allows the hand to better conform to the shape of various objects and improve grasp

palpation: the use of physical touch to identify, assess, or provide intervention to a specific part of the body

paranasal sinuses: hollow, air-filled spaces within the skull that decrease the weight of the skull and contribute to vocal quality

parasympathetic nervous system: the portion of the autonomic nervous system responsible primarily for processes that conserve energy (rest and digest)

Parkinsonian gait: a gait pattern affected by impaired perception and modulation of motor movements associated with Parkinson's disease; involves small, shuffling steps

passive insufficiency: the inability of an antagonist muscle to elongate enough to allow a joint to move through its full range of a desired movement

pelvic floor (diaphragm): the muscles that form the inferior muscular wall of the pelvic cavity

pelvic obliquity: the position of the pelvis in the frontal plane

pelvic organ prolapse: herniation of the uterus, rectum, or bladder into the vagina

pelvic rotation: the position of the pelvis in the transverse plane

pelvic tilt: the position of the pelvis in the sagittal plane

performance patterns: the habits, routines, rituals, and roles that form the rhythms and expectations of daily life

performance skills: the goal-directed actions that contribute to occupational performance, including motor, process, and social interaction skills

peripheral nerve injury: an injury to a specific nerve or nerves in the peripheral nervous system

peripheral nervous system (PNS): the nerves of the body including the cranial nerves

peripheral neuropathy: a general term for disorders that contribute to damage to the peripheral nerves of the body

pes cavus: a higher than normal arch of the foot

pes planus: a flatter than normal arch of the foot

pharyngeal phase: the phase of swallowing in which the bolus passes into the oropharynx, triggering a reflexive response to advance the bolus into the esophagus

phonemes: distinct units of sound as components of speech

planes of motion: the fixed planes that segments of the human body move through or parallel to; include the sagittal, frontal, and transverse planes

plantar fasciitis: an inflammatory condition of the fascia on the plantar surface of the foot related to overuse

posterior pelvic tilt: the position of the pelvis in which its anterior portion is elevated relative to its posterior portion

postural alignment: the collective position of the segments of the body at any given moment

postural control: the ability to achieve or maintain a balanced body position for a given activity

posture: the relative position of the segments of the body

pressure sore: an injury to the skin or underlying tissue due to prolonged pressure

primary curve: a single kyphotic curvature of the entire vertebral column that is present at birth

prime mover: an individual muscle contributing the most force for a desired movement

pronator teres syndrome: a condition in which the median nerve is compressed between the two heads of the pronator teres as it enters the forearm

proprioception: the perception of the position and movement of the joints and body in space

purposeful movement: meaningful, goal-directed motion

quiet standing: an upright posture in which the body is vertically aligned with a degree of postural sway above the ankles

radiculopathy: compression of a spinal nerve root

rotator cuff: an anatomical cuff around the proximal humerus formed by the supraspinatus, infraspinatus, subscapularis, and teres minor muscles to provide stability and movement

sacral plexus: an interconnected network of nerves from which primary nerves emanate to innervate the lower extremity

sarcomere: the contractile unit of a muscle

scaption: the plane of motion for humeral elevation that lies midway between the sagittal and frontal planes; often a functional plane of movement

scapular dyskinesis: an alteration in the resting or active position of the scapula

scapular plane: a plane of motion that aligns with the resting position of the glenoid fossa relative to the frontal plane, typically 30°–40° anterior to the frontal plane

scapular winging: tilting of the medial border of the scapula posteriorly, away from the rib cage, often associated with weakness of the serratus anterior; interrupts scapulohumeral rhythm

scapulohumeral rhythm: the proportional scapular and humeral motion that maintains optimal anatomical alignment of the bones of the shoulder complex

sciatica: a condition involving pain and paresthesia in the leg due to compression of the sciatic nerve on the posterior aspect of the hip

scissor gait: a gait pattern that demonstrates a narrowing, or even crossing-over, of the legs with walking; associated with tightness or spasticity of the hip adductor muscles

scoliosis: an abnormal curvature of the spine

screw-home mechanism: an arthrokinematic pattern of the knee that involves rotation of the femur and tibia to stabilize the joint in full extension

second-class lever: a lever arranged with the exerted and resistive forces on the same side of an axis, with the resistive force closer to the axis

secondary curve: lordotic curvature of the lumbar or cervical spine that forms in children as they begin to sit, stand, and walk

sensorimotor system: a feedback loop of the sensory and motor systems that guides purposeful movement and function

sensory cortex: the part of the brain that receives sensory information

sensory nerves: the peripheral nerves that transmit afferent sensory information

shoulder separation: an informal term for dislocation of the acromioclavicular joint

sliding board transfer: a transfer technique involving a stable board placed between two functional surfaces to serve as a bridge; may be completed independently or with assistance

soft palate: the posterior aspect of the roof of the mouth formed by soft tissue

somatosensation: all forms of sensation from the skin, limbs, and joints

spherical grasp: a pattern of grasp involving varied flexion of the digits around a rounded object

spinal cord injury (SCI): an injury to the spinal cord that blocks transmission of neurological signals between the brain and body

spinal nerve: a nerve that originates in the spinal cord and connects peripheral nerves to the central nervous system

spinal tract: an axonal pathway in the spinal cord that transmits specific types of information to and from the brain

squat-pivot transfer: a modified stand-pivot transfer in which the individual being transferred does not come to a full stand but maintains some hip and knee flexion throughout the transfer

stability: the ability to maintain control over the position or movement of the body

stagger stance: standing with one foot in front of the other with hips and knees somewhat flexed; facilitates functional weight-shifting

stand-pivot transfer: a transfer technique that includes an assisted stand with some degree of weight-bearing through the legs, pivoting, and sitting on a surface positioned next to the original surface

static stability: the stability of a joint at rest; passive stability

step: the distance the foot advances in relation to the other, measured as the distance from the same point on opposite feet

stereognosis: the ability to identify an object based on tactile sensation alone

strain: the amount of material displacement under a specific amount of stress

stress: the amount of applied force per area

stride: a single stance and swing phase for each lower extremity, measured from the point at which the foot comes into contact with the ground to the next point of initial contact from the same foot

subacromial impingement: compression of the soft tissues between the acromion and humeral head

surface anatomy: the features of anatomy that are palpable or visible on the surface of the skin

swallowing: a complex mechanism that involves both voluntary and involuntary muscle function to propel food from the mouth to the esophagus

swan-neck deformity: a deformity of the finger involving hyperextension of the proximal interphalangeal joint and flexion of the distal interphalangeal joint

sympathetic nervous system: the portion of the autonomic nervous system responsible primarily for processes that expend energy (fight or flight)

synergist: a muscle that assists a prime mover in producing a desired movement

synovial joint: a joint with a capsule that contains a layer of lubricating fluid and permits motion

tenodesis: passive flexion of the fingers with active extension of the wrist due to increased passive tension on the flexor muscles of the fingers; may be a compensatory method for light grasp for someone with loss of active finger flexion

therapeutic use of self: the integration of empathetic communication and the therapist's unique personality into the therapeutic relationship

third-class lever: a lever arranged with the exerted and resistive forces on the same side of an axis, with the exerted force closer to the axis

thoracic outlet syndrome (TOS): a condition in which the brachial plexus and/or adjacent vascular structures are compressed in the neck or axilla area

thoracic spine: the middle portion of the vertebral column, formed by twelve thoracic vertebrae

three-jaw chuck pinch: a pinch pattern involving the tip of the thumb pressed against the tips of the index and middle fingers

tip pinch: a pinch pattern used for precision, involving the distal tips of the thumb and index finger

torque: the turning effect of a force or its ability to rotate an object

total hip arthroplasty (THA): the surgical replacement of the entire hip joint with a prosthetic implant

total knee arthroplasty (TKA): the surgical replacement of the entire knee joint with a prosthetic implant

transfer: movement from one functional surface to another; requires specific techniques depending on the functional ability of the individual being transferred and the level of assistance needed

Trendelenburg gait: a gait pattern involving excessive dropping of the pelvis on the swing side leg; associated with weakness of the gluteus medius

trigger finger: a condition that involves painful or limited movement of a finger or the thumb due to inflammatory thickening of the synovial lining of a flexor tendon pulley

trunk: the core of the body, including the back, abdomen, thorax (chest), and pelvis

trunk control: the voluntary ability to position and stabilize the body's core to support function

two-person squat-pivot transfer: a transfer technique involving two individuals to facilitate a modified stand-pivot transfer in which the individual does not fully extend the hips and knees

upper limb amputation: the loss of a portion of or the entire upper extremity due to disease process, trauma, or surgical removal

ventral nerve root: the portion of a spinal nerve that connects directly to the spinal cord via nerve rootlets and transmits motor information

vertebral (spinal) column: the vertebrae that form the skeletal structure of the spine

weight-shifting: moving the weight of the body from one leg to another to facilitate functional alignment and positioning

wrist drop: a deficit in the hand limiting extension of the wrist, digits, and/or thumb; associated with a radial nerve injury

Young's modulus: a method for measuring and representing the relative stiffness of a particular material

Figure Credits

Index

bold denotes photo; *f* denotes figure; *t* denotes table

A

AA (atlantoaxial) joint, 71–72, 71*f*

abdominal aorta, 88*f*, 373*f*

abdominal muscles, 17, 75*f*, 85–89, 97, 291

abdominal wall, 85, 86, 87

abducent nerve, 40, 40*f*

abduction
  of carpometacarpal joint of thumb, 225
  of ellipsoid joint, 29
  of fingers, 245, 250*f*, 256, 257
  of foot, 317
  of GHJ, 154, 161, 168*f*, 169*f*
  of hip, 278, 290*f*
  of metacarpophalangeal joints, 224
  of scapulothoracic joint, 150, 151*f*
  of shoulder complex, 173, 205
  of thumb CMC, 251*f*
  of wrist, 238, 249*f*

abductor digiti minimi (ADM), 46*f*, 242, 242*t*, 325*f*, 329

abductor hallucis, 325*f*

abductor opponens, 241*f*

abductor pollicis brevis (APB), 46*f*, 240, 241*f*, 241*t*, 244*f*, 251

abductor pollicis longus (APL), 46*f*, 226, 234, 238, 238*f*, 239*f*, 239*t*, 240, 248, 248*f*, 249, 251

abnormal muscle tone, 61, 99, 294, 351, 364

above-knee amputation (AKA), 308, 377

AC (acromioclavicular) joints. *See* acromioclavicular (AC) joints

acceleration (in gait), 358, 359*f*

accessory motions, 31

acetabular component, 297*f*

acetabular labrum, 278*f*

acetabulum, 273*f*, 274, 275*f*, 296

Achilles tendon, 322

ACL (anterior cruciate ligament). *See* anterior cruciate ligament (ACL)

acquired amputation, 191, 377

acromioclavicular (AC) joints, 145*f*, 150, 151*f*, 153, 153*f*

acromioclavicular ligament, 153*f*, 154*f*, 176*f*

acromion, 146*f*, 147, 147*f*, 154*f*, 155*f*, 165, 175*f*, 176*f*, 345*f*

actin, 19, 21*f*

action, defined, 11

active insufficiency, 27, 28, 252, 254, 377

active range of motion (AROM), 216

activities of daily living (ADLs), 5, 10, 23, 27, 37, 45, 95, 100, 131, 133, 134, 135, 150, 171, 172, 175, 176, 186, 191, 192, 195, 204, 208, 253, 259, 297, 317, 332, 345, 350, 366

activity analysis, 6, 9, 202, 317

adapted dressing, **100***f*

adaptive equipment (AE), 10, 14, 16, 62, 100–101, 179, 259, 261, 296, 332, 349, 355, 377

adaptive jar opener, **14***f*

adaptive shortening, 16, 23, 146, 207, 256, 377

adaptive utensils, **133***f*

adduction
  of carpometacarpal joint of thumb, 225
  of ellipsoid joint, 29
  of fingers, 245, 250*f*, 256, 257
  of foot, 317
  of GHJ, 154, 168, 169*f*
  of hip, 278, 290*f*
  of metacarpophalangeal joints, 224
  of palmar interossei, 243
  of scapulothoracic joint, 150, 151*f*
  of teres major, 168
  of thumb CMC, 252*f*

adductor brevis, 48*f*, 284, 284*f*, 285*f*, 285*t*, 288, 289, 290

adductor hallucis, 325*f*

adductor hiatus, 284*f*

adductor longus, 48*f*, 284, 284*f*, 285*f*, 285*t*, 288, 289, 290, 320*f*

adductor magnus, 48*f*, 49*f*, 284, 284*f*, 284*t*, 288, 289, 290

adductor pollicis (AP), 46*f*, 240, 244, 244*f*, 244*t*, 251, 252

adductor tubercle, 276*f*, 284*f*, 306*f*

adhesive capsulitis, 154, 377

ADLs (activities of daily living). *See* activities of daily living (ADLs)

ADM (abductor digiti minimi). *See* abductor digiti minimi (ADM)

AE (adaptive equipment). *See* adaptive equipment (AE)

afferent, 38, 377

AFO (ankle-foot orthosis), **331***f*, 363, **363***f*

aggregated lymphatic follicle (Peyer's patch), 375*f*

agonist, 24, 377

AIIS (anterior inferior iliac spine), 274, 275*f*, 278*f*

AKA (above-knee amputation). *See* above-knee amputation (AKA)

ala, 273, 274*f*

alar ligaments, 71*f*

alimentary (digestive) tract, 115

ALL (anterior longitudinal ligament). *See* anterior longitudinal ligament (ALL)

alveolar process, 109

ambulation, 304, 353, 360*f*, 361*f*, **362***f*, 377

amputation, 191, 308, 368

anatomical neck (of humerus), 149, 149*f*

anatomical position, 7, 8, 377

anatomical snuffbox, 219, 238*f*, 240*f*

anatomical stability, 342, **343***f*

anatomical terminology, 7–10

anatomical terms of location, 7*f*

anconeus, 46*f*, 195*f*, 199, 199*f*, 199*t*, 203

angle of inclination, 276, 377

ankle
  bones of, 308–309
  dorsiflexors of. *See* dorsiflexion, of ankle
  as example of second-class lever, 12*f*
  guide to goniometry & MMT on, 329
  as interconnecting segment of body, 340*f*
  joints of, 313–317
  as link for functional mobility, 304–305
  medial view of, 323*f*
  musculature and movement of knee, ankle, and foot, 318–329
  plantar flexors of, 322–324, 322*f*
  purposeful movement of, 326–329

ankle-foot orthosis (AFO), **331***f*, 363, **363***f*

ankylosing spondylitis, 278, 377

annular ligament, 193*f*, 194, 194*f*

annular pulley, 232, 232*f*, 247*f*

annulus fibrosus, 64

anococcygeal ligament, 279*f*

anococcygeal nerve, 48*f*

anococcygeal raphe, 279*f*

anorectal hiatus, 279, 279*f*

coracoacromial ligament, 147f, 153, 153f, 154f, 176f, 177f

coracoclavicular ligaments, 147f, 153

coracohumeral ligament, 153f

costoclavicular ligament, 73f, 152f

costotransverse ligament, 73f

cruciform ligament, 71f

deep transverse metacarpal ligament, 224, 225f

deltoid ligament, 314, 314f

distal intercarpal ligaments, 223f

dorsal calcaneocuboid ligaments, 316f

dorsal cuboideonavicular ligament, 316f

dorsal cuneocuboid ligament, 316f

dorsal cuneonavicular ligaments, 316f

dorsal intercarpal ligaments, 223f

dorsal intercuneiform ligaments, 316f

dorsal metatarsal ligaments, 317f

dorsal radioulnar ligament, 221, 223f

dorsal tarsometatarsal ligaments, 317f

dorsoradial ligament, 225

fibular collateral ligament, 17f, 312f

glenohumeral ligaments, 154

iliofemoral ligament, 278

iliolumbar ligament, 277f

inferior glenohumeral ligament, 155f

inguinal ligament, 85f, 275, 277f, 280f, 320f

interarticular ligament, 73f

intercarpal ligaments, 223f

interclavicular ligament, 73f, 152, 152f

intermetacarpal ligaments, 225

interspinous ligaments, 72, 72f

intertransverse ligaments, 72

ischiofemoral ligament, 278

lateral collateral ligament (LCL), 312

lateral costotransverse ligament, 73f

lateral temporomandibular ligament, 116f

ligament of Osborne, 200f

ligamentum capitis femoris, 278f

ligamentum flavum, 72, 72f, 73f

long plantar ligament, 310f

lunotriquetral ligament, 223f

medial collateral ligament (MCL), 27, 312

middle glenohumeral ligament, 155f

nuchal ligament, 66, 67f, 71f, 80f

oblique retinacular ligament (ORL), 236f, 237

palmar radiocarpal ligament, 223f

patellar ligament, 17f, 26f, 308, 312f, 313f

pisohamate ligament, 223f

plantar calcaneocuboid ligament, 310f

plantar calcaneonavicular ligament, 310f

plantar cuboideonavicular ligament, 310f

plantar ligaments, 309

plantar metatarsal ligaments, 310f

posterior cruciate ligament (PCL), 17f, 311–312, 311f

posterior longitudinal ligament (PLL), 71f, 72, 72f

posterior meniscofemoral ligament, 311f, 312f

posterior oblique ligament, 225

posterior sacrococcygeal ligaments, 277f

posterior sacroiliac ligament, 277, 277f

posterior talocalcaneal ligament, 314f

posterior talofibular ligament, 314, 314f

posterior tibiofibular ligament, 314, 314f

pubofemoral ligament, 278

radial collateral ligament (RCL), 192, 192f, 193f, 194f, 223f

radiate ligament, 152f

radiocapitate part (of palmar radiocarpal ligament), 223f

radioscapholunate part of palmar radiocarpal ligament, 223f

radiotriquetral part (of palmar radiocarpal ligament), 223f

round ligament, 278

sacrospinous ligament, 277, 279f

sacrotuberous ligament, 277, 277f, 279f

scapholunate ligament, 223f

sphenomandibular ligament, 116, 116f, 117f

stylomandibular ligament, 116, 116f

superior costotransverse ligament, 73f

superior glenohumeral ligament, 155f

suprascapular ligament, 153

supraspinous ligament, 277f

temporomandibular ligament, 116, 116f

thyrohyoid ligament, 113f

tibial collateral ligament, 17f, 312f

transverse acetabular ligament, 278f

transverse carpal ligament, 246

transverse ligament, of atlas (C-1), 71f

transverse ligament, of forearm, 248

transverse ligament, of knee, 312f

transverse retinacular ligament, 236f

triangular ligament, 236f

ulnar collateral ligament (UCL), 192, 192f, 193f, 223f

ulnar collateral ligament (UCL) injury, 207

ulnolunate part (of palmar ulnocarpal ligament), 223f

ulnotriquetral part (of palmar ulnocarpal ligament), 223f

volar radioulnar ligament, 221

ligamentum capitis femoris, 278f

ligamentum flavum, 72, 72f, 73f

light bulb, muscles used in changing overhead light bulb, **206f**

line of gravity (LOG), 342, 344, 347f, 379

line of pull, 11f

linea alba, 17f, 85f

linea aspera, 276f, 306f

Lister's tubercle, 218, 218f, 223f

LL (lower limb) amputation, 308, 379

load rate, 27

load to failure, 14

LOG (line of gravity). *See* line of gravity (LOG)

logroll, 354, **354f**, 379

long head (triceps brachii), 199f

long plantar ligament, 310f

longissimus, 76, 77f, 78f, 93

longissimus capitis, 75f, 76, 78f, 79f, 91, 92

longissimus cervicis, 76, 78f, 91, 92

longissimus thoracis, 78f

longitudinal arch, 220, 220f, 256f

longus capitis, 90, 92

longus colli, 90, 92

low back pain (LBP), 100, 379

lower cervical spine, 66

lower extremities

    adaptive equipment for dressing of, 100

    functional mobility of, 317, 330

    musculoskeletal injuries of, 331–333

    neurological impairment of, 330–331

    occupational and clinical perspectives of, 330–333

    osteology of, 305–310

    use of prosthesis on, **308f**

lower limb (LL) amputation, 308, 379

lower subscapular, 44f

lower thorax, 69f

LRTI (ligament reconstruction and tendon interposition) procedure, 226

lumbar lordosis, 63f

lumbar plexus, 47, 47f, 48f, 379

lumbar spinal nerves (L1–L5), 40, 41f, 42f

lumbar spine, 69, 340f, 380

lumbar vertebrae, 63, 69, 69f, 88f, 273f

About the Authors

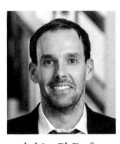

Nathan (Nate) Short, PhD, OTD, OTR/L, CHT, is an associate professor of occupational therapy at Huntington University in Fort Wayne, Indiana. He received his OTD from Belmont University in Nashville, Tennessee, in 2009 and his PhD from Kingston University in London, England, in 2020. He began his career serving with the Indian Health Service (IHS) in Gallup, New Mexico, and has worked across the spectrum of practice including in acute care, rehabilitation, early intervention, and outpatient settings. He remains clinically active, primarily in occupation-based hand and upper extremity rehabilitation. Additionally, he leads a partnership between Huntington University and the Joni and Friends International Disability Center, providing seating and mobility services in developing countries. His research interests include technology, international service learning (ISL) as pedagogy, and hand and upper extremity rehabilitation, and he has published numerous research articles related to these topics. He enjoys traveling with his wife and daughter and is also a mediocre tennis player, scuba diver, and cyclist.

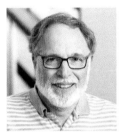

Joel Vilensky, PhD, received his PhD in 1979 from the University of Wisconsin. After a postdoctoral fellowship at the University of Iowa, he became an assistant professor of anatomy at Indiana University. He retired as a professor after thirty-four years of teaching medical gross anatomy at Indiana University. He now teaches anatomy part-time within the OTD program at Huntington University. He has published more than one hundred peer-reviewed articles and has coauthored three textbooks related to anatomy and radiology.

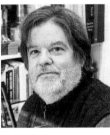

Carlos A. Suárez-Quian, PhD, graduated from the University of North Carolina at Chapel Hill and earned his PhD at Harvard University in 1983. After postdoctoral training at the National Institute of Child Health, he joined the Department of Cell Biology at Georgetown University Medical Center in 1987. He has published more than sixty peer-reviewed manuscripts and chapters and eight e-products that focus on gross anatomy. His teaching expertise is in medical gross anatomy, and he teaches at the high school, college, medical school, and professional levels. He was inducted into the MAGIS Society of Master Teachers, the highest award Georgetown bestows on a faculty member at the School of Medicine.

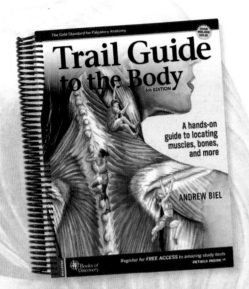
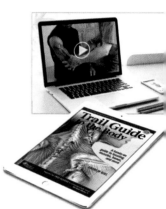
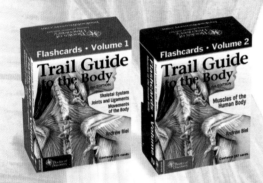
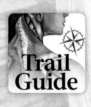
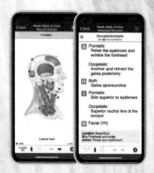
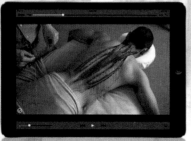

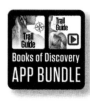